MW00674045

Delmar's Textbook of Basic Pediatric Nursing

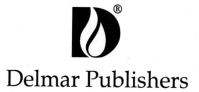

Delmar Publishers

an International Thomson Publishing company I(T)P®

Albany • Bonn • Boston • Cincinnati • Detroit • London • Madrid
Melbourne • Mexico City • New York • Pacific Grove • Paris • San Francisco
Singapore • Tokyo • Toronto • Washington

NOTICE TO THE READER

Publisher does not warrant or guarantee any of the products described herein or perform any independent analysis in connection with any of the product information contained herein. Publisher does not assume, and expressly disclaims, any obligation to obtain and include information other than that provided to it by the manufacturer.

The reader is expressly warned to consider and adopt all safety precautions that might be indicated by the activities described herein and to avoid all potential hazards. By following the instructions contained herein, the reader willingly assumes all risks in connection with such instructions.

The publisher makes no representations or warranties of any kind, including but not limited to, the warranties of fitness for particular purpose or merchantability, nor are any such representations implied with respect to the material set forth herein, and the publisher takes no responsibility with respect to such material. The publisher shall not be liable for any special, consequential, or exemplary damages resulting, in whole or in part, from the readers' use of, or reliance upon, this material.

Cover Illustration: Sergio J. Sericolo

Delmar Staff

Publisher: Susan Simpfenderfer
Acquisitions Editor: Marion Waldman
Developmental Editor: Jill Rembetski
Project Editor: William Trudell
Art and Design Coordinator: Rich Killar
Production Coordinator: John Mickelbank
Editorial Assistant: Sarah Holle
Marketing Manager: Darryl L. Caron

Copyright © 1997
By Delmar Publishers Inc.
a division of Internation Thomson Publishing Inc.

The ITP logo is a trademark under license.

Printed in the United States of America

For more information, contact:
Delmar Publishers
3 Columbia Circle, Box 15015
Albany, New York 12212-5015

International Thomson Publishing Europe
Berkshire House 168-173
High Holborn
London WC1V 7AA
England

Thomas Nelson Australia
102 Dodds Street
South Melbourne, 3205
Victoria, Australia

Nelson Canada
1120 Birchmount Road
Scarborough, Ontario
Canada, M1K 5G4

International Thomson Editores
Campos Eliseos 385, Piso 7
Col Polanco
11560 Mexico D F Mexico

International Thomson Publishing GmbH
Konigswinterer Strasse 418
53227 Bonn
Germany

International Thomson Publishing Asia
221 Henderson Road
#05-10 Henderson Building
Singapore 0315

International Thomson Publishing—Japan
Hirakawacho Kyowa Building, 3F
2-2-1 Hirakawacho
Chiyoda-ku, Tokyo 102
Japan

Online Services

Delmar Online
To access a wide variety of Delmar products and services on the World Wide Web, point your browser to:
    http://www.delmar.com/delmar.html
    or email: info@delmar.com

thomson.com
To access International Thomson Publishing's home site for information on more than 34 publishers and 20,000 products, point your browser to:
    http://www.thomson.com
    or email: findit@kiosk.thomson.com

A service of I(T)P®

All rights reserved. No part of this work covered by the copyright hereon may be reproduced or used in any form or by any means — graphic, electronic, or mechanical, including photocopying, recording, taping or information storage and retrieval systems — without written permission of the publisher.

10 9 8 7 6 5 4 3 2   xxx 02 01 00 99 98 97

Library of Congress Cataloging-in-Publication Data

Basic pediatric nursing.
    p.   cm.
  Includes bibliographical references and index.
  ISBN 0-8273-7717-7
  1. Pediatric nursing.
  [DNLM: 1. Pediatric Nursing. WY 159 B311 1996]
RJ245.B35 1996
610.73'62—dc20
DNLM/DLC
for Library of Congress

96-21917
CIP

Contents

Preface

The licensed practical nurse is in a unique position. Few professions provide so much responsibility and challenge to recent graduates. The licensed practical nurse who serves as a first line manager must exert leadership and management skills. He or she must be able to make decisions and accept responsibility in the provision of hands-on care to clients of all ages in a variety of settings.

This text explores the role of the licensed practical nurse in the pediatric setting. The pediatric nurse faces special challenges. In addition to providing pediatric clients with high quality nursing care, he or she may serve in a number of capacities, such as counselor, teacher, health promoter, and resource person. Pediatric nurses play a critical role as patient advocates and must be up to date and proactive in ensuring that their clients' legal rights are protected. They must also be aware of the role the family plays in pediatric health. This is an essential component of family-centered care, in which the health care team treats the child as part of a family, community, and culture—not as an isolated clinical case.

Delmar's Textbook of Basic Pediatric Nursing expands on the pediatric content of *Basic Maternal/Pediatric Nursing*. Relevant chapters from this text have been revised, updated, and expanded to reflect current information on pediatric nursing. We have continued our time-proven philosophy that complicated material can be presented in a straightforward and friendly manner. Chapters are short and readable. Each chapter includes learning objectives and key terms. Charts and tables highlight important information, and the use of photographs to support and illustrate textural content is extensive. Detailed nursing care sections, including nursing care plans, emphasize the nursing process. Review questions and suggested activities reinforce learning.

The text is divided into six units. Units 1 and 2 introduce the specialty of pediatrics, focus on the newborn, and present an overview of the growth and development process. Unit 3 explores pediatric health promotion, including a detailed presentation of physical examinations, immunizations, and adolescent self-examinations. Unit 4 focuses on hospitalization of the pediatric patient, with a separate chapter on fluid and electrolyte therapy. Unit 5 explores psychological aspects of caring for the dying child, with special focus on dealing with the child's parents and siblings. This unit also includes a separate chapter on sudden infant death syndrome. Finally, Unit 6 presents common pediatric disorders of each body system, including a separate chapter on conditions of the reproductive system. The appendices include growth charts, NANDA nursing diagnoses, and conversion charts.

An instructor's manual containing answers to all the review questions is also available. The instructor may be interested in the two related textbooks in this series, *Basic Maternal/Pediatric Nursing* by Pamela Shapiro and *Basic Maternal/Pediatric Nursing, 6E* by Barbara Anderson and Pamela Shapiro.

Acknowledgments

Delmar Publishers would like to acknowledge the contributions of the following reviewers throughout the development of this project.

Colleen Booth, RN, MSN
Westchester Community College
Valhalla, New York

Mary S. Lewin
Health Occupations Educator
New York State BOCES
Lockport, New York

Kathleen L. Miller, ARNP, PhD
University of South Florida
Tampa, Florida

Jane Powhida, RN, MS, OCN
Hocking College School of Nursing
Nelsonville, Ohio

Carol Ann Stacy
State of Michigan, Department of Education
Health Occupations Educator
Portage, Michigan

The following individuals contributed to *Basic Maternal/Pediatric Nursing*. A portion of this textbook was adapted in the development of *Delmar's Textbook of Basic Pediatric Nursing*.

Molly Allison, MSN, RN
Assistant Professor
Department of Nursing
Angelo State University
San Angelo, Texas
(Chapter 31 — The Pediatric Surgical Patient)

Ruth Bindler, MS, RNC
Associate Professor
Intercollegiate Center for Nursing Education
Washington State University
Spokane, Washington
(Chapter 23 — Developmental Stages; co-author)

Donna Marie Frassetto
Senior Developmental Editor
Cracom Corporation
Maryland Heights, Missouri
(Chapter 22 — Physical Growth; co-author)
(Chapter 23 — Developmental Stages; co-author)
(Chapters 26, 28, 30, 34–36, 39, 40; co-author)

P. K. Holmes
Advising Coordinator
Department of Nursing
University of South Dakota
Vermillion, South Dakota
(Chapter 24 — Basic Nutrition)

Peggy Larsen, MS, RN
Assistant Professor
Nursing Department
University of South Dakota
Vermillion, South Dakota
(Chapter 41 — Musculoskeletal Conditions; primary author)

June Peterson Larson, MS, RN
Associate Professor, Assistant Director, Department of Nursing
Director, Vermillion Campus
University of South Dakota
Vermillion, South Dakota
(Chapter 29 — The Hospitalized Child; primary author)
(Chapter 32 — Caring for the Dying Child)

Stephanie G. Metzger, MS, RN, C
Clinical Nurse Specialist
Children's Hospital
Richmond, Virginia
(Chapter 42 — Neurological Conditions)

Barbara Ellen Norwitz, BSN, RN, PNP
Publisher and Editorial Director
Cracom Corporation
Maryland Heights, Missouri;
formerly Pediatric Nurse Practitioner
Johns Hopkins Hospital
Baltimore, Maryland
(Chapter 22 — Physical Growth)
(Chapter 23 — Developmental Stages; primary author)
(Chapter 26 — Child Safety)
(Chapter 28 — Assessment)
(Chapter 30 — Routine Pediatric Procedures)
(Chapter 34 — Communicable and Infectious Diseases)
(Chapter 35 — Integumentary Conditions)
(Chapter 36 — Conditions of the Eyes and Ears)
(Chapter 39 — Digestive and Metabolic Conditions)
(Chapter 40 — Genitourinary Conditions)

Nancy O'Donnell, BSN, MS, RN
Associate Professor
J. Sargeant Reynolds Community College
Richmond, Virginia
(Chapter 43 — Conditions of the Blood and
    Blood-Forming Organs)

Joann F. Pieronek, PhD, RN
Director of Nursing
Wayne County Community College
Detroit, Michigan
(Chapter 27 — Preparing for Hospitalization)

Carla Ries
Assistant Professor
Department of Nursing
University of South Dakota
Vermillion, South Dakota
(Chapter 29 — The Hospitalized Child; co-author)
(Chapter 41 — Musculoskeletal Conditions; co-author)

Ann G. Ross, MN, ARNP, CS
Professor of Nursing
Health Occupations Division
Shorelines Community College
Seattle, Washington
(Chapter 44 — Emotional and Behavioral Conditions)

Mary Ann Scoloveno, EdD, RN
Associate Professor
Rutgers, The State University of New Jersey
College of Nursing
Newark, New Jersey
(Chapter 21 — Principles of Growth and Development)
(Chapter 25 — Immunizations)

Pamela J. Shapiro, BSN, ARNP
OB-GYN Nurse Practitioner
Kirkland, Washington
(Chapters 1–20 — Maternal/Newborn Chapters)

Lisa Shaver
Assistant Professor
J. Sargeant Reynolds Community College
Richmond, Virginia
(Chapter 37 — Cardiovascular Conditions)

Rosemarie C. Westberg, MSN, RN
Associate Professor, Nursing
Northern Virginia Community College
Annandale, Virginia
(Chapter 33 — Sudden Infant Death Syndrome)
(Chapter 38 — Respiratory Conditions)

Special thanks also goes to the staff of Visual Education Corporation, especially Teresa Moore, for their excellent work on the development of this text.

UNIT

Pediatrics and the Newborn

1

CHAPTER

1

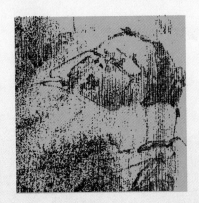

Introduction to Pediatrics

OBJECTIVES

AFTER STUDYING THIS CHAPTER, THE STUDENT SHOULD BE ABLE TO:

- TRACE THE HISTORY OF CHILD HEALTH CARE.
- EXPLAIN ETHICAL PRINCIPLES IN NURSING.
- DISCUSS FAMILY FUNCTIONS RELATED TO CHILDREN.
- DESCRIBE THE ROLES OF THE PEDIATRIC NURSE.
- EXPLAIN EACH STEP OF THE NURSING PROCESS.

KEY TERMS

PEDIATRIC NURSING	EXTENDED FAMILY
RESPECT FOR PERSONS	SINGLE-PARENT FAMILY
FIDELITY	TWO-CAREER FAMILY
BENEFICENCE	STEPFAMILY
JUSTICE	BLENDED FAMILY
NUCLEAR FAMILY	SOCIALIZATION

ediatrics refers to the medical specialty that deals with child development and care, including childhood diseases. **Pediatric nursing** is the health care profession that blends the science of health promotion and illness prevention with the art of caring for children and their families.

HISTORICAL PERSPECTIVE

During early Western civilization, people had no concept of childhood as a separate stage of development. They believed infancy lasted until age 7. After that age, children were considered miniature adults, valued for their contribution to the family income and rarely sent to school. Even when sick, children were treated as adults.

Toward the end of the Middle Ages, families began to view childhood as a separate growth stage. By the mid-1800s, a greater number of children attended school. Pediatrics developed as a medical specialty. In 1853, the Children's Aid Society for homeless children was founded in New York City. Two years later, The Children's Hospital of Philadelphia opened. Sadly, most early institutions were unsanitary, and their mortality rates ranged from 50% to 100%.

In the early 1900s, institutions tried to reduce mortality by following strict asepsis. They placed infants in separate cubicles, discouraged staff and parents from holding them, removed toys, and strictly limited parental visits to one hour every week. Yet mortality rates remained high.

Beginning in 1932, a series of studies found that maternal deprivation and lack of stimulation caused stuporousness and other symptoms in infants, and had possible long-term effects on families. In response, hospitals gradually liberalized visitation policies, relaxed isolation restrictions, and encouraged play. From 1935 to 1960, infant mortality fell from 70 deaths per 1,000 live births to about 25.

Today, Americans think of children as individuals who are growing and developing physically, mentally, emotionally, and spiritually. We view childhood as a distinct stage of life that emphasizes learning. Our laws and customs protect children's rights.

Child health care now focuses on promoting optimal growth and development, as well as on treating illnesses. It also centers on the child as a member of the family. Hospitalized children now receive care in cheerful, homelike children's units, as shown in Figure 1–1. In addition, children may receive care in special pediatric diagnostic and treatment centers and

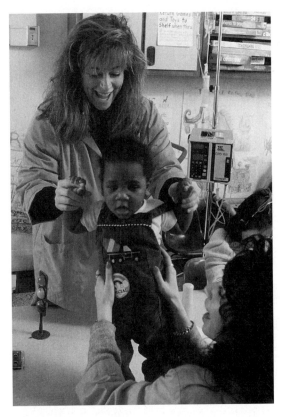

Figure 1–1   *Children's unit in a hospital. (Courtesy Carl Howard and Albany Medical Center.)*

from many new health care specialists, such as pediatric surgeons. Despite improvements in infant and child health, however, the United States lags behind 18 nations in infant mortality.

CHILD HEALTH CARE
LEGISLATION

Throughout the twentieth century, federal laws and programs improved the health of American children. In the early 1900s, the Children's Bureau studied infant and maternal mortality, prompting interest in the improvement of maternal and child health. During the Depression, the government passed the Social Security Act (1935), which funded programs for maternal and child care, care for crippled children, and preventive health care. It also passed the Fair Labor Standards Act (1938), which set the minimum working age at 16 years (18 years for hazardous jobs) and established minimum standards for child labor. (Before this law, many children worked in coal mines, textile mills, and at other unsanitary or dangerous sites.) Since then, the government has implemented many child health care programs, which are summarized in Figure 1–2.

LEGAL AND ETHICAL ISSUES

In pediatric nursing, legal and ethical issues often arise. When facing an ethical dilemma, the nurse should identify the conflict, note pertinent laws and facts, consider each option and its consequences, and apply the following ethical principles to decide on a course of action:

• **Respect for persons**: Supporting a patient's right to autonomy (self-determination), confidentiality (respect of privacy), refusal of treatment, and truthfulness.
• **Fidelity**: Remaining faithful to promises and duties.
• **Beneficence**: Trying to do good and to avoid or prevent harm.
• **Justice**: Treating all patients fairly in providing care and allocating resources.

To face ethical issues confidently and to reduce the risk of liability, the nurse should also know the law. The chief legal resource for nurses is the relevant state practice act, which provides general guidelines for legal conduct. The Code for Nurses, Figure 1–3, provides more specific guidance.

SELECTED FEDERAL PROGRAMS AFFECTING CHILD HEALTH

Year	Law or Program	Description
1965	Medicaid Early and Periodic Screening, Diagnosis, and Treatment (EPSDT)	Provides for early and periodic screening, diagnosis, and treatment for children up to age 21, in low-income or inaccessible areas.
1965	Crippled Children's Service	Provides services to children under age 21.
1965	Head Start	Addresses health and education needs of economically disadvantaged preschool children.
1966	National School Lunch Act and Child Nutrition Act	Provides free or reduced-rate meals to children from low-income families.
1972	Consumer Product Safety Commission	Develops safety regulations for toys, cribs, children's clothing, and related products.
1974	Special Supplemental Food Program for Women, Infants, and Children (WIC)	Provides nutritious food and nutrition education to low-income perinatal women and their children under age 5.
1975	Education of All Handicapped Children	Provides free public education (and related support services) to handicapped children ages 5 to 21.
1982	Community Mental Health Centers	Increases the availability of mental health centers to low-income families.
1993	Family and Medical Leave Act	Provides 12 weeks of unpaid leave for maternity or care for a sick family member.
1993	Vaccines for Children Program	Provides free vaccines to children who are Medicaid-eligible, Native American, uninsured, or underinsured.

Figure 1–2

ROLES OF FAMILIES AND PARENTS

Because the family affects a child's health, the nurse should understand family structures and functions as well as parenting styles. The functions of families are basically similar. Family structures and parenting styles, however, vary widely.

FAMILY STRUCTURES

Traditional family structures include nuclear and extended families. In a **nuclear family**, a father, mother, and children share the same household. Once standard, this structure now accounts for less than one-third of U.S. families. An **extended family** consists of a nuclear family and other relatives, such as aunts,

CODE FOR NURSES

1. The nurse provides services with respect for human dignity and the uniqueness of the client, unrestricted by considerations of social or economic status, personal attributes, or the nature of health problems.

2. The nurse safeguards the client's right to privacy by judiciously protecting information of a confidential nature.

3. The nurse acts to safeguard the client and the public when health care and safety are affected by the incompetent, unethical, or illegal practice of any person.

4. The nurse assumes responsibility and accountability for individual nursing judgments and actions.

5. The nurse maintains competence in nursing.

6. The nurse exercises informed judgment and uses individual competence and qualifications as criteria in seeking consultation, accepting responsibilities, and in delegating nursing activities to others.

7. The nurse participates in activities that contribute to the ongoing development of the profession's body of knowledge.

8. The nurse participates in the profession's efforts to implement and improve standards of nursing.

9. The nurse participates in the profession's efforts to establish and maintain conditions of employment conducive to high quality nursing care.

10. The nurse participates in the profession's effort to protect the public from misinformation and misrepresentation and to maintain the integrity of nursing.

11. The nurse collaborates with members of the health professions and other citizens in promoting community and national efforts to meet the health needs of the public.

Figure 1–3   *American Nurses Association (ANA)*

uncles, and grandparents, who often assist with childrearing.

Among the many modified family structures are single-parent, two-career, step-, and blended families. About 23% of U.S. households are **single-parent families**. In these families, one parent assumes virtually all of the responsibilities for maintaining a home and raising children. A **two-career family** consists of two parents who work outside the home. One parent may also be the homemaker, or both may share the task. In a **stepfamily**, the custodial parent and children live in a household with the parent's new spouse. Two custodial parents who bring children from previous marriages into one new household form a **blended family**. By the year 2000, these and other types of modified-structure families will account for more than half of the households in America.

FAMILY FUNCTIONS

As the most basic social unit, the family's primary goal is to ensure the survival of the family, its members, and its culture. Its child-related functions include providing physical care, socialization, and emotional development. By providing physical care, the family meets each child's basic needs for food, clothing, and

patient goals represent desired outcomes of nursing care, they should include measurable patient behaviors and criteria, such as verbalization and time. A goal for the preschooler might be "The child will report reduced ear pain within 24 hours."

The diagnoses, goals, and interventions are integral parts of the **nursing care plan**. This is a written guide that directs individualized nursing care. (Care plans appear throughout this book.)

During the **implementation** step, the nurs-ing care plan is put into action. For each intervention, the nurse monitors and documents the child's responses. For the preschooler, the nurse might administer an analgesic and antibiotic as prescribed, apply heat, and monitor the child's pain level.

By determining if the patient has achieved the goals, the **evaluation** step measures the care plan's success. If the preschooler's goals were met, the nurse might document "The child reports no ear pain." If the goals were not met, the nurse would begin the process again.

REVIEW QUESTIONS

A. Multiple choice. Select the best answer.

1. Pediatrics became a medical specialty in
   a. the early seventeenth century
   b. the mid-1800s
   c. the early twentieth century
   d. the mid-1900s

2. Which federal program provides food to low-income women and their children?
   a. Medicaid ESPDT
   b. Community Mental Health Centers
   c. Head Start
   d. WIC

3. A nurse is describing treatment options to an adolescent with AIDS. This action reflects the ethical principle of
   a. respect for persons
   b. beneficence
   c. justice
   d. fidelity

4. A 10-year-old girl lives with her mother, her mother's new husband, and his 2 children. This is an example of a
   a. stepfamily
   b. blended family
   c. nuclear family
   d. extended family

5. When showing parents how to feed their new infant, the nurse assumes the role of
   a. direct caregiver
   b. health promoter
   c. counselor
   d. teacher

B. Match the term in column I to the correct description in column II.

Column I	Column II
1. nursing diagnosis	a. performing nursing interventions
2. assessment	b. determining if goals have been met
3. evaluation	c. stating a health problem
4. implementation	d. collecting objective and subjective data
5. planning	e. setting goals and selecting interventions

SUGGESTED ACTIVITIES

• Discuss the ethical issues involved in caring for a premature infant with HIV (human immunodeficiency virus).

• Describe how patient goals are used in later steps of the nursing process.

BIBLIOGRAPHY

Betz, C. L., M. Hunsberger, and S. Wright. *Family-Centered Nursing Care of Children*, 2nd ed. Philadelphia: W. B. Saunders, 1994.

Burns, M., and C. Thornam. "Broadening the scope of nursing practice: Federal Programs for Children." *Pediatric Nursing*, 19, no. 6 (November–December, 1993): 546–552.

Cohen, S., C. Kenner, and A. Hollingsworth. *Maternal, Neonatal, and Women's Health Nursing*. Springhouse, PA: Springhouse, 1991.

Jackson, D. *Child Health Nursing: A Comprehensive Approach to the Care of Children and Their Families*. Philadelphia: J. B. Lippincott, 1993.

Wong, D. L. *Whaley & Wong's Nursing Care of Infants and Children*, 5th ed. St. Louis, MO: Mosby–Year Book, 1995.

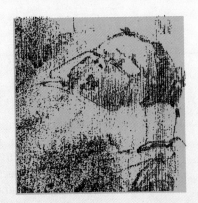

The Newborn

OBJECTIVES

AFTER STUDYING THIS CHAPTER, THE STUDENT SHOULD BE ABLE TO:

- DESCRIBE THE TRANSITION TO EXTRAUTERINE LIFE.
- EXPLAIN APGAR SCORING.
- IDENTIFY CHARACTERISTICS OF THE NEWBORN.
- LIST SIX FACTORS THAT INFLUENCE BONDING.
- DISCUSS KEY ASPECTS OF NEWBORN CARE.
- COMPARE BREAST-FEEDING WITH BOTTLE-FEEDING.
- DISCUSS TOPICS TO TEACH PARENTS ABOUT A NEWBORN.

Key Terms

the birth of a newborn is an exciting event for the parents and for everyone attending the birth. It is also a critical time for nursing care. The nurse must assist in the newborn's transition to extrauterine life. Then the nurse must provide skillful care and assess the newborn's immediate responses and general characteristics. The nurse must also teach the parents so that they can care for the infant at home.

TRANSITION TO EXTRAUTERINE LIFE

The transition to **extrauterine life** (life outside the uterus) is a critical time for the newborn. At birth, the newborn makes its first sound— a lusty cry—and takes its first breath. The birth cry serves two purposes: it supplies the blood with sufficient oxygen and inflates the unexpanded lungs. With this cry, the dormant respiratory system begins to function, Figure 2–1. If the newborn does not breathe immediately, the doctor may stimulate the cry by holding the head down and rubbing the newborn's back or by flicking the soles of the feet. The doctor wipes or suctions mucus from the newborn's mouth, and checks its respiratory status.

The doctor clamps the umbilical cord in two places—about 1½ inches and 2½ inches from the newborn's body. Then the doctor cuts the cord between the clamps, physically separating the newborn from the mother. With this action, the newborn establishes a circulatory system independent from the mother's. The cord stump should be examined closely. If only one artery is present instead of two, the newborn must be evaluated closely for internal organ defects. After this, if no respiratory problems are present, the doctor may hand the newborn to the nurse and return to care of the mother.

11

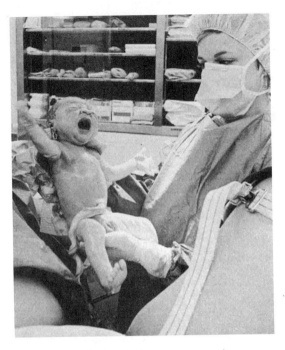

Figure 2–1 Newborn's first vigorous cry after delivery

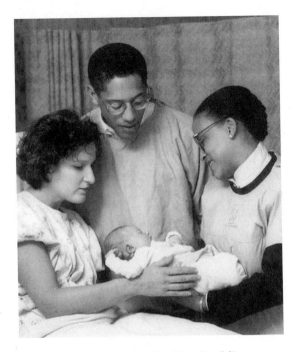

Figure 2–2 Parent-infant bonding after delivery

The nurse should then dry the newborn and wrap the infant snugly in a warm, dry blanket to ensure warmth before handing it to the parents to promote **bonding** (development of an enduring affectional tie between two people). Bonding occurs at birth, as the parents and newborn exchange messages and feelings through eye contact, skin-to-skin contact, smell, and sound. The first few minutes and hours after birth are especially critical to bonding. During this time, the newborn is alert and ready to respond to the environment. The mother and father are physically and emotionally attracted to their newborn, and these reciprocal feelings may have long-lasting effects on the parent-child relationship, Figure 2–2.

The role of touch in maternal-infant bonding is vital. The mother may want to place the newborn on her abdomen immediately after

birth. To help keep the newborn warm, the nurse may cover the mother and newborn with a blanket. Giving the newborn to the mother permits skin-to-skin contact and helps the uterus become firm by stimulating hormone release.

IMMEDIATE CARE AND NEWBORN RESPONSES

The first minutes of extrauterine life are key to the newborn's survival. Because the nurse is usually the first health care professional available to assess the newborn's adjustment to this transition, the nurse must be able to perform Apgar scoring and provide basic immediate care.

APGAR SCORING

The nurse assesses the newborn's general condition with the **Apgar scoring system**, Figure 2–3. At 1 and 5 minutes after birth, the newborn's condition is evaluated on 5 signs: heart rate, respiratory effort, muscle tone, reflex response, and color. Each sign is graded as 0, 1, or 2. A perfect total score is 10.

After observing a number of births, the nurse can do the scoring almost at a glance. A newborn who is pink all over, howling, and clenching his fists scores a 10 almost automatically. A quiet, limp newborn probably scores 0 to 1. A zero-rated newborn has a better than 50% chance of survival. A stillborn has no score at all.

RESUSCITATION OF THE NEWBORN

After an infant is born, the nurse's most important responsibility is to observe the newborn closely and continuously for signs of respiratory or circulatory depression. Some infants who cry at birth subsequently develop apnea

APGAR SCORING SYSTEM

Sign	0	1	2
Heart Rate	Absent (begin resuscitation)	Slow (below 100 bpm)	Good (over 100 bpm)
Respiratory Effort	Absent (begin resuscitation)	Weak cry; hypoventilation	Good strong cry; established respirations
Muscle Tone	Limp	Some flexion of extremities; weak or floppy resistance	Well flexed; strong resistance; active motion
Reflex response			
1. Response to catheter in nostril (tested after oropharynx is clear)	No response	Grimace	Cough or sneeze
2. Tangential foot slap	No response	Grimace	Strong cry and foot withdrawal
Color	Blue; pale	Body pink; extremities blue	Completely pink

Total Score— Condition

    0 to 3 – poor, critical, severely depressed

    4 to 6 – moderately depressed

    7 to 10 – good

Figure 2–3   *(Adapted from Nursing Inservice Aid, No. 2, Courtesy Ross Laboratories, published with permission of Dr. Virginia Apgar)*

(temporary loss of breath) and may die unless they receive resuscitation (restoration to life). Therefore, the nurse should observe a newborn continuously for at least 5 minutes after delivery and report any signs of depression to the obstetrician.

The anesthetist and obstetrician are responsible for resuscitating a newborn. The degree to which a nurse is involved varies from hospital to hospital. The nurse may perform routine measures, such as aspirating the mouth, nose, and pharynx; flicking the feet; and administering oxygen. Resuscitating a newborn in distress is detailed in Chapter 3. Providing cardiopulmonary resuscitation for an infant is discussed in Chapter 10.

EYE CARE

After gently wiping the newborn's eyes, the nurse instills erythromycin or tetracycline ointment or drops, as ordered. This treatment protects the newborn from gonococcus and Chlamydia organisms that may have been in the birth canal and could cause blindness. About 15 minutes after application, the nurse gently wipes away excess medication. Because the medication may temporarily blur the newborn's vision, parents may ask to delay the treatment for up to 1 hour so that they may have eye contact with their newborn.

THERMOREGULATION

The newborn's unstable heat-regulating system causes the infant's body temperature to change with the environmental temperature. If the room is cold, so is the newborn's body. If the infant is covered with too many blankets, the body temperature rises. Therefore, the nurse should prevent heat loss or overheating by drying the newborn thoroughly, placing the baby directly on the mother's abdomen or under a radiant warmer, and providing blankets as well as clothes and a cap for the infant as needed.

IDENTIFICATION AND DOCUMENTATION

The nurse should fill out and attach Identabands before the mother and newborn leave the delivery room. Identabands consist of three bands, printed with the same number. One wristband is used for the mother, and a wristband and an ankleband are used for the newborn. A record of the mother's name, doctor's name, sex of the newborn, and date and time of birth is inserted into each band. Some hospitals take footprints of the newborn and fingerprints of the mother for further identification. Complete the newborn record before the newborn is taken to the nursery.

GENERAL CHARACTERISTICS OF THE NEWBORN

After respirations are sustained, the nurse can perform a more detailed examination. Although every newborn is unique, the nurse should remember averages and the range of normality so that a newborn who deviates too far from the average may receive medical care.

GENERAL APPEARANCE, WEIGHT, AND LENGTH

Observe the newborn's overall appearance. Typically, a newborn looks surprisingly complete despite its small size. The hands, for example, resemble those of an adult with fingerprints, fingernails, and palm creases.

Record the newborn's weight and length. Although the weight of normal newborns varies, about two-thirds of all full-term infants weigh 6 to 8½ lb (2,700 to 3,850 g). During the

PROCEDURE

Initial Assessment and Care of the Newborn

1. As soon as the newborn is delivered, record the exact time of birth.

2. With a sterile towel, receive the newborn from the doctor.

3. Rate the newborn according to the Apgar scoring system (discussed in this chapter); record the score.

4. Wipe the newborn dry and wrap him or her in a warm blanket. It is vital that the newborn be kept warm. Protect the newborn from thermal stress, preferably by using a radiant warmer.

5. If the condition of the mother and newborn permit, take the newborn to the head of the table for the mother and father to see and hold for a time. This is an important time in establishing the parent-infant bond.

6. Place the newborn on its side in the heated incubator or crib, with the head of the crib lowered; this position promotes mucus drainage.

7. Suction the newborn with a bulb syringe to remove mucus or other secretions from the mouth, nose, and pharynx. Positioning and suctioning are necessary so the infant does not aspirate this material. (*Caution:* Squeeze the bulb and expel all the air from the syringe before inserting it gently. Otherwise, the material in the oropharynx will be forced into the bronchi and lungs when the bulb is collapsed.) Gentle suction is provided as the bulb regains its original shape, as shown at right.

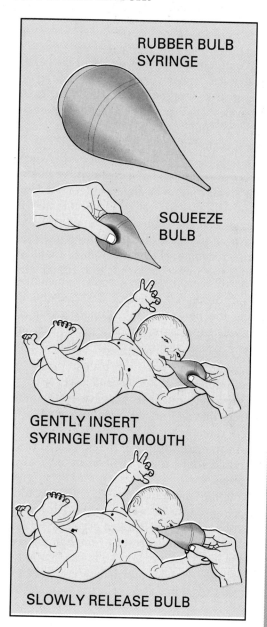

RUBBER BULB SYRINGE

SQUEEZE BULB

GENTLY INSERT SYRINGE INTO MOUTH

SLOWLY RELEASE BULB

Figure 2-4   *Bulb syringe suctioning*

first few days after birth, the infant may lose 6 to 10 oz (217 to 311 g) or 5% to 10% of the birth weight. The newborn's length normally ranges from 19 to 21½ in. (47.5 to 53.75 cm).

HEAD AND NECK

Observe for obvious malformation of the head, such as microcephaly, anencephaly, cleft lip or palate, and malformed ears. The head normally appears too large for the body. It may be temporarily out of shape—lopsided or elongated—because of pressure during birth.

Palpate the **fontanels** (spaces between skull bones that have not yet grown together), which should feel soft and not depressed or swollen. The anterior fontanel is located above the brow, and the posterior fontanel is at the crown near the back of the head, Figure 2–5. The anterior fontanel closes within 18 months; the posterior fontanel takes 2 to 6 months to close.

Measure the head circumference, which is usually about 1 to 2 in. larger than the chest circumference. Evaluate the face for symmetry. Facial characteristics commonly include round cheeks, a broad flat nose with a slight bridge, a receding chin, and an undersized lower jaw.

Check the mouth for excessive, frothy oral secretions that may suggest esophageal atresia. Observe the eyes for shape, position, size, and the appearance of pupils. If the newborn cries, you should see no tears. The lids are normally edematous.

Note the length of the neck, which should be short, as well as its relationship to the body, mobility, and the presence of webbing or fat pads. Goiters and cystic lymphangiomas (tumors consisting of lymphatic vessels) may compromise the airway, making immediate tracheal intubation necessary.

CHEST AND ABDOMEN

Measure the newborn's chest circumference, which should be smaller than the head circum-

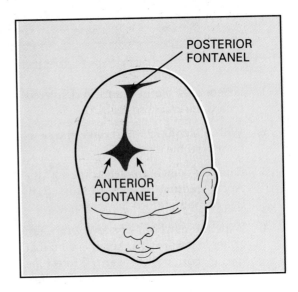

Figure 2–5   *Fontanels*

ference. Palpate the clavicles, which should be intact and have no masses. A fracture of the clavicle may occur during delivery. Inspect the size, symmetry, and shape of the chest and the shape of the abdomen, which usually appears large and rounded. Palpate the liver, spleen, and kidneys. Observe the umbilical cord, which should have one vein and two arteries.

Note the breasts of male and female neonates, which may be swollen because of maternal hormone exposure before birth. Some neonates leak drops of milk from the nipples (witches' milk). This condition disappears without treatment.

CARDIOVASCULAR SYSTEM

Note the heart rate and rhythm. The pulse is usually rapid—around 120 to 160 beats per minute—and irregular. If the newborn is startled or cries, the pulse rate increases and becomes more irregular. A rate over 160 or under 120 beats per minute usually requires further examination. Evaluate the peripheral pulses and compare the strength of the upper pulses with that of the lower pulses.

Measure blood pressure in both the upper and lower extremities. The newborn's blood pressure, which is usually about 80/46 mmHg, is difficult to measure accurately. Care should be taken to ensure that the size of the cuff used is correct.

RESPIRATORY SYSTEM

Check the respiratory rate, which varies from 30 to 60 breaths per minute and is irregular in depth and rhythm. Like the pulse rate, it is easily altered by internal or external stimuli.

When auscultating the chest, note coarse rales, which usually disappear in the first hours after birth. Unilateral absence of breath sounds suggests pneumothorax or diaphragmatic hernia.

Watch for signs of respiratory distress, which include tachypnea (more than 60 breaths per minute), chest wall and sternal retractions, nasal flaring, and grunting. They indicate a need for close observation. Slow, shallow respirations (fewer than 30 breaths per minute) may suggest central nervous system (CNS) depression or respiratory distress.

GASTROINTESTINAL SYSTEM

Observe for elimination of **meconium** (the first stools, which are sticky and greenish black). This usually occurs 8 to 24 hours after birth and confirms anal patency.

TEMPERATURE

Take the newborn's temperature by axilla. Refer to Chapter 12 for the procedure for taking an axillary temperature. Be sure that the infant's arm is close to the trunk. Be careful not to chill the infant. The newborn's temperature, although unstable, is usually about 37.5°C (99.5°F).

URINARY SYSTEM

Particularly note the first urination, which confirms urinary tract function. The newborn generally urinates within 24 hours of birth. Observe males for the position of the urethral opening.

REPRODUCTIVE SYSTEM

Observe the appropriateness of the visible genitals for the newborn's stated sex. The genitals may seem relatively large. Observe females for maturation of the labia and for vaginal discharge. A slight milky or bloody vaginal discharge may occur. Observe males for the presence of testes and maturation of the scrotum.

MUSCULOSKELETAL SYSTEM

Palpate and inspect the spinal column. The vertebrae should be symmetrical and there should be no dimple or masses. Count the digits on the hands and feet. The hands should have finely lined palms, thin nails, and deep bracelet creases at the wrist.

Note the symmetry and mobility of all extremities. The legs may be drawn up to the abdomen and usually appear slightly bowed. The knees stay slightly bent. Normally, the muscles are weak and uncontrolled, making the newborn's movements random and uncoordinated. The newborn wiggles and stretches. Because the newborn lacks muscle strength, the back and head must be supported when the infant is picked up.

Evaluate hip rotation by abducting the thighs and rotating the hips through the full range of motion. Watch the leg creases, which should be symmetrical. The pelvis and hips should appear slender and narrow.

Nervous System

Observe and evaluate muscle tone, tremulousness, and jitteriness; and assess common newborn reflexes, Figure 2–6. If the infant is floppy, suspect a spinal cord injury or CNS depression. An absent, weak, or asymmetrical reflex is abnormal and requires further examination.

Moro Reflex. To elicit the **Moro reflex**, suddenly but gently drop the newborn's head back, relative to the body. Normally, the newborn responds by tensing, throwing the arms out in an embracing motion, and crying loudly. The index finger and thumb form a C. The Moro reflex disappears by 6 months of age.

Startle Reflex. After a loud noise is made nearby, the newborn should cry and abduct and flex the arms and legs. Absence of this reflex may indicate a hearing deficit. The startle reflex disappears by 4 months of age.

Galant Reflex. Stroke one side of the back while the newborn is lying on his or her stomach. The whole trunk should curve toward the stroked side. This reaction disappears by the end of the second month.

Tonic Neck (Fencing) Reflex. With the newborn lying on his or her back, quickly turn the head to one side. In response, the newborn should extend the arm and leg on the side to which the head is turned and should flex the other arm and leg. This reflex disappears at age 5 to 6 months.

Primary Standing Reflex. If held upright on both feet, the newborn should stand, support-

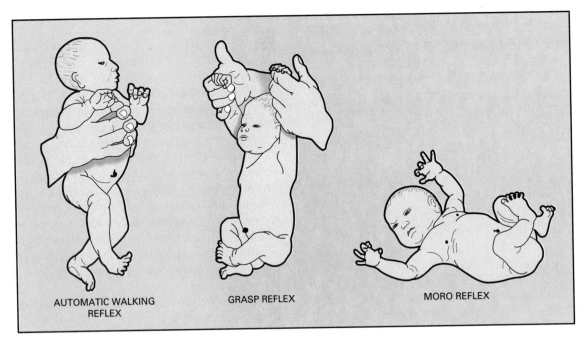

AUTOMATIC WALKING REFLEX GRASP REFLEX MORO REFLEX

Figure 2–6   Common newborn reflexes

ing some of his or her body weight. This reflex disappears by the end of the second month.

Automatic Walking (Stepping) Reflex. When the newborn is supported upright, the legs make walking motions. This ability also disappears at the end of the second month.

Grasp Reflex. To elicit the palmar grasp reflex, place a finger in the newborn's palm. The infant should grasp it firmly enough and hold it long enough to allow his or her body to be lifted. This reflex is gone by the end of the fourth month, when the grasp becomes purposeful.

To elicit the plantar reflex, place a finger at the bottom of the newborn's toes. The infant's toes should curl down to try to grasp the finger. This reflex does not disappear until the eighth month.

Sucking Reflex. When a finger or nipple is placed near the newborn's mouth, the infant should be able to grasp it and suck on it vigorously. Sucking continues until the child can drink from a cup.

Rooting Reflex. The newborn reacts to being touched on the cheek by turning his or her head in the direction of the touch to search for the nipple to feed. This reflex continues for as long as the newborn is nursing.

Placing Reflex. When the newborn's shins are placed against an edge, the newborn steps up to the top of the surface. This reflex disappears at the end of the second month.

Protective Reflexes. Certain reflexes are absolutely essential to the infant's life. These protective reflexes include the blinking reflex, which is aroused when the infant is subjected to a bright light, and the coughing and sneezing reflexes, which clear the respiratory tract.

The yawn reflex is protective because the infant draws in added oxygen by yawning. The swallowing reflex allows the newborn to swallow, and the gag reflex enables the infant to gag when taking more into the mouth than can be swallowed.

SPECIAL SENSES

Assess the newborn's sight, hearing, smell, taste, and touch. Normally, the newborn reacts to light by blinking, frowning, or closing the eyes. The eyes are unfocused, and the newborn may appear cross-eyed or wall-eyed because the infant cannot control eye movement. At birth, the infant can see most clearly from a distance of about 7 to 12 inches. The eyes are blue or gray and change to the permanent color at approximately 3 to 6 months. Although the sense of smell is not highly developed, the newborn can taste and usually prefers sweet fluids and resists sour or bitter fluids. The newborn normally reacts to loud or sudden sounds and responds to soothing sounds.

INTEGUMENTARY SYSTEM

Check for **vernix caseosa**, a white cheesy substance on the skin. It normally appears in preterm infants, but not in postterm infants and only in the skin folds of term infants.

Inspect the skin, which is commonly dark pink, soft, thin, dry, and covered with **lanugo** (fine, downy hair distributed over the body). Lanugo is most pronounced in the premature infant. In the newborn, veins may be visible through the skin; when the infant cries, a deep flush may spread over the entire body and veins on the head may swell and throb. Skin on the hands and feet is loose and wrinkled.

Note the skin color. **Cyanosis** (bluish skin discoloration) of the feet and hands, known as acrocyanosis, can persist for some time after respirations have been adequately established.

To assess oxygenation in a newborn with highly pigmented skin, look at the mucous membranes (gums). Pallor (lack of color) may indicate anemia, resulting from hemolysis or hemorrhage, or may suggest shock with inadequate cardiac output. Jaundice (yellowish skin) that appears 3 to 5 days after birth is common and usually disappears by the end of the first week. Jaundice that appears earlier may indicate disease. (Refer to Chapter 4 for additional information about jaundice in the newborn.) Mongolian spots (bluish black pigmentation) may appear at the base of the spine or on the buttocks of newborns of African, Hispanic, Mediterranean, or Native American descent.

Finally, check for blemishes. **Milia** (tiny white pimples, particularly on the nose and chin) may be present. These normal markings are caused by obstructed sweat and oil glands. Petechiae (small reddish spots due to broken capillaries) may be seen over the newborn's head and neck after a rapid or difficult delivery. A premature newborn may display ecchymosis (bruising) in areas that were grasped firmly during delivery.

Newborn Care

If the newborn's condition is good, many hospitals allow the newborn to remain in the mother's room. Some hospitals admit the newborn to the nursery. No matter where the newborn is, the nurse must promote bonding and provide routine care.

Promotion of Bonding

Research has shown that newborns are in a heightened state of alertness and responsiveness in the first hours after birth. During this time, many mothers wish to nurse their newborn, and parents may want to cuddle, hold, talk to, and get to know their infant. The infant may nuzzle or suck at the mother's breast, make eye contact with the parents, and respond to their sound and touch. This reciprocal responsiveness is the first step in bonding, which was first identified by Klaus and Kennel in 1972.

Many factors can influence bonding. These factors include the parents' cultural and socioeconomic backgrounds; their education, personalities, ages, and number of children; their previous experience with pregnancy; their attitudes toward pregnancy, parenting, and the newborn; obstetric complications; and their childbirth experience. The mother's physical and mental health before and during pregnancy can affect fetal health and development and the capacity for the mother and newborn to interact at birth.

The nurse can promote bonding by giving the parents at least 15 to 20 minutes alone with their newborn in a comfortable room after birth, encouraging the mother to hold the newborn naked against her bare chest in a warm area. Have the newborn stay with the mother continuously (rooming-in) or for long periods (at least 5 hours a day), and let the mother be the newborn's primary care provider. The nurse should also point out and reinforce the parents' perceptions of their newborn's abilities and should encourage the father to touch, hold, and interact with his newborn. Because early father-newborn interactions may be important to the development of a strong father-child relationship later in life, the nurse's support of the father's role in childbearing and child care is essential.

Routine Care

Place the newborn in the Trendelenburg position in the bassinet with the infant's head lower than the body. This position allows mucus to drain out of the nose and mouth. Fill out the appropriate-color crib card and place it on the newborn's bassinet. Remove the cord clamp after 24 hours if the cord has dried.

Apply alcohol several times a day until the stump falls off.

Assessment. To identify problems early, the newborn needs continued assessment. If the initial findings were normal, assess the following:

- vital signs (except for temperature, which may be checked every 4 hours)
- weight (compared with birth weight)
- fontanels
- general changes in color or activity
- mucus production
- feeding status
- elimination
- umbilical cord stump
- parent-newborn interactions

Infection prevention. When assessing or caring for the newborn, the nurse should take measures to prevent infection. For example, the nurse should wear gloves during all contact with the newborn until the infant has had the first bath. After the first bath, the nurse should handwash thoroughly for 30 seconds before touching the newborn. The nurse should also perform all care (except weighing) inside the bassinet. To weigh the newborn, the nurse should cover the scale with a disposable liner. Observe universal precautions; gloves should be worn when changing diapers.

Vitamin K Administration. The pediatrician may order a vitamin K injection for the newborn to protect against hemorrhage. In adults, normal bacteria in the intestines help produce vitamin K, which is needed for blood clotting. However, the newborn's intestines are sterile at birth and cannot manufacture sufficient vitamin K until after oral feeding has begun and normal intestinal flora are produced.

Phenylketonuria (PKU) Testing. A simple urine test or a blood test for PKU is performed after the newborn has ingested some protein but before hospital discharge. If the mother and newborn are discharged early, instruct the mother to return to the nursery or her pediatrician's office for a PKU test. **Phenylketonuria** results from a congenital defect in phenylalanine metabolism, which allows phenylalanine to accumulate and prevents normal brain development. If the disorder is detected early, brain damage can be prevented by a special diet for the newborn. (For details, see Chapter 4.)

Bathing the Newborn. The doctor or hospital policy determines the kind of bath the newborn receives. Usually, the newborn receives a sponge bath with water and a bacteriostatic agent until the cord has fallen off. During the bath, observe the newborn for irritation to the eyes, skin, and umbilical cord. Weigh the infant and take an axillary temperature after the bath.

Feeding. Unless contraindicated, the mother feeds the newborn in her room when the infant is hungry. Before taking the newborn from the nursery bassinet, check the bassinet card and Identabands. Check the identification of the mother and newborn again in the mother's room. If the newborn is bottle-feeding, check the formula to be sure it is the one prescribed for this child. Occasionally, the breast-fed newborn is weighed before and after nursing. Feeding time is an excellent time to teach the mother how to care for her newborn and to answer any questions.

Circumcision Care. If a male newborn has undergone **circumcision** (surgical removal of the foreskin of the penis), provide appropriate care. Record the first voiding. Gently cleanse the penis with a moist cotton ball at bath time. Petrolatum gauze may be used to prevent the penis from sticking to the diaper. Note any bleeding. Advise the parents that the wound usually heals in 2 or 3 days.

FEEDING

Successful infant feeding requires cooperation between the mother and her newborn, starting with the initial feeding experience. Feeding time should be pleasant and pleasurable for the mother and infant. Maternal feelings are readily transmitted to the newborn and can affect the feeding. If a mother is anxious, irritable, or easily upset, she may have difficulty with feeding. If she is comfortable, she and her newborn are likely to have a satisfying feeding experience.

The emptying time of the infant's stomach may vary from 1 to 4 or more hours. Therefore, there may be considerable differences in the desire for food at different times of the day. Ideally, the feeding schedule should be based on self-regulation by the infant. This approach is called **demand feeding**. Most healthy infants will want 8 to 12 feedings in 24 hours and will take enough at one feeding to

COMPARING BREAST-FEEDING WITH FORMULA-FEEDING

Breast-Feeding/Breast Milk

- Supplies all nutrients and sufficient water, as well as antibodies
- Is allergen-free
- Is always the right temperature
- Is readily available
- Is inexpensive
- May enhance maternal-infant bonding
- Promotes development of the infant's jaws, teeth, and facial muscles
- Often results in short gastric emptying time (1 to 4 hours)
- Requires mother to consume extra fluids and possibly nutritional supplements
- Lets drugs and certain foods that may adversely affect the infant enter the milk supply
- May provide less milk a few months into a new pregnancy; mother may need nutritional supplements to breast-feed
- Can be collected via breast pump for feeding by others
- Is contraindicated if the mother has certain conditions or illnesses

Formula-Feeding/Formula

- Supplies specified nutrients in ready-to-feed preparations, canned liquid concentrates, or powders
- Requires supplementation with water
- May cause allergies
- Must be warmed to the proper temperature
- Requires purchase, preparation, refrigeration, and storage
- Is more expensive than breast milk
- Allows mother and others to bond with the infant
- Allows more accurate measurement of the infant's intake
- Lengthens gastric emptying time—and time between feedings
- Requires no change in the mother's diet
- Is unaffected by the mother's diet or use of drugs, alcohol, or tobacco
- Is unaffected by pregnancy
- Is easily performed by caregivers
- Poses no contraindications for the mother

Figure 2–7

satisfy them for 2 to 3 hours. Smaller infants, with more rapid gastric emptying, will want milk more frequently than larger ones. Infants may not eat on a regular schedule; they nurse 4 or 5 times in 5 to 6 hours and then sleep for a long time. To ensure adequate nourishment, the nurse should suggest frequent daytime feeding if the newborn sleeps for long periods at night.

At around 3 weeks, 6 weeks, 3 months, and 6 months, the infant may suddenly want to feed at more frequent intervals. He may also be fretful, irritable, and more sensitive to stimuli. These behaviors reflect a growth spurt and an attempt to stimulate the breasts to produce more milk to meet increasing needs.

It is important to establish that an infant may cry for reasons other than hunger (such as a soiled diaper, desire to be held, or pain) and that the infant need not be fed every time he or she cries. The newborn may sleep 15 to 20 hours each day. The infant is usually awakened by hunger.

For most newborns, the mother may choose to breast-feed or bottle-feed. Both techniques have advantages and disadvantages, Figure 2–7. For newborns with special needs, other feeding techniques may be required, as described in Chapter 3.

BREAST-FEEDING

For the first few days after delivery, the breasts release colostrum. **Colostrum** is a thin, yellowish fluid composed chiefly of white blood cells and serum. It is rich in antibodies, salt, protein, and fat. Colostrum has a laxative effect that helps the newborn expel meconium from the intestinal tract. About 3 days after delivery, it is replaced by breast milk, which is bluish-white.

Breast-feeding Techniques. Breast-feeding has certain health benefits over bottle-feeding.

Therefore, the American Academy of Pediatrics recommends its use, whenever possible.

To breast-feed, the mother may sit up or lie on her side. (To protect the incision after a cesarean delivery, the mother may sit up with the newborn on a pillow in her lap, support the newborn on pillows in a football hold, or lie on her side.) Proper newborn positioning is essential, Figure 2–8. The mother's supporting arm should be under the newborn's buttocks. She should lift the newborn to the height of the breast and then turn the infant to face her, with their abdomens touching. Her other hand should support the breast with the thumb above and index finger below and behind the areola, compressing it to make the nipple thrust out. The mother must avoid blocking the newborn's nasal passage with breast tissue so that the infant can breathe well while feeding.

To get the newborn to take the nipple and areola into the mouth, the mother tickles the infant's lip with her nipple. When feeding is finished, the mother breaks the suction by placing a finger at the corner of the newborn's mouth before removing the infant from the breast. She should not pull the infant from one breast to feed from the other. The newborn usually nurses at least 10 to 15 minutes. When the infant takes a break, the mother can change breasts.

The mother should offer both breasts at each feeding because emptying the breasts stimulates milk production and prevents engorgement. The length of time the infant nurses varies widely from feeding to feeding and from infant to infant. Once a woman's milk supply is well established, a newborn gets most of the milk from the breast in the first 10 minutes. A woman may want to allow the infant this amount of time on the first breast and let the newborn nurse on the second breast as long as desired. Infants continue to derive pleasure from sucking and contact with their mothers long after satisfying their hunger.

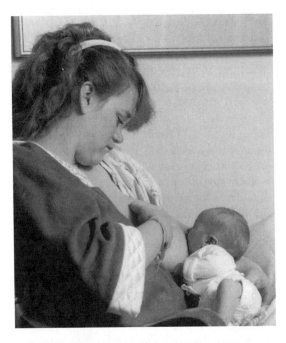

a.

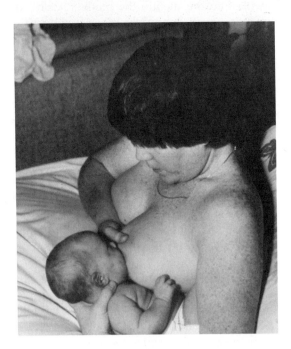

b.

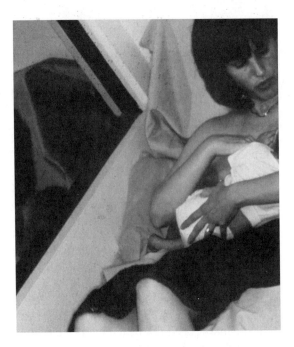

c.

Figure 2-8   *Proper positions for breast-feeding include (a) the sitting position for a mother after vaginal delivery, and the (b) clutch or football position and (c) semi Fowler's for a mother after cesarean delivery (b & c used with permission of Chele Marmet, MA, IBCLC and Lactation Institute, 818-995-1913, USA).*

To be sure the newborn is getting enough milk, the mother should look for these things:

- feeding well every 2 hours or so for a total of 20 to 40 minutes
- 6 to 8 wet diapers a day
- loose stool after each feeding or three or more stools a day for the first month
- contentment after feeding
- expected weight gain

The mother should burp the newborn frequently during breast-feeding to release air that may have been swallowed during the feeding. Otherwise, the newborn will be uncomfortable and may burp spontaneously, regurgitating the entire feeding. Two methods of burping are shown in Figure 2–9.

Weaning. **Weaning** means transferring a newborn from dependence on mother's milk to dependence on another form of nourishment. A mother can wean her breast-fed infant whenever she wants. Some mothers want to breast-feed for a few weeks, others for more than a year. However long a newborn is breast-fed, weaning should be done gradually. Generally, replacing one breast-feeding at a time with a substitute feeding is a good way to wean. When the infant is used to one substitute feeding, a second substitute feeding can be given after a few days. This process continues until the newborn is no longer feeding at the breast.

BOTTLE-FEEDING

Mothers who breast-feed as well as those who bottle-feed should learn bottle-feeding techniques. The pediatrician may order

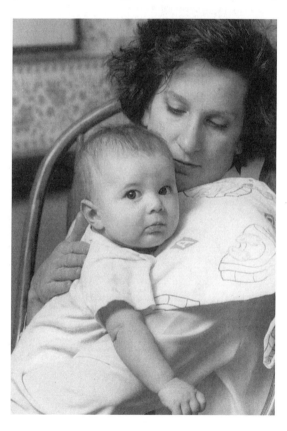
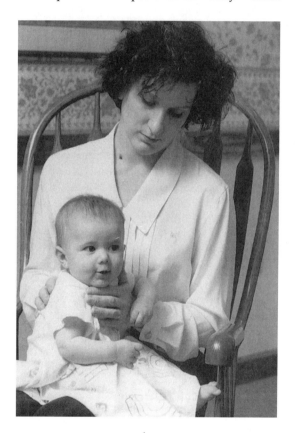

a. *b.*

Figure 2-9 *Burping an infant. (a) Hold the infant so that the infant's chin rests against a covered shoulder. Gently stroke the back. (b) Hold the infant upright, leaning slightly forward. Support the head and chest with one hand and stroke the back with the other hand.*

supplementary bottle-feedings if the infant's need is greater than the mother's milk supply. After breast-feeding is well established, the nursing mother may want to give her newborn an occasional bottle when her schedule does not allow her to breast-feed.

On discharge from the hospital, the mother should receive instructions about the formula. These instructions tell her the type of formula to use and how to prepare it. She should follow the instructions exactly.

The mother should select a nipple with the proper size hole. The hole is the right size if the formula drips out when the bottle is held upside down. If the milk comes out in a stream, the newborn will get too much formula too quickly. If it drips too slowly or not at all, the newborn will swallow too much air, will tire, and will not get enough formula.

The infant should be held in a semi-reclining position during bottle-feeding. If the infant's head is too low, the milk may pool back in the throat around the eustachian tubes, which could cause a middle ear infection. To promote normal eye muscle development in the newborn, the mother should use one arm and then the other to hold the infant. When feeding, the bottle should be held so that the nipple is full of milk. This prevents the newborn from swallowing air.

A young infant should be burped after consuming 1 to 2 oz of formula; as the infant matures, the mother should burp the baby about half-way through each feeding. The infant may not consume the same amount of formula at every feeding. The baby should not be coaxed to empty the bottle at each feeding if the infant seems satisfied with less. Encourage the mother to make feeding a special time and never to prop the bottle and leave the newborn during a feeding.

After feeding, the newborn should be placed on his or her back or side. The side position is recommended if the newborn tends to regurgitate and the right side is preferred over the left side. If the newborn is placed on the right side, the milk passes more easily into the stomach because the stomach contour is to the right. This reduces the chance of aspiration.

Besides formula, 1 or 2 oz of water should be given twice daily. During hot weather, 2 or 3 oz of water may be given twice daily. If the newborn is constipated, an increased amount of water should remedy the situation.

EDUCATING THE FAMILY

New parents need guidelines for helping them evaluate the unfamiliar and unexpected situations that may arise when caring for a newborn. They also need reassurance that normal behavior varies greatly.

TEACHING DURING ASSESSMENTS

The nurse is in an ideal position to help parents focus on their newborn's personality and develop effective parenting skills. One way to do this is to perform assessments in the parents' presence and to use them as an opportunity for discussion and teaching.

To help parents understand their newborn's uniqueness, the nurse may use the **neonatal behavioral assessment scale (NBAS)**, which was developed by Dr. T. Berry Brazelton. The scale contains 27 characteristics of newborns grouped into four categories: irritability, social responsiveness, activity level and physical responsiveness, and response to stress. Every newborn scores differently. The newborn's responses can reveal ways to approach the infant's care.

Irritability. **Irritability** focuses on behaviors that frequently distress new parents. Parents of the irritable, fussy newborn feel helpless;

their attempts to calm and console their newborn are ineffective. Using scale items in this category can help determine whether the parents have a quiet, calm newborn, a fairly well-organized newborn who gets upset only occasionally, or a very irritable newborn who naturally spends a lot of time crying. The evaluation cannot assess parents' skill at consoling their newborn, but it can demonstrate what personality traits the newborn brings to the situation. The point is to show parents that a newborn's unique behavior and responses to irritation are derived from the infant's personality, not from their abilities as parents. Items on the scale that determine how quickly a newborn gets used to a light or a noise help evaluate how the infant controls his or her own behavior. A flashlight is shone briefly in a newborn's eyes 10 times or a bell is rung 4 times. Many infants are startled by these activities at first. Then they gradually stop all eye and body movement as if they were unaware of anything happening in their environment. Other infants seem to have no response to the bell or light at first and later are startled by it. These infants may need a little help to remain calm, such as a reassuring pat. Still other infants seem unable to tune out stimuli; in response to it, they get more and more upset. These infants need a lot of help from parents to calm down. Such infants may benefit from living in a quiet home where extra environmental stimuli are kept to a minimum.

Social Responsiveness. One of the most satisfying aspects of a relationship with a newborn is **social responsiveness**. The NBAS gives parents a good idea of how easily they can get a social response from their newborn, how long the newborn sustains the response, and whether the newborn prefers auditory or visual interactions with people and things.

When a shiny object, such as a ball, is moved in front of the newborn's face slowly, the infant may or may not follow the ball with his or her eyes. If a rattle is shaken out of sight, the newborn may or may not turn toward the rattle. A minimal response is for the newborn to become still and alert. Sometimes parents have difficulty sustaining a response, or they stop trying. Parents can be taught to move the object more slowly and to return it to the newborn's line of vision, or to repeat the rattle sound. These exercises increase the opportunity for parent-infant exchanges and increase the parents' insight into their newborn's unique personality.

Consolability, an aspect of social responsiveness, is a measure of the infant's ability to calm down after fussiness. Newborns quiet themselves by sucking on a fist or finger or by looking at or listening to something interesting. Parents watch the crying newborn for 10 seconds and slowly introduce a small amount of consolation such as talking soothingly. If this does not work, parents can try gentle restraint, such as laying a hand on the newborn's trunk or holding one or both arms. The next step is holding the newborn, then rocking, then swaddling, or giving the infant a pacifier. These methods give parents strategies to quiet a fussy newborn. Some babies can calm themselves when fussing but need help to stop crying. The benefit to parents is the discovery that consolability is not related to the effectiveness of their intervention but rather to some internal process that the newborn cannot yet control.

Activity Level and Physical Responsiveness. Observing activity level and physical responsiveness can help parents learn whether they have an active, alert newborn or a passive, quiet one. Parents learn that their newborn is unique and cannot be changed or molded to conform to expectations. Using information from the scale, parents may learn that their newborn is happier in a large crib rather than a small cradle. Or they may find that the infant prefers to be carried facing outward and to be visually stimulated instead of being carried on a shoulder.

Response to Stress. This category includes physical changes such as startles, chin and limb tremors, and skin color changes. Some infants are rarely startled; others are startled for no apparent reason. If a newborn is easily startled and demonstrates frequent skin color changes, the parents can expect that the infant needs some restraint. Many parents mistakenly interpret normal newborn tremors as shivering caused by cold.

Discharge Teaching. Before discharge, the nurse should help the parents make appoint-

ments for follow-up visits and immunizations. As early as possible, the nurse should also begin teaching them about:

- feeding patterns and techniques
- bathing and skin care
- cord care
- circumcision care, if appropriate
- elimination patterns and diaper changes
- temperature measurement
- expected growth and development
- expected parent, sibling, and infant adjustments
- safety precautions, including the use of car seats
- infection prevention measures
- cradle cap removal
- any treatments to be done at home
- additional topics based on the newborn's individual needs

PROCEDURE

Infant Bathing

1. Gather these items: a washcloth, towel, basin of warm (100° to 105°F) water, mild unscented soap, cotton balls, a comb, clean infant clothes, and a blanket.
2. Wash the infant's face with water only. Then dry it.
3. Wash the eyelids from the inner to outer corner with a washcloth wrapped around one finger and no ends dangling.
4. Wash the external part of the ears with the washcloth wrapped around one finger.
5. Clean each nostril with a separate dampened cotton ball.

6. Gently wash the scalp with soap lather. Holding the head over the basin, rinse with warm water. Dry the head quickly but gently.
7. Remove the diaper and wash the perineal area from front to back, using a clean cotton ball for each stroke.
8. Remove other clothes. Then wash and rinse the rest of the body, carefully cleaning folds, creases, and genitals.
9. Pat dry, dress the infant, and comb the infant's hair.
10. Cover the infant with a clean blanket to maintain warmth.

REVIEW QUESTIONS

A. Multiple choice. Select the best answer.

1. Evaluation of the newborn using the Apgar system must *first* be done at
    a. 1 minute after delivery
    b. 5 minutes after delivery
    c. any time before the newborn is taken to the nursery
    d. 24 hours after delivery

2. The purpose of instilling an antibiotic ointment in the newborn's eyes is to
    a. help the newborn see better
    b. prevent infection and blindness
    c. promote parent-infant bonding
    d. help prevent jaundice

3. Immediate newborn care includes
    a. recording the weight and length
    b. palpating the fontanels
    c. bathing the newborn
    d. instilling eye drops or ointment

4. An average full-term newborn weighs
    a. 4 to 5½ lb
    b. 5 to 7 lb
    c. 6 to 8½ lb
    d. 8 to 9 lb

5. Which reflex should a loud, nearby noise elicit in the newborn?
    a. Galant reflex
    b. startle reflex
    c. fencing reflex
    d. plantar reflex

6. The success of breast-feeding may depend on
    a. vaginal delivery of the newborn
    b. careful scheduling of feedings
    c. size of the mother's breasts
    d. the mother's diet

7. To break the oral suction of a breast-feeding newborn, the mother should
    a. pull the newborn away gently
    b. squeeze the nipple together
    c. place a finger at the corner of the newborn's mouth
    d. squeeze the newborn's cheeks

8. The NBAS groups newborn characteristics into categories in order to
    a. measure a newborn's susceptibility to mental disease
    b. help parents understand their newborn's personality traits
    c. evaluate parental skills in caring for their newborn
    d. provide a means of rating a newborn's physical and mental abilities

B. Briefly answer the following questions.

1. Name the five items assessed in the Apgar scoring system.

2. List six factors that may influence parent-infant bonding.

3. Identify the advantages and disadvantages of bottle-feeding and breast-feeding.

SUGGESTED ACTIVITIES

- Discuss the respiratory and circulatory effects of the transition to extrauterine life.
- Role play assisting with immediate care of the newborn.
- Describe and chart normal and abnormal findings in the neonate.
- Describe parental and newborn behaviors that reflect bonding.
- In groups, debate the advantages and disadvantages of breast-feeding and bottle-feeding.
- Explain how to use the NBAS as a teaching tool for new parents.

BIBLIOGRAPHY

Betz, C., M. Hunsberger, and S. Wright. *Family-Centered Nursing Care of Children*, 2nd ed. Philadelphia: W. B. Saunders, 1994.

Cohen, S., C. Kenner, and A. Hollingsworth. *Maternal, Neonatal, and Women's Health Nursing*. Springhouse, PA: Springhouse, 1991.

Jackson, D., and R. Saunders. *Child Health Nursing: A Comprehensive Approach to the Care of Children and Their Families*. Philadelphia: J. B. Lippincott, 1993.

Lawrence, R. *Breast Feeding: A Guide for the Medical Profession*, 3rd ed. St. Louis, MO: C. V. Mosby, 1989.

Reeder, S., L. Mastroianni, Jr., and L. Martin. *Maternity Nursing*, 16th ed. New York: J. B. Lippincott, 1987.

Tucker, S., et al. *Patient Care Standards: Nursing Process, Diagnosis, and Outcome*, 5th ed. St. Louis, MO: C. V. Mosby, 1992.

Wong, D. L. *Whaley & Wong's Nursing Care of Infants and Children*, 5th ed. St. Louis, MO: Mosby–Year Book, 1995.

CHAPTER

3

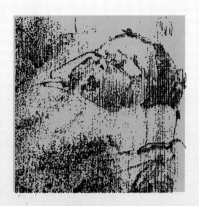

*T*he High-Risk
Newborn

OBJECTIVES

AFTER STUDYING THIS CHAPTER, THE STUDENT SHOULD BE ABLE TO:

- DESCRIBE THE CHARACTERISTICS AND CARE OF A PRETERM NEW-
BORN.
- DISCUSS THE CHARACTERISTICS AND CARE OF A POSTTERM
INFANT.
- EXPLAIN THE TREATMENT FOR HYPOGLYCEMIA IN AN INFANT OF
A DIABETIC MOTHER.
- IDENTIFY THE SIGNS OF FETAL ALCOHOL SYNDROME.
- DESCRIBE THE EFFECTS OF MATERNAL SUBSTANCE ABUSE ON THE
NEWBORN.

Key Terms

HIGH-RISK NEWBORN

NEONATAL INTENSIVE CARE UNIT (NICU)

PRETERM INFANT

SMALL-FOR-GESTATIONAL-AGE INFANT

LOW-BIRTH-WEIGHT INFANT

VERY-LOW-BIRTH-WEIGHT INFANT

BALLARD SCALE

APNEA

RESPIRATORY DISTRESS SYNDROME (RDS)

SURFACTANT DEFICIENCY

DYSPNEA

HYPERBILIRUBINEMIA

INCUBATOR

GAVAGE FEEDING

PHOTOTHERAPY

POSTTERM INFANT

LARGE-FOR-GESTATIONAL-AGE INFANT (LGA)

HYPOGLYCEMIA

SUBSTANCE ABUSE

FETAL ALCOHOL SYNDROME (FAS)

a **high-risk newborn** is any neonate who is at risk for a serious condition or illness, or death. Such a newborn requires high-tech care by expert health care professionals. The nurse needs to be able to assess a high-risk newborn and to provide care.

Most high-risk newborns are premature or have a low birth weight. The less a newborn weighs at birth, the greater the chance of physical problems or death. Postterm newborns and those born to diabetic or substance-abusing mothers are also considered high-risk newborns.

Besides the infant's physical problems, a high-risk newborn and the parents may face other problems. For example, the infant may have to be transferred to a **neonatal intensive care unit (NICU)** or regional care center. This can interfere with parent-infant bonding and with providing for the infant's emotional needs, making the infant irritable. Parents may feel increased stress not only because of the infant's physical condition but because of the lack of parent-infant interactions. Therefore, NICU nurses and other caregivers must have expert clinical and interpersonal skills when dealing with high-risk newborns and their families.

PRETERM NEWBORN

A small newborn may be preterm (premature), small for his or her gestational age, low in birth weight, or very low birth weight. A **preterm infant** is one born at less than 37 weeks' gestation. In comparison, a full-term infant is born between 38 and 42 weeks' gestation. A **small-for-gestational-age infant** is one in the lowest 10th percentile of weight for his or her gestational age. Regardless of gestational age, a **low-birth-weight infant** weighs less than 2,500 g, and a **very-low-birth-weight infant** weighs less than 1,500 g. Prematurity and low birth weight commonly coexist.

Only 7% to 10% of all live births are preterm. Yet, prematurity is the most common cause of death in infants. Premature birth may be caused by maternal illness, multiple pregnancy, or pregnancy problems, such as toxemia and placental abnormalities. In most cases, the cause is unknown.

CHARACTERISTICS

Premature birth produces distinctive characteristics in the newborn, Figure 3–1. In general, the newborn appears similar to a fetus at 7 months' gestation. The infant is listless and inactive, weighs less than 5½ lb (2,500 g), and measures less than 18 in. (45 cm) long. The cry is feeble, and the newborn's reflexes may be weak or absent. The head is disproportionately large, has large fontanels (soft spaces between skull bones) and prominent sutures (lines of closure), and may be flattened on the sides. The ears have little cartilage and are soft. The skin is thin, dull red, wrinkled, and covered with lanugo (downy fine hair) and thick vernix caseosa (cheeselike substance). Typically, the abdomen is abnormally large, with visible veins. In male infants, the testes are undescended; in females, the clitoris may be prominent. The arms and legs appear thin. The soles and palms display few creases and short nails. Respirations are shallow and irregular. Body temperature is unstable and subnormal, often between 34° and 36°C (94° and 96°F). The suck and swallow reflexes may be weak.

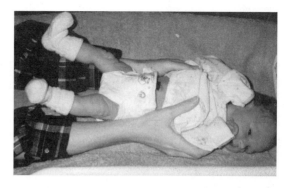

a.

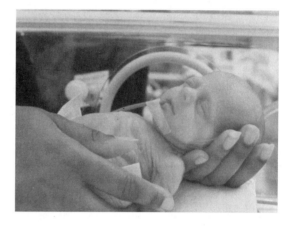

b.

Figure 3–1   *Compared with a full-term newborn (a), a preterm newborn (b) is much smaller and thinner, and has a larger head and looser skin. (b. Courtesy Carl Howard and Albany Medical Center)*

The nurse may estimate the infant's gestational age quickly by looking at the sole creases, breast nodules, scalp hair, ear lobes, and posture. For a more detailed gestational age estimation, the **Ballard scale** may be used, Figure 3–2. The examiner assesses and scores aspects of neuromuscular and physical maturity, totals the scores, and finds gestational age (in weeks) across from the total score under "Maturity Rating."

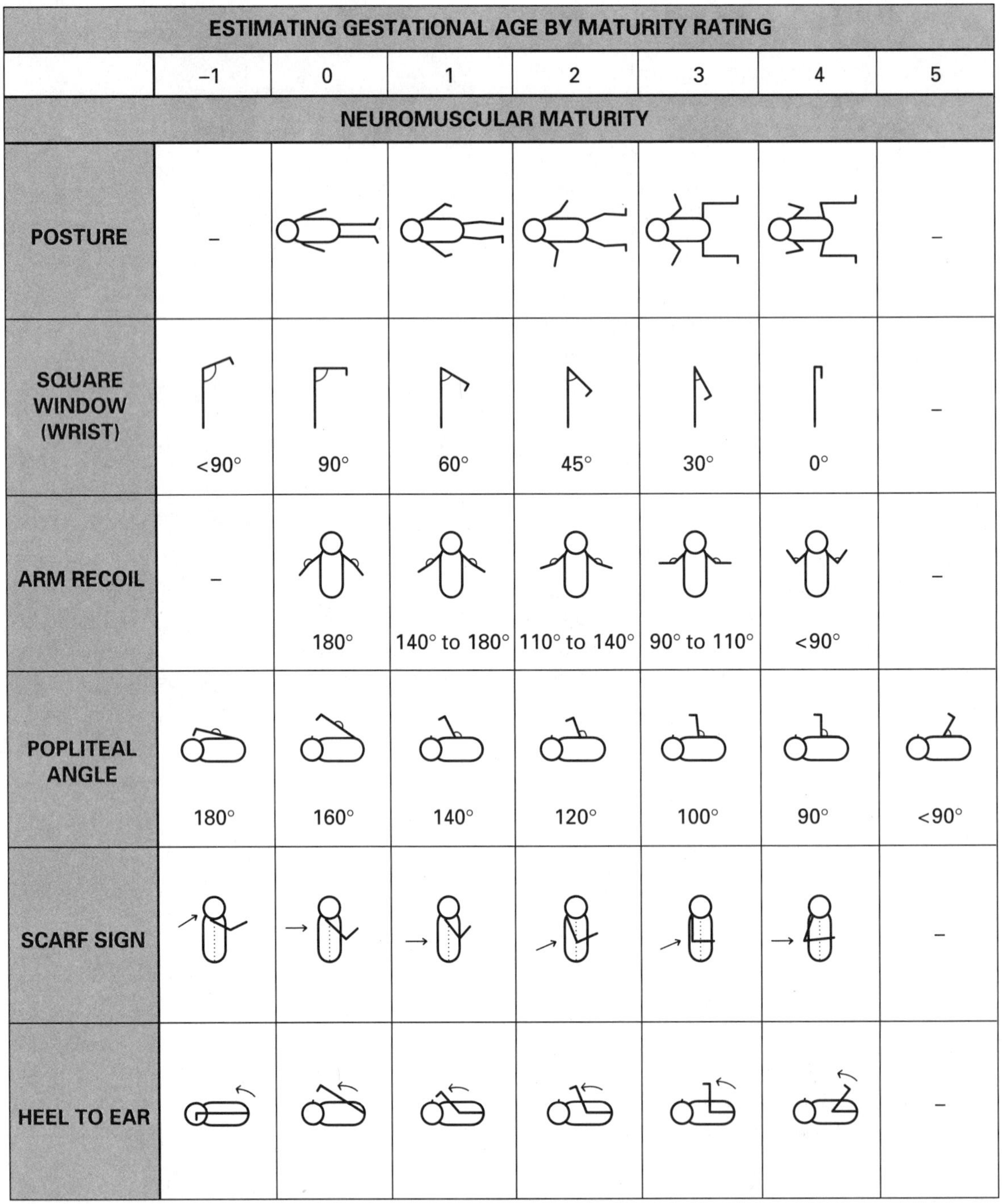

ESTIMATING GESTATIONAL AGE BY MATURITY RATING							
	−1	0	1	2	3	4	5
NEUROMUSCULAR MATURITY							
POSTURE	–						–
SQUARE WINDOW (WRIST)	<90°	90°	60°	45°	30°	0°	–
ARM RECOIL	–	180°	140° to 180°	110° to 140°	90° to 110°	<90°	–
POPLITEAL ANGLE	180°	160°	140°	120°	100°	90°	<90°
SCARF SIGN							–
HEEL TO EAR							–

Figure 3–2   *Ballard scale for estimating a newborn's gestational age based on maturity rating. (With permission from Ballard, J.L., et al. New Ballard Score, expanded to include extremely premature infants. Journal of Pediatrics, 119:417–423, 1991.)*

	−1	0	1	2	3	4	5
PHYSICAL MATURITY							
SKIN	Sticky, friable, transparent	Gelatinous, red, translucent	Smooth, pink; visible veins	Superficial peeling and/or rash; few visible veins	Cracking; pale areas; rare visible veins	Parchment-like; deep cracking; no visible veins	Leathery, wrinkled, cracked
LANUGO	None	Sparse	Abundant	Thinning	Bald areas	Mostly bald	–
PLANTAR SURFACE	Heel-to-toe 40–50mm: −1 <40mm: −2	<50 mm; no crease	Faint red marks	Anterior transverse crease only	Creases over anterior two-thirds	Creases over entire sole	–
BREAST	Imperceptible	Barely perceptible	Flat areola; no bud	Stippled areola; 1– to 2–mm bud	Raised areola; 3– to 4–mm bud	Full areola; 5– to 10– mm bud	–
EYES AND EARS	Lids fused, loosely: −1 tightly: −2	Lids open; pinna flat, stays folded	Slightly curved pinna; soft, slow recoil	Well-curved pinna; soft but ready recoil	Formed and firm; instant recoil	Thick cartilage; ear stiff	–
GENITALIA, MALE	Scrotum flat, smooth	Scrotum empty, faint rugae	Testes in upper canal; rare rugae	Testes descending; few rugae	Testes down; good rugae	Testes pendulous; deep rugae	–
GENITALIA, FEMALE	Prominent clitoris; labia flat	Prominent clitoris; small labia minora	Prominent clitoris; enlarging minora	Majora and minora equally prominent	Majora large; minora small	Majora cover clitoris and minora	–

MATURITY RATING													
SCORE	−10	−5	0	5	10	15	20	25	30	35	40	45	50
WEEKS	20	22	24	26	28	30	32	34	36	38	40	42	44

Figure 3–2   *continued*

Risks

The preterm newborn is at greatest risk for respiratory problems. Shallow, irregular respirations may be interrupted by **apnea** (temporary cessation of breathing) or may be accompanied by chest wall and sternal retractions. Because life-threatening respiratory distress can occur, the nurse must be prepared to perform resuscitation, Figure 3–3.

Respiratory distress syndrome (RDS) affects about one-fifth of all premature infants in the United States. Formerly called hyaline membrane disease, RDS may result from a **surfactant deficiency**. Lack of this substance inhibits complete alveolar expansion in the lungs. As a result, the lungs lose their elasticity, and gas exchange is blocked. The main symptoms of RDS are **dyspnea** (difficult breathing), tachypnea (abnormally rapid respiration), and cyanosis (bluish tinge to the skin).

RDS treatment may include administration of surfactant replacement and oxygen, and use of continuous positive airway pressure (CPAP) to assist in ventilation. To help prevent RDS, the pregnant mother may undergo amniocentesis to assess the amount of sphingomyelin and lecithin (surfactant's major component). The ratio of lecithin to sphingomyelin in a fetus with mature lungs is at least 2:1. If the amniotic fluid has insufficient lecithin 24 to 48 hours before delivery, the mother may receive the glucocorticoid drug betamethasone, which stimulates surfactant production.

Preterm newborns are also at high risk for hypothermia (abnormally low body temperature) because these infants have immature temperature-regulating centers, decreased fat stores, an inability to sweat or shiver, and low metabolic reserves. Exposure of such a newborn to a cool environment may produce cold stress and increased oxygen requirements.

The preterm newborn may experience nutrient and fluid deficits. The immature gastrointestinal system, small stomach capacity (1 to 2 oz), and weak sucking and swallowing reflexes may make it difficult for the newborn to obtain sufficient nutrition. In addition, the immature stomach sphincters may cause regurgitation or vomiting of feedings.

The preterm newborn's risk for infection results from insufficient transfer of the mother's antibodies and from the newborn's inability to produce antibodies. Muscle weakness contributes to the newborn's nutritional and respiratory problems as well as to fatigue or exhaustion from such simple activities as eating and breathing.

Because of liver immaturity, the preterm newborn is at high risk for **hyperbilirubinemia** (high blood bilirubin levels). This occurs because the liver cannot process bilirubin, causing it to accumulate. Hyperbilirubinemia may cause jaundice and in severe cases may result in brain damage. Phototherapy is used to treat newborns with hyperbilirubinemia.

Care

The premature infant's survival depends on the nurse's skillful care, judgment, and devotion. Besides frequently monitoring vital signs, the basics of preterm newborn care include:

- maintaining the airway and adequate oxygen intake
- maintaining body temperature
- ensuring adequate nutrient and fluid intake
- providing protection from infection
- conserving the infant's energy
- providing phototherapy, if needed

Maintaining the Airway and Adequate Oxygen Intake. Maintaining respiratory function takes top priority when caring for a preterm newborn. The head of the bed is generally raised 4 to 6 in. to ease the effort of breathing. Suction equipment should be kept nearby to clear the airway if needed.

PROCEDURE

Resuscitation of the Newborn

Purpose: The purpose of resuscitation is to establish or reestablish regular breathing patterns in the infant (see Figure 3–3).

1. Establish an open airway by wiping or suctioning any mucus from the mouth.
2. Tilt the infant's head back slightly by placing your hand at the base of the infant's neck. The breathing passages may be obstructed if the head is too far back.
3. Place your mouth over the infant's nose and mouth to establish an airtight seal.
4. Gently blow air from your cheeks into the infant's nose and mouth at the rate of about 3 puffs per second. The infant's chest should rise and fall after each breath. If it does not, reposition the infant's head so that the tongue is not resting on the back of the throat, or resuction to establish a clear airway.
5. After each puff of air, raise your mouth and turn your head to the side. This allows air to escape back out of the infant's lungs and gives you a chance to take a breath.
6. Continue rescue breathing until proper medical equipment can help ventilation.
7. Observe for signs that the infant is breathing on his or her own.

Equipment:

- Radiant heat source
- Bulb syringe
- Oxygen tank and liter gauge
- Oxygen tubing
- Infant oxygen mask

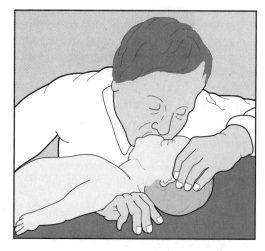

Figure 3–3   *Resuscitation of the newborn*

- Pen-Lon valve bag
- Ambu bag
- Wall suction tubing
- Suction catheters #6.5 and #8
- Bottle of sterile water
- Laryngoscope with two blades
- Portex blue-line endotracheal tubes #2.5, #3.0, #3.5
- Stylette
- Clean scissors
- Connector adaptor
- Closed system bag with water manometer
- Stethoscope

Precautions:

1. Keep the infant warm to minimize oxygen demands during resuscitation. The infant's axillary temperature should be maintained at 98° to 98.6° F (36.7° to 37° C).

PROCEDURE

Resuscitation of the Newborn *continued*

2. Quickly establish an open airway. Ten to fifteen seconds of gentle suctioning with a bulb syringe is all that is usually needed. Delay in clearing the airway can result in brain damage.

3. Suction the oropharynx before the nose. If the nose is suctioned first, the infant may aspirate mucus or amniotic fluid.

Procedure:

1. Briefly flick the infant's feet or rub the infant's back gently.

2. If breathing does not begin immediately, give 5 positive breaths of oxygen-enriched air by mask.

3. Maintain the first 5 inspirations for 4 to 5 seconds at a water pressure of 30 cm on the manometer. Use this high pressure for the first few breaths only to clear excess fetal lung liquid and to open collapsed alveoli.

4. Check for chest movement and breath sounds.

5. If breathing does not start, suction and/or intubate.

6. If breathing begins, expect the heart rate, color, and tone to improve immediately.

7. If breathing does not start, continue bag breathing at a rate of 40 breaths per minute with water pressures that do not exceed 20 to 25 cm.

8. Check the infant's apical pulse.

9. If the apical pulse falls below 100 beats per minute in spite of assisted ventilation, initiate cardiac massage.

10. To give cardiac massage, place one hand under the baby's back.

11. With the tips of the index and middle fingers of the other hand, depress the midsternum about ½ to ¾ in.

12. Gently but forcibly do this at a rate of 80 to 100 compressions per minute (a little more than once per second). To avoid injuring the infant, do not push too hard.

13. Ventilate once after every 5 compressions. Do not interrupt the compressions while ventilating, but avoid compressing the chest and giving a breath at the same time.

If the Apgar score is less than 6 at 3 to 5 minutes of age, the infant may need to be transferred to the intensive care unit. Resuscitation must continue during transport to the unit.

If extra oxygen is needed, the preterm infant may be placed in an incubator that can supply humidified oxygen in concentrations higher than 20%. Or a clear plastic hood may be placed over the newborn's head to provide humidified oxygen, as ordered.

Whenever the newborn receives oxygen, oxygen saturation should be monitored by pulse oximetry, or oxygen and carbon dioxide levels should be checked by transcutaneous monitoring. Monitoring is vital because a preterm infant who maintains oxygen saturations greater than 90 to 95% for a prolonged period may develop blindness.

The preterm infant who is receiving oxygen should also have his or her respiratory rate assessed, any retractions noted, and any signs of respiratory distress—especially tachypnea or apnea—observed. An electronic apnea alarm may be used, which automatically triggers a visual or audio alarm if the respiratory rate changes greatly or if apnea occurs. If apnea is detected, provide gentle stimulation, such as rubbing the chest. If this is not effective, assist respirations with a bag and mask: (1) extend the newborn's neck slightly, (2) place the mask over the newborn's mouth and nose to form a tight seal, and (3) quickly squeeze the small bag filled with oxygen or air.

Maintaining Body Temperature. An **incubator** or radiant warmer helps maintain the infant's body heat. Unlike radiant warmers, incubators can be regulated to control heat and humidity and to administer oxygen. Some incubators have hand holes in each side that permit care of the infant, Figure 3–4. The thermostat of an incubator or radiant warmer should be controlled by a temperature-sensitive probe attached to the infant's skin.

While in the incubator, the newborn wears only a diaper. When removed from the incubator, the newborn may be dressed in a shirt and diaper, wrapped in blankets, and possibly dressed in a cotton cap to prevent heat loss from the head.

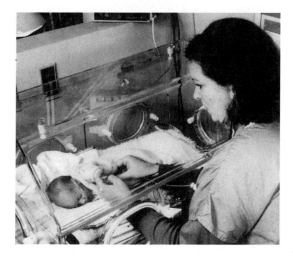

Figure 3–4 *Caring for the premature infant requires special attention.*

The infant's temperature should be taken every 2 to 3 hours until it stabilizes, then every 3 to 4 hours after that. Temperature is taken by axilla. The infant's axillary temperature is commonly taken even if the infant is in an incubator or under a radiant warmer and body temperature is being automatically monitored. In addition, the infant's color, respiratory rhythm, and ease of breathing should be checked frequently.

Ensuring Adequate Nutrition and Hydration. An infant who weighs 3 lb 5 oz (1,500 g), has a gestational age of 34 to 35 weeks or more, and can suck and swallow may be fed with a regular bottle and soft nipple. Enteral feeding (through the gastrointestinal tract) is begun on an individual basis depending upon the infant's condition and needs. Because a premature infant is prone to deficiency diseases, vitamins and iron are added after the seventh day of age.

An infant who cannot suck or swallow may have to be fed by **gavage** (tube) **feeding**, medicine dropper, or IV line. In gavage feeding, a tube is placed through the infant's mouth or nose into the stomach, Figure 3–5. A syringe is attached to the tube, and the formula or feeding is poured into the syringe. Care must be taken to ensure that the tube is actually in the infant's stomach.

Intermittent gavage feeding is often preferred to indwelling gavage feedings because of the risk of stomach perforation, nasal airway obstruction, ulceration, irritation to the mucous membrane, and nosebleed.

IV fluids are given to an infant via a catheter placed in the umbilical vein or a peripheral vein, or through a central venous catheter. Because a preterm infant requires very small amounts of fluid (10 mL/h or less), an infusion pump should be used for accurate administration. IV fluid intake should be accurately recorded. In addition, urine output should be measured. (To determine urine

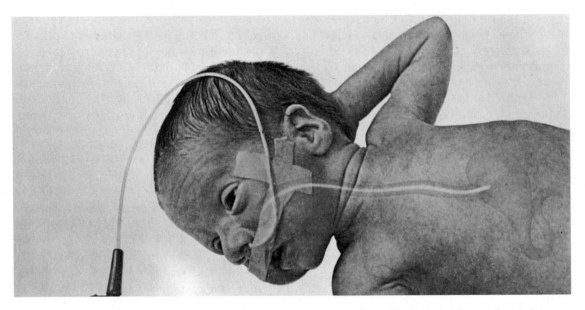

Figure 3–5   *Plastic indwelling catheter inserted through the nose for gavage feeding (Courtesy Ross Laboratories)*

output, weigh each diaper before and after use.) For the first few days after birth, urine output normally ranges from 35 to 40 mL/kg per 24 hours. After that, it increases to 50 to 100 mL/kg per 24 hours. The number of voidings, urine color, and signs of edema should also be documented.

Preventing Infection.   To protect the preterm newborn from infection, an incubator should be used. All nursery personnel must be free of respiratory infections. Routine checkups are given, and masks may be worn. In addition, personnel are required to wear special uniforms and scrub their hands meticulously before handling each premature infant.

Several other practices help prevent infection in preterm newborns. These include physical separation of the high-risk nursery from the normal newborn nursery as well as frequent changing or cleaning of humidifier water; IV tubing; and suctioning, respiratory, and monitoring equipment.

Conserving the Infant's Energy.   To conserve the newborn's energy, handling is kept to a minimum. The newborn is left in bed for baths, feedings, and examinations until the infant's weight reaches 4 lb 7 oz (about 2,000 g). Only the newborn's face and perineal area are cleaned. The newborn's weight is taken at the same time daily, and formula requirements are calculated every 24 to 48 hours. In addition, the newborn is dressed only in a diaper to conserve energy and allow better observation.

Providing Phototherapy.   A preterm newborn with hyperbilirubinemia is treated with **phototherapy** (exposure to special fluorescent lights). This treatment prevents the bilirubin level from reaching 20 mg/dL, which increases the danger of severe brain damage. The naked newborn is placed in the incubator, and the lights are arranged above. Figure 3–6 is a nursing care plan for a newborn receiving phototherapy.

NURSING CARE PLAN: Newborn Receiving Phototherapy

NURSING DIAGNOSIS	GOAL(S)	NURSING INTERVENTION	RATIONALE
High risk for injury to the eyes	Infant will not sustain injury to the eyes.	Cover infant's eyes during phototherapy with a soft bandage or eye patches that are clean and fit properly. Apply correctly and securely. Check for signs of irritation, infection, and exposure to ultraviolet light.	Correctly applying a soft bandage or eye patches protects the eyes from ultraviolet light and injury such as corneal irritation. Clean eye patches help prevent infection.
High risk for fluid volume deficit	Infant will maintain hydration.	Increase fluid intake up to 25%. Monitor fluid input and output and infant's weight. Check for signs of dehydration such as dryness and loss of skin turgor.	Increasing fluid intake helps prevent dehydration as a result of phototherapy, which increases water loss. Monitoring weight and fluid input and output helps ensure that proper hydration is maintained.
High risk for altered body temperature, hyperthermia	The infant will maintain a normal body temperature (approximately 37.5°C, or 99.5°F).	Monitor the infant's body temperature. Monitor and, if necessary, adjust the temperature inside an incubator.	Monitoring body temperature and, if necessary, adjusting temperature inside the incubator helps maintain the infant's normal body temperature, which can be affected by the radiant heat of phototherapy.

Figure 3–6   *Nursing care plan for a newborn receiving phototherapy*

RELATED CARE

Handling and sensory stimulation should be limited and planned for the preterm newborn to allow for rest and growth. To provide sensory stimulation, a mobile can be hung above the incubator or an audiotape of the family's voices or soft music can be played. To supply tactile stimulation, the newborn can be bathed, held, and cuddled. To prevent skin breakdown and to improve sensory stimulation, the newborn should be positioned from one side to the other, unless directed otherwise.

To promote bonding, parents should be encouraged to visit the special care nursery, to touch and hold their infant, and to participate in infant care if possible. Parents should be taught about other aspects of care and should be reassured that the preterm newborn's growth usually catches up to that of full-term newborns by age 2.

Because the birth of a preterm newborn is a significant stress on the family, the nurse should be prepared to provide emotional support and appropriate information. To help relieve the parents' anxiety about caring for their preterm newborn, the nurse may refer them to parent aides and to other types of home support and assistance.

POSTTERM NEWBORN

A **postterm infant** (postmature infant) is one born after 42 weeks' gestation. Although such an infant may appear large, he or she is not necessarily a **large-for-gestational-age (LGA) infant** (one in the highest 10th percentile of weight for his or her gestational age). By the same token, an LGA infant, such as a diabetic mother's infant, may not be postterm. Such a newborn's unusually large size is due to abnormally rapid fetal growth.

Although it affects about 12% of all infants, the cause of postmaturity is unknown. It is clear that the problems of postterm infants stem from inadequate functioning of the aging placenta. For these infants, the mortality rate is up to three times greater than it is for full-term infants.

CHARACTERISTICS

Some postterm infants look like full-term ones; others appear similar to infants up to 3 weeks old. Typically, these infants appear long and thin, with the loose skin suggestive of weight loss. They have minimal lanugo, and their lack of vernix caseosa leaves the skin extremely dry and fragile.

Postterm infants have abundant scalp hair, long fingernails that may be stained with meconium due to fetal distress, and alert expressions. They need close monitoring for the effects of being dependent on a failing placenta in the last weeks of gestation.

RISKS AND CARE

A failing placenta places a postterm fetus at risk for intrauterine hypoxia, particularly during labor and delivery. If delivery is significantly delayed, labor may be induced or the infant delivered by cesarean section.

During fetal distress, meconium is expelled in utero. The stressed postterm infant may take meconium into the lungs at birth, causing meconium aspiration syndrome or pneumonia. If meconium-stained amniotic fluid appears during delivery, the newborn's mouth and nose are suctioned as soon as the head emerges from the birth canal. Gastric lavage may be performed after delivery if it appears that the newborn may have swallowed meconium, which could later be aspirated from vomitus.

INFANT OF A DIABETIC MOTHER

A diabetic woman has an increased risk of abortion, stillbirth, and premature labor, and of having an LGA infant or one with a congenital defect. The severity of her disease determines the degree of risk. If she closely controls her blood glucose level before and during pregnancy, she reduces the risk of congenital defects in her infant.

A full-term infant of a diabetic mother has a higher mortality rate than an infant delivered earlier because vascular changes in the placenta compromise the fetus and because the fetus's larger size can complicate the delivery. That is why early delivery may be scheduled, at about 36 to 38 weeks' gestation.

CHARACTERISTICS

The infant of a mother with poorly controlled blood glucose levels has certain characteristic features. Typically, the infant is LGA and plump. The infant's face apppears large and puffy, the body is covered with vernix caseosa, and the umbilical cord is large.

RISKS AND CARE

If a mother has high blood glucose levels during pregnancy, her infant can develop **hypoglycemia** (abnormally low blood glucose level) shortly after birth. During pregnancy, the fetus obtains glucose from maternal blood by diffusion through the placenta. High maternal glucose levels produce high fetal levels that stimulate insulin production by the fetal pancreas. Once the umbilical cord is severed, the newborn's excessive supply of glucose is cut off, but the high level of insulin remains until the fetal pancreas can adjust. Meanwhile, the newborn's blood glucose level may fall dangerously low. Signs of hypoglycemia include:

- apnea or tachypnea
- rapid, irregular respirations
- tremors, jitters, twitches, or convulsions
- decreased level of consciousness
- abrupt pallor, cyanosis, or gray shock
- sweating
- upward rolling of the eyes
- weak or high-pitched cry
- refusal to feed
- inability to regulate temperature

Administration of oral or IV glucose should raise the infant's blood glucose level and make these signs subside quickly. If they do not subside, hypoglycemia was not the cause. Other treatments may include administration of IV fluids and early feedings. Frequent blood glucose monitoring may be performed by heel stick.

Normal blood glucose levels range from 45 to 125 mg/dL in full-term infants who weigh over 2,500 g (5 1/2 lb) and from 20 to 100 mg/dL in infants who weigh less than 2,500 g. Prolonged hypoglycemia (below 30 mg/dL) can lead to brain damage and death.

Infants of diabetic mothers may display other problems, such as perinatal asphyxia, birth trauma, congenital anomalies, hypocalcemia, hyperbilirubinemia, polycythemia, and respiratory distress syndrome. Malformations are more likely to affect infants of women with uncontrolled type I or type II diabetes than infants of women with gestational diabetes.

INFANT OF A SUBSTANCE ABUSING MOTHER

Substance abuse is the use of any mind-altering substance in socially inappropriate ways or in ways that impair the ability to function. Such substances include alcohol, prescription drugs (such as amphetamines and barbiturates), and illicit drugs (such as marijuana, cocaine, crack, heroin, and LSD).

ALCOHOL

Alcohol has a direct toxic effect on the developing fetus. It quickly passes through the placenta and enters the fetus's blood. In the first trimester, alcohol may affect the cell membrane and alter embryonic tissue. Throughout pregnancy, alcohol may interfere with the metabolism of carbohydrates, lipids, and proteins, and thus retard cell growth and division. The central nervous system may be most vulnerable in the third trimester, when rapid brain growth occurs. Alcohol use also is associated with premature delivery, which poses additional risks.

While alcohol use is classified by amount, Figure 3–7, no amount of alcohol is considered safe. Consumption of more than 1½ oz of absolute alcohol (3 to 4 drinks) per day is likely

ALCOHOL CONSUMPTION

Heavy drinker	More than 45 drinks per month, or more than 5 drinks per occasion
Moderate drinker	Between 1 and 45 drinks per month, never more than 5 drinks per occasion
Light or rare drinker	Fewer than 1 drink per month

One drink is equal to ½ ounce of alcohol, or:
- One beer
- 4 ounces of wine
- 1.2 ounces of liquor

Figure 3–7 Medical classification of alcohol consumption

to produce an adverse effect. Moderate drinking may also have negative effects. Infants born to alcoholic mothers are at greatest risk.

The most serious adverse effect associated with alcohol is **fetal alcohol syndrome (FAS)**. It can occur even in infants of mothers who are low to moderate drinkers. FAS is diagnosed when abnormalities occur in each of the following categories:

- prenatal or postnatal growth retardation
- neurological abnormality, developmental delay, or intellectual impairment
- characteristic facial dysmorphology (abnormal shape) with at least two of these signs: microcephaly (small head), microphthalmia (small eyes), short palpebral (eyelid) fissures, poorly developed philtrum (groove on upper lip), thin upper lip, or flattening of the maxillary area

Other signs may include a flattened nasal bridge and reduced ocular growth, Figure 3–8. Infants with FAS are susceptible to respiratory problems, hyperbilirubinemia, hypocalcemia, and hypoglycemia. In spite of adequate nutrition and skilled care, their physical and mental development is slow.

To help prevent FAS, women should be counseled to stop all alcohol consumption for at least 3 months before becoming pregnant. To deal with FAS in a newborn, monitor for hypoglycemia and other problems, and provide appropriate care. A quiet, nonstimulating environment should be provided in addition to IV fluids and anticonvulsant drugs as prescribed.

DRUGS

If a mother is addicted to cocaine, heroin, or other narcotics, her infant will be born addicted. Shortly after birth, her infant can experience such withdrawal symptoms as:

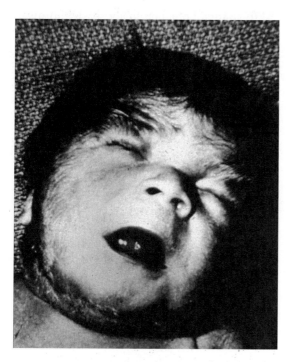

Figure 3–8 Infant with fetal alcohol syndrome. *(Reprinted with permission. Streissguth, A. P., Landesman-Dwyer, S., Martin, J. C., & Smith, D. W. (1980). Teratogenic effects of alcohol in humans and laboratory animals.* Science, *209(18):353–361)*

- tachypnea
- weak or poorly organized reflexes
- tremors, restlessness, or hyperactivity
- increased muscle tone
- sneezing
- a high-pitched cry
- regurgitation and vomiting of feedings

Depending on the amount and type of drug exposure, the infant of a substance abuser may be born prematurely or have intrauterine growth retardation, congenital anomalies, or other problems. For example, an infant exposed to cocaine may have difficulty responding to the human voice and face and exhibit depressed interactions and poor responses to environmental stimuli.

Although prevention is important, it can be difficult to achieve because pregnant substance abusers often have little or no prenatal care. Treatment for an infant with withdrawal symptoms typically includes oral or intramuscular administration of diazepam, chlorpromazine, paregoric, or phenobarbital; close body contact with caregivers; and secure wrapping in a small blanket with the arms folded across the chest.

REVIEW QUESTIONS

A. Multiple choice. Select the best answer.

1. Nursing care for a preterm newborn includes
   a. placing the infant in an incubator to help regulate body temperature
   b. providing abundant visual and tactile stimulation
   c. adding infant cereal to the formula to increase the nutritive value
   d. giving the infant a regular bath daily

2. A preterm newborn typically weighs
   a. less than 4,000 g
   b. less than 3,500 g
   c. less than 3,000 g
   d. less than 2,500 g

3. A postterm infant is one born after
   a. 44 weeks' gestation
   b. 42 weeks' gestation
   c. 40 weeks' gestation
   d. 38 weeks' gestation

4. The biggest health problem for infants of diabetic mothers is
   a. hypoglycemia
   b. hypercalcemia
   c. hyperglycemia
   d. hypokalemia

5. In an infant of a heroin abuser, withdrawal symptoms include
   a. respiratory arrest
   b. hypotonicity of muscles
   c. tremors
   d. abrupt pallor

B. Briefly answer the following questions.

1. How is betamethasone used to treat RDS?

2. How is hyperbilirubinemia treated?

3. What problem can occur if a preterm infant maintains oxygen saturations greater than 90 to 95% for a prolonged period of time?

4. What treatments are usually prescribed for a newborn with hypoglycemia?

5. What characteristics typify an infant with FAS?

SUGGESTED ACTIVITIES

- Explain how the health risks for preterm newborns determine their nursing care.
- Observe an NICU nurse use the Ballard scale to assess a high-risk newborn.

- Develop a list of substance abuse prevention programs for pregnant women in your community.

BIBLIOGRAPHY

Ballard, J. L., et al. New Ballard Score, expanded to include extremely premature infants. *Journal of Pediatrics* 119 (1991):417–423.

Beckman, C. Postterm pregnancy: Effects on temperature and glucose regulation. *Nursing Research* 39, no. 1 (1990): 21–24.

Betz, C., M. Hunsberger, and S. Wright. *Family-Centered Nursing Care of Children*, 2nd ed. Philadelphia: W. B. Saunders, 1994.

Cohen, S., C. Kenner, and A. Hollingsworth. *Maternal, Neonatal, and Women's Health Nursing.* Springhouse, PA: Springhouse, 1991.

Neonatal Network: Journal of Neonatal Nursing. Fetal alcohol syndrome (reprinted from *Alcohol Alert*). *Neonatal Network: Journal of Neonatal Nursing* 11, no. 3 (1992): 47–49.

Jackson, D., and R. Saunders. *Child Health Nursing: A Comprehensive Approach to the Care of Children and Their Families.* Philadelphia: J. B. Lippincott, 1993.

Nolan, E. Infants at risk: A time for action. *Pediatric Nursing* 17, no. 2 (1991): 175–178.

Rotondo, L. Diabetes mellitus: Impact on pregnancy. *NAACOG'S Clinical Issues in Perinatal and Women's Health Nursing* 1, no. 2 (1990), 133–145.

Tanner, M. Fetal alcohol syndrome: A nursing concern. *Minnesota Nursing Accent* 64, no. 5 (1992): 7.

Wong, D. L. *Whaley & Wong's Nursing Care of Infants and Children,* 5th ed. St. Louis, MO: Mosby—Year Book, 1995.

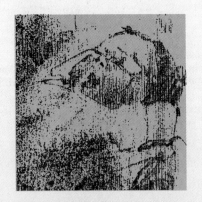

*D*isorders of the Newborn

OBJECTIVES

AFTER STUDYING THIS CHAPTER, THE STUDENT SHOULD BE ABLE TO:

- NAME THREE CAUSES OF ASPHYXIA NEONATORUM.
- DESCRIBE THE SIGNS OF RESPIRATORY DISTRESS.
- IDENTIFY PRINCIPLES TO FOLLOW WHEN TREATING A NEWBORN WITH BREATHING DIFFICULTY.
- LIST ONE DISORDER OF THE NEWBORN FOR EACH BODY SYSTEM DESCRIBED IN THIS CHAPTER.
- DESCRIBE THE CAUSES AND TREATMENTS OF SPECIFIC DISORDERS OF THE NEWBORN.

Key Terms

CONGENITAL

ASPHYXIA NEONATORUM

ANOXIA

CEREBRAL INJURY

NARCOSIS

CONTINUOUS POSITIVE AIRWAY PRESSURE (CPAP)

CHEST RETRACTION

SILVERMAN-ANDERSON INDEX

PHYSIOLOGICAL JAUNDICE

BILIRUBIN

ERYTHROBLASTOSIS FETALIS

RHOGAM

ABO INCOMPATIBILITY

CLEFT LIP

CLEFT PALATE

THRUSH

PYLORIC STENOSIS

DIAPHRAGMATIC HERNIA

HIATAL HERNIA

INGUINAL HERNIA

UMBILICAL HERNIA

OMPHALOCELE

IMPERFORATE ANUS

SPINA BIFIDA OCCULTA

MENINGOCELE

MENINGOMYELOCELE

DOWN SYNDROME

HYDROCEPHALUS

TALIPES

CONGENITAL HIP DYSPLASIA

TORTICOLLIS

ERB'S PALSY

EXSTROPHY OF THE BLADDER

HYPOSPADIAS

EPISPADIAS

CRYPTORCHIDISM

PSEUDOHERMAPHRODITISM

HERMAPHRODITISM

GALACTOSEMIA

CONGENITAL HYPOTHYROIDISM

ecoming a parent is a major event, a turning point in life, particularly for the parents of a newborn with a disorder. Some parents can cope and adapt to the situation with increased maturity; others react with distress, which leaves them emotionally drained. When an infant is born with a disorder, the health care team members are responsible for understanding the psychodynamics that take place in both the parents and themselves. By assuming this responsibility, they can deal with the situation constructively and therapeutically.

ATTITUDES OF THE STAFF

The delivery of a newborn with a disorder is difficult for the entire health care team. The mother may sense their frustration and misinterpret it as hostility. She may feel sadness rather than the expected joyfulness. All of this distress comes at a time when the mother may be physically and emotionally exhausted. The importance of the nurse's presence should never be underestimated. The mother needs to feel that someone understands. By simply holding the mother's hand or encouraging her to express her feelings, the nurse renders tremendous emotional support.

The nurse should provide realistic reassurance to the mother and father. The parents need to feel that their newborn is accepted and treated like any other newborn and that the hospital staff will give any assistance possible. The nurse can help by cuddling the newborn and calling the infant by name. The nurse can also encourage the parents to talk about their feelings openly. The hospital staff should avoid offering the mother helpful platitudes such as "You can always have other children" or "Don't feel so bad." Such statements simply convey a lack of understanding and empathy.

ETIOLOGY AND TREATMENT

Observation of the newborn is one of the nurse's most important duties in the delivery room and the nursery. Through careful observation, serious threats to the infant's health may be averted. Early treatment of congenital anomalies and diseases may be initiated when a nurse reports unusual signs and symptoms. These observations alert the physician or supervising nurse to the fact that a condition may exist for which medical attention is necessary.

Most infants are born mature and healthy. A small percentage, however, are born with a disease or defect. Such disorders of the newborn may be acquired during development in the uterus (**congenital**), during the birth process, or as a result of medical conditions.

Disorders may affect any one of the following body systems or may overlap and involve more than one system:

- respiratory system
- cardiovascular system
- gastrointestinal system
- nervous system
- musculoskeletal system
- urinary system
- reproductive system

Disorders may also include inborn errors of metabolism. This chapter will discuss some of the most common birth disorders of newborns.

RESPIRATORY SYSTEM OF THE NEWBORN

ASPHYXIA NEONATORUM

Normally, the newborn's respirations are slightly irregular and may range from 30 to 60 breaths per minute. If respirations do not begin within 30 seconds after birth, the newborn has a condition called **asphyxia neonatorum**. Failure of the newborn to breathe spontaneously is usually due to one or a combination of three causes:

- deprivation of oxygen (**anoxia**)
- damage to brain tissue (**cerebral injury**)
- unconscious or stuporous state caused by drugs (**narcosis**)

Anoxia. Any interference with the function of the placenta or the umbilical cord, which supplies oxygen to the fetus, puts the infant in great danger of anoxia. A prolapsed cord, nuchal cord, premature separation of the placenta (placenta abruptio), or extremely severe uterine contractions could all produce intrauterine asphyxia. The fetus may literally suffocate while in the uterus because of the lack of oxygen.

Cerebral Injury. Cerebral injury is a common cause of apnea at birth when the delivery is particularly difficult. Brain hemorrhage may damage the respiratory center and injure other vital centers. A disproportion between the size of the infant's head and the size of the mother's pelvis can cause compression of the skull during birth. This compression may be severe enough to damage the brain.

Narcosis. A state of unconsciousness or stupor may be produced in the infant by analgesic and anesthetic drugs given to the mother during labor. Although with narcosis the newborn's respirations may be sluggish at first, the infant usually does quite well when the effects of the medication have worn off.

RESPIRATORY DISTRESS SYNDROME

Formerly called hyaline membrane disease, respiratory distress syndrome (RDS) often occurs within minutes to several hours after birth, Figure 4–1. The cause of RDS is unknown, but the disorder may be due to a surfactant deficiency in the infant's system. The lack of this phospholipid inhibits the complete expansion of the alveoli in the lungs. As a result, the lungs lose their elasticity.

The main signs and symptoms of RDS are cyanosis (bluish color of nails, lips, and skin), dyspnea (difficulty breathing) with retractions, and tachypnea. The disorder more frequently affects premature newborns and those born by cesarean section than it affects full-term or vaginal-birth newborns. Observation and the recording of respiratory signs and symptoms are important. Treatment consists of providing humidified oxygen. **Continuous positive airway pressure (CPAP)**, or air provided at a constant pressure to assist in ventilation, can be given. Antibiotics are often administered in addition to intravenous feedings.

SIGNS OF RESPIRATORY DISTRESS

The nurse should be alert for the following signs of respiratory distress, which may be evident at birth or may develop several days later:

* nasal flaring
* excessive mucus
* increased respiratory rate, possibly with apneic periods
* **chest retraction** upon inspiration (see-saw type of respirations)
* expiratory grunt or feeble cry
* cyanosis, except in the hands and feet

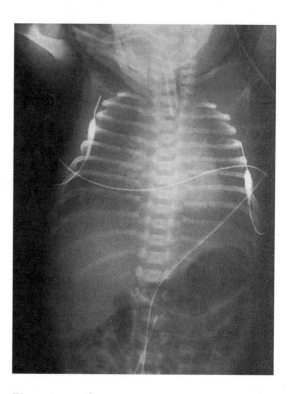

Figure 4–1   *Chest x-ray of an infant with respiratory distress syndrome*

At birth, the newborn is normally slightly blue because the lungs have not yet expanded. As soon as breathing begins, the newborn's skin becomes rosy pink. The nurse should immediately report the development of cyanosis because it is a sign of respiratory or circulatory difficulty.

When an infant who does not breathe spontaneously at birth is being treated, five considerations are:

- gentleness
- provision of warmth
- management of mucus
- positioning
- artificial respiration

Because the newborn is likely to be in a state of shock, gentleness is essential in all procedures. Physical stimulation should be limited to rubbing the newborn's back or flicking the soles of the infant's feet. Because the temperature of the room may aggravate the state of shock, the newborn must be kept warm. Excessive mucus should be reported immediately and emergency measures taken if necessary. Mucus may be removed with a suction catheter or with a bulb syringe. The infant should be placed in the Trendelenburg position with the head turned to one side. If the infant does not respond, additional resuscitation measures are initiated. Once the infant begins to breathe spontaneously, continued close observation is vital. See the procedure for resuscitation of the newborn in Chapter 3.

SILVERMAN-ANDERSON INDEX

The **Silverman-Anderson Index** is designed to provide a continuous evaluation of the infant's respiratory status, Figure 4–2. The index assigns values to five categories: upper chest, lower chest, xiphoid retractions, nares dilation, and expiratory grunt. A score of 0 indicates no respiratory distress; a score of 10 indicates severe respiratory distress.

CARDIOVASCULAR SYSTEM OF THE NEWBORN

The heart, blood vessels, lymph vessels, and lymph nodes make up the cardiovascular system. Blood is pumped to all body tissues. The circulating blood carries oxygen, nutrients, and chemicals to the body's cells and removes waste materials from those cells.

JAUNDICE

As the circulatory pattern adapts to extrauterine life, many newborns develop mild jaundice. This normal characteristic, which appears in up to 50% of full-term infants and 80% of premature newborns, is called **physiological jaundice**. It is caused by the liver's failure to cope with the breakdown of red blood cells no longer needed by the newborn. This liver failure causes increased amounts of **bilirubin** (a product of red blood cell destruction) to appear in the bloodstream, resulting in a yellowish tint to the skin. This type of jaundice appears 3 to 5 days after birth and subsides around the eighth day; it has little medical significance. Jaundice can and frequently does occur in breast-fed infants because of a compound in some mothers' milk that inhibits bilirubin breakdown. If the bilirubin level is too high, the mother may be asked to interrupt her breast-feeding for 24 to 48 hours and to pump her breasts to maintain the milk supply. Breast-feeding can be tried later and the bilirubin level monitored. The mother should always be assured that nothing is wrong with her breast milk.

If jaundice appears within the first 24 hours after birth, the nurse should promptly report it to the physician. Jaundice at this time could indicate a hemolytic disease, such as erythroblastosis fetalis or ABO incompatibility.

A blood test to determine the bilirubin level is done to assess the degree of jaundice in

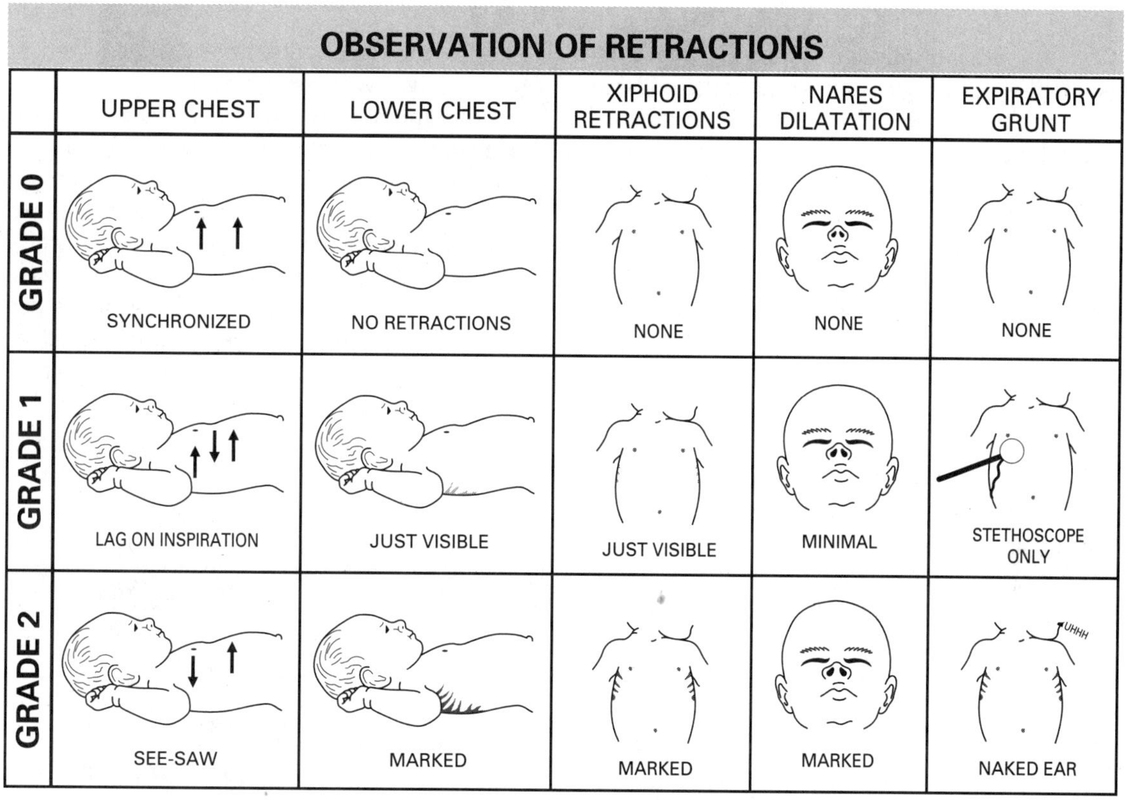

OBSERVATION OF RETRACTIONS

	UPPER CHEST	LOWER CHEST	XIPHOID RETRACTIONS	NARES DILATATION	EXPIRATORY GRUNT
GRADE 0	SYNCHRONIZED	NO RETRACTIONS	NONE	NONE	NONE
GRADE 1	LAG ON INSPIRATION	JUST VISIBLE	JUST VISIBLE	MINIMAL	STETHOSCOPE ONLY
GRADE 2	SEE-SAW	MARKED	MARKED	MARKED	NAKED EAR

Figure 4–2   *The Silverman-Anderson Index for the evaluation of respiratory status*

the infant. The pediatrician may order phototherapy (exposure of the infant to fluorescent blue light). To treat hyperbilirubinemia, the infant is placed unclothed under the light, which helps to remove the yellow or jaundice from the skin by helping the body break down the bilirubin more efficiently. The nurse must protect the infant's eyes with eye patches or a soft bandage. The infant's body temperature should be monitored carefully, and the infant should receive extra fluids. A newer form of phototherapy uses a plastic body wrap and fiberoptic lights. The infant does not need eye patches and may be fed and held without interrupting treatment.

CONGENITAL HEART DISEASE

Congenital heart disease ranks second, after prematurity, as the leading cause of death during the first year of life. Most congenital heart diseases develop during the fourth through eighth weeks of fetal life, because this is when the heart is developing. Common causes include maternal alcoholism, rubella during pregnancy, maternal insulin-dependent diabetes mellitus, maternal ingestion of certain drugs during pregnancy, and maternal age over 40. Many congenital heart diseases can be successfully treated with surgery. (For more information, see Chapter 22.)

Congestive Heart Failure

Congestive heart failure results when the heart is unable to pump enough blood to the body to meet its metabolic demands. In infants, congenital heart disease causes most congestive heart failure. The right or left side of the heart may be affected, or both sides of the heart may be involved. An infant with congestive heart failure usually has both left- and right-sided heart failure. Treatment requires medication and expert nursing care. (For more information, see Chapter 22.)

Erythroblastosis Fetalis

The Rh incompatibility that results when an Rh-negative woman gives birth to an Rh-positive infant may cause a disease known as **erythroblastosis fetalis**, Figure 4–3. In this condition, the infant's red blood cells are destroyed by Rh antibodies. Antibodies are proteins that are made as a response to foreign antigens. When Rh-positive red blood cells enter the bloodstream of an Rh-negative person, the recipient produces antibodies that can destroy Rh-positive cells. Some of the fetus's

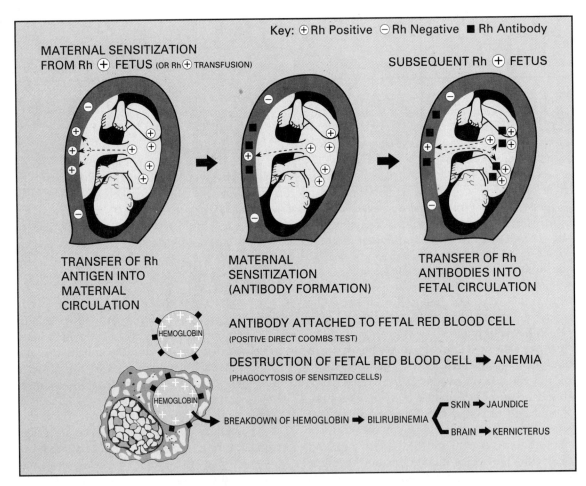

Figure 4–3   *Erythroblastosis fetalis (Adapted from Nursing Education Aid, No. 9, Ross Laboratories)*

Rh-positive red blood cells may spill into the pregnant woman's bloodstream—especially during a spontaneous or an induced abortion or delivery. If this occurs, the Rh-negative woman develops Rh antibodies. The process is not instantaneous, so it rarely affects the first Rh-positive fetus. However, since Rh antibody production increases with each exposure, every additional Rh-positive fetus is more likely to develop the disease. Destruction of the fetus's red blood cells is indicated by increased levels of bilirubin in the infant's blood. Erythroblastosis fetalis is characterized by anemia, jaundice, enlargement of the liver and spleen, and generalized edema of the newborn. If the anemia is severe enough, brain damage, heart failure, or death can occur.

Treatment of this disorder usually consists of giving the newborn exchange transfusions of Rh-negative blood during the first weeks after birth. Phototherapy is a simple and safe way to treat mild hemolytic disease and greatly reduces the need for exchange transfusions. However, it is relatively ineffective in severe cases when serum bilirubin rises rapidly.

A specific gamma globulin, **RhoGAM**, has made erythroblastosis fetalis rare. RhoGAM is a specially prepared gamma globulin that contains a concentration of Rh antibodies. These antibodies suppress the Rh-negative mother's immune response by destroying any Rh-positive red blood cells that enter her bloodstream. RhoGAM provides virtually complete protection by preventing the woman from producing her own permanent Rh antibodies. It is administered intramuscularly within 3 days after delivery of an Rh-positive infant. Studies have shown that RhoGAM administration, once between 28 and 32 weeks' gestation and once after delivery, further decreases the risk of antibody production. RhoGAM should also be administered to an Rh-negative woman who has had a miscarriage or abortion after 12 weeks of pregnancy, even though the Rh type of the fetus cannot be confirmed. MICRhoGAM is a reduced dose of RhoGAM and is administered to the Rh-negative woman if she aborts within the first 12 weeks of pregnancy.

ABO INCOMPATIBILITY

In **ABO incompatibility**, the etiology is similar to that of Rh incompatibility. The difficulty is caused by the presence of naturally occurring maternal antibodies that attack the fetal blood cells of group A, B, or AB, Figure 4–4. ABO

POSSIBLE ABO INCOMPATIBILITIES THAT MAY LEAD TO HEMOLYSIS IN NEWBORNS

Maternal Blood Type	Maternal Antigens	Maternal Antibodies	Fetal Blood Type
A	A	B	B or AB
B	B	A	A or AB
O	None	A & B	A or B

Figure 4–4

incompatibility occurs most frequently when the mother has type O blood and the infant has either type A or type B blood. Hemolytic disease due to A or B incompatibility is not usually anticipated unless previous children in the family have had this problem. The disease in the newborn is usually mild and may even pass unnoticed. It should be treated, however, if signs are well developed:

- mild jaundice during the first 24 hours after birth
- enlargement of the liver and spleen
- central nervous system complications (rare)
- varying degrees of anemia or erythroblastosis

Treatment consists of phototherapy or an exchange transfusion using group O blood of the appropriate Rh type if the newborn's serum bilirubin level approaches 20 mg per 100 mL. Most affected newborns need no treatment but should be observed carefully with special attention to respirations, pulse, temperature, and increasing lethargy. The nurse should also watch for and report any increased jaundice, urine pigmentation, edema, cyanosis, convulsions, and any vital sign changes.

Gastrointestinal System of the Newborn

The gastrointestinal system is made up of all the body's organs involved in taking food, converting it into substances that the body can use, and discarding those elements that are considered waste. The gastrointestinal system includes the mouth, teeth, pharynx, and the alimentary or gastrointestinal tract (esophagus, stomach, intestines, and other organs, such as the liver, gallbladder, and pancreas).

Cleft Lip and Cleft Palate

A **cleft lip** is a vertical cleft or split in the upper lip, Figure 4–5. It is also known as a harelip. A **cleft palate** is a fissure in the roof of the mouth and nasal cavities. A cleft lip, or a cleft lip associated with a cleft palate, may be unilateral or bilateral.

In infants with cleft lip or palate, feeding is usually the most immediate problem. It is best accomplished by placing the infant in an upright position and directing the flow of milk against the side of the mouth. This method decreases the amount of air swallowed. The infant should be bubbled or burped frequently. Various nipples may be tried, including cleft palate nipples and regular nipples with enlarged holes. Breast-feeding may be tried as well.

Cleft lip and cleft palate can occur separately or together. Both conditions result from failure of the soft or bony tissues or both of the upper jaw and palate to unite between 8 and 12 weeks' gestation. Surgical repair is the usual treatment. Depending on the severity, treatment may be immediate or may be delayed until the second year of life. The parents often require a great deal of support, as this disorder can be quite disfiguring. Repair is generally successful; it is helpful if the parents know and understand this fact. Speech therapy may be necessary. Figure 4–6 summarizes nursing care for the infant with a cleft lip and palate.

Thrush

Thrush, or oral candidiasis, is an infection caused by the fungus *Candida (Monilia) albicans*, which is generally found in the vagina of the mother. Spores grow on the delicate tissue of the newborn's mouth. A newborn can also be infected by improperly cleaned nipples or breasts of the mother.

Thrush appears as pearly white, elevated

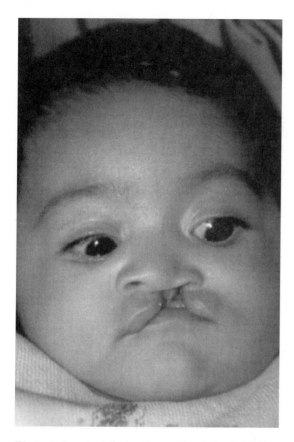

Figure 4–5 *An infant with a right unilateral cleft lip and palate. (Photo courtesy of Janet Salomonson , M.D. Reprinted with permission from the Cleft Palate Foundation. 1-800-24-CLEFT)*

lesions resembling milk curds. It is usually found on the tongue margins, inside the lips and cheeks, and on the hard palate. Prognosis with treatment is good, and recovery usually takes place in 3 to 4 days. Nystatin or aqueous gentian violet (1% solution) may be used to treat thrush.

PYLORIC STENOSIS

Pyloric stenosis is a common condition of the intestinal tract. The circular musculature of the pylorus (the junction of the stomach and the small intestine) increases in size. The musculature is greatly thickened. The mass constricts the pyloric opening and impedes stomach emptying.

Symptoms usually appear within 2 to 4 weeks after birth. Vomiting is the initial symptom and may be mild at first, becoming more forceful until it is projectile. Because little of the feeding is retained, the newborn is always hungry. The infant fails to gain weight and begins to appear starved. Because little food passes through the pylorus, bowel movements decrease in frequency and amount.

The signs of pyloric stenosis are dehydration, poor skin turgor, peristaltic waves visible on the abdomen, and a palpable olive-shaped mass in the right upper quadrant of the abdomen. Surgical intervention is usually necessary. If surgery is performed early, the prognosis is excellent. The nurse should provide parental support and reassurance. Vomiting may occur after surgery because of gastric irritation as well as anesthesia. Position the infant to prevent aspiration of vomitus. Feedings are administered frequently, slowly, and in small amounts, as ordered. The infant should be burped frequently. Encourage the parents to participate in the infant's care.

HERNIAS

A hernia is the protrusion of part of an organ through the wall of the cavity in which it is normally contained. If large enough, a hernia can disrupt the functioning of other nearby organs.

In a **diaphragmatic hernia**, some abdominal organs protrude through the diaphragm into the chest cavity. This usually occurs in the left chest, displacing the heart to the right and compressing the left lung. The newborn may display signs of respiratory distress, dyspnea, cyanosis, and a boat-shaped abdomen.

NURSING CARE PLAN: CLEFT LIP AND PALATE

Nursing Diagnosis	Goal(s)	Nursing Intervention	Rationale
High risk for altered nutrition: less than body requirements, related to impaired ability to feed	The infant will gain 1 oz (28 g) per day (after usual loss of 10% of birth weight).	If the mother plans to breast-feed, arrange for speacial teaching, such as with a member of La Leche League.	Knowledge helps decrease anxiety about feeding and should make feedings as effective as possible.
		If the mother does not breast-feed, teach the parents how to use a bottle or large syringe for feedings. Show them how to hold the infant almost upright, place a long soft nipple (or tubing attached to a syringe on the side of the mouth opposite the cleft, and let the milk drip slowly, allowing the infant to swallow small amounts.	
		Instruct the parents to burp the infant frequently—about every 0.5 oz of feeding.	Infants with cleft lip and palate usually swallow more air than other infants. Frequent burping helps prevent regurgitation and loss of feeding.
		Record the infant's fluid intake, urine output, and daily weight.	Tracking these factors helps in determining the need for more or different formula and in evaluating the effectiveness of feedings.
High risk for injury to infection	The infant will have a temperature below 100°F and healthy, pink pink skin and mucous membranes at the cleft.	Instruct the parents to give the infant water after each feeding to rinse milk from the cleft.	These techniques help prevent aspiration as well as pooling of milk or formula in the mouth, which could lead to infection.
		Instruct the parents to feed the infant for no more than 30 minutesat each sitting.	

Figure 4-6   *Nursing care plan for an infant with cleft lip and palate*

NURSING CARE PLAN: CLEFT LIP AND PALATE

Nursing Diagnosis	Goal(s)	Nursing Intervention	Rationale
High risk for altered parenting related to impaired bonding with infant who has an obvious defect.	The parents will describe positive feelings about their infant.	Advise the parents to place the infant in a semisitting position and on the right side after feeding.	Parents who can express their feelings of disappointment are more likely to move beyond them and begin bonding with the infant.
		Encourage the parents to discuss their feelings about their newborn's defect. Demonstrate acceptance of their feelings.	
		Demonstrate your positive reaction to the infant, emphasizing the infant's good qualities, such as beautiful eyes.	Positive modeling helps parents adopt more positive behaviors.
	The parents will demonstrate bonding behaviors.	Urge the parents to participate in the infant's feeding and care as soon as possible.	Early, frequent interactions with the infant help parents get used to the defect and appreciate the infant's other qualities.
		Reinforce bonding behaviors, such as cuddling and eye contact.	Reinforcement promotes the adoption of appropriate behaviors.
Anxiety (parental) related to their infant's surgery	Before surgery, the parents will demonstrate minimal anxiety.	Before the surgery, explain the procedure for cleft lip and palate repair. gives parents a chance	Such teaching decreases anxiety and to ask questions and discuss concerns.
		Orient the parents to the medical-surgical surgical unit. Explain where their infant will be at all times.	Orientation familiarizes the parents with the sights and sounds of the unit, which helps reduce anxiety.
		Provide written information about cleft lip and palate repair.	Written information reinforces teaching sessions and is useful for later referral at home.

Figure 4–6   *Continued*

A diaphragmatic hernia may be detected in utero by ultrasound and may be confirmed after birth by chest x-ray. To correct this serious defect, surgery is performed to remove the abdominal organs from the chest and to close the diaphragmatic opening.

A **hiatal hernia** is actually a type of diaphragmatic hernia. In a hiatal hernia, part of the stomach pushes through the esophageal hiatus. This defect may result in gastric reflux and regurgitation or may cause pain and gastric obstruction. It may be managed with upright positioning and alternative feeding techniques. If these measures are not sufficient, surgery is required.

An **inguinal hernia** occurs when the peritoneum, the membrane lining of the abdominal wall, admits abdominal contents into the groin through the inguinal canal. It is more common in males, resulting from failure of the proximal part of the peritoneal sac that precedes the testes into the scrotum to atrophy and close after the testes descend. When this occurs, the intestine is displaced into the inguinal canal and becomes swollen. Symptoms also include irritability and constipation. If intestinal obstruction occurs, vomiting and severe abdominal pain may be present. Generally, an inguinal hernia is surgically corrected as soon as possible.

An **umbilical hernia** is caused by a weakness or an incomplete closure of the umbilical ring, allowing a portion of the small intestine or omentum to protrude. The omentum is a double fold of peritoneum attached to the stomach that connects it to the abdominal viscera. An umbilical hernia is indicated by a soft swelling at the site of the umbilicus. The swelling may disappear when pressure is applied and reappear when pressure is removed or when the infant cries. The condition often disappears by itself when the abdominal muscles become stronger—usually when the child learns to stand or walk. If the hernia does not disappear spontaneously, it can be repaired surgically.

Although rare, an **omphalocele** results from herniation of some abdominal contents into the umbilical cord's root. This forms an external sac covered with peritoneal membrane on the abdomen. Treatment calls for surgery to place the organs back into the abdomen.

COLIC AND DIARRHEA

Colic is most common during the first 3 to 4 months and is characterized by intestinal cramping. The infant may pass gas from the anus or belch it up from the stomach. The infant draws up his or her knees and cries loudly in pain. The exact cause of colic is unknown, but predisposing factors may include excessive air swallowing, too much excitement, too rapid feeding, or a tense mother who communicates this tenseness to the infant.

The treatment is to bubble or burp the newborn frequently, holding the infant upright to get rid of the air in the intestinal tract. Letting the infant suck on a pacifier, breast, or finger; walking and rocking the infant; swaddling the infant; or holding the infant by lying him or her, facing outward, on the arm may also help comfort a colicky baby. Colic is not a serious condition, and infants usually gain weight despite periods of pain.

Diarrhea is a symptom of various conditions and can range from mild to severe. Diarrhea can be difficult to detect because of the varied appearance of stools in infants, Figure 4–7. Faulty preparation of formula, overfeeding, an unbalanced diet (excessive sugar), infection, antibiotics, and spoiled food may all cause diarrhea. A diagnosis is made from the health history and clinical evaluations. Weight loss and dehydration may

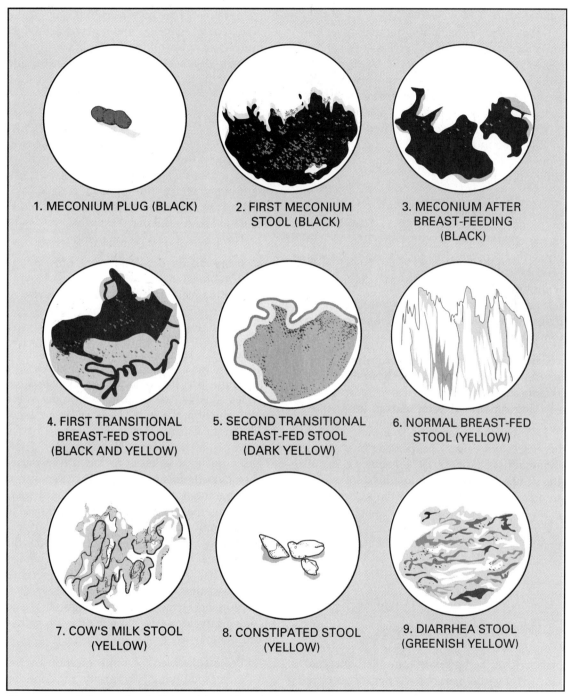

1. MECONIUM PLUG (BLACK)

2. FIRST MECONIUM STOOL (BLACK)

3. MECONIUM AFTER BREAST-FEEDING (BLACK)

4. FIRST TRANSITIONAL BREAST-FED STOOL (BLACK AND YELLOW)

5. SECOND TRANSITIONAL BREAST-FED STOOL (DARK YELLOW)

6. NORMAL BREAST-FED STOOL (YELLOW)

7. COW'S MILK STOOL (YELLOW)

8. CONSTIPATED STOOL (YELLOW)

9. DIARRHEA STOOL (GREENISH YELLOW)

Figure 4–7   *Infant stool cycle (Adapted from Clinical Education Aid, No. 3, courtesy Ross Laboratories)*

follow.

Treatment is usually a reduction in formula feedings in order to put less stress on the gastrointestinal tract. Fluid (5% glucose in saline solution) is increased and given orally every 3 to 4 hours until the diarrhea subsides. Diarrhea can be a serious problem. Infants with diarrhea are generally isolated from other infants. The mother should be encouraged to report continued episodes of diarrhea to the baby's physician.

IMPERFORATE ANUS

In the eighth week of embryonic life, a membrane that separates the rectum from the anus is usually absorbed, leaving a continuous canal whose outlet is the anus. If this membrane is not absorbed, an **imperforate anus** results. A diagnosis is made when the following symptoms appear:

- no anal opening is found on examination
- no stool is passed within the first 24 hours after birth
- later abdominal distention occurs

Obstruction must be relieved at once because stool cannot be passed. In a female infant, a fistula (opening) sometimes exits into the vagina or perineum, allowing stool to pass. In a male infant, a fistula to the bladder may exist. Surgical correction is necessary; the procedure depends on the anomaly. Prognosis is good with early detection and surgical correction.

NERVOUS SYSTEM OF THE NEWBORN

All parts of the body are controlled and coordinated by the nervous system. The brain, spinal cord, and nerves make up the nervous system. The sensory organs are also part of this system. They receive stimuli by sight, touch, taste, smell, and hearing. When impulses are transmitted to the brain through the sense organs, the body responds through action by the brain, spinal cord, and nerves.

SPINA BIFIDA

Spina bifida is a malformation of the spine in which the posterior portion of the laminae of the vertebrae fails to close, Figure 4–8. It can occur in any area of the spine but is most common in the lumbosacral region. Spina bifida occurs in about 1 out of 1,000 births.

Three basic types of spina bifida exist:

- **spina bifida occulta** (defect only of the vertebrae)
- **meningocele** (meninges protrude through the opening of the spinal cavity)
- **meningomyelocele** (spinal cord and meninges protrude through the defect in the bony rings of the spinal canal)

With spina bifida occulta, treatment is not needed unless neurological symptoms show involvement of the spinal cord. With meningocele, surgical correction is necessary, but the prognosis is excellent. Generally, this defect causes no leg weakness or lack of sphincter control. With meningomyelocele (also called myelomeningocele), the newborn may display symptoms that range from slight weakness to flaccid paralysis of the legs and absence of sensation in the feet. With surgical correction, the neurological deficit can be improved. Therapy may further improve function as the nervous system matures.

Nursing care in meningocele and meningomyelocele is mainly of a protective nature until surgery:

- Protect the bladder from infection by frequent emptying. To empty the bladder, apply firm, gentle pressure starting at the umbilical area and progressing downward

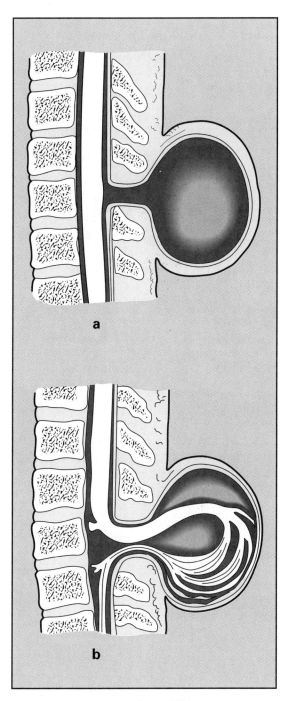

Figure 4–8 *Two types of spina bifida.*
(a) Meningocele. (b) Meningomyelocele.

(the Credé's method).

- Protect the protruding sac from pressure.
- Protect the sac from infection caused by urine and feces.
- Protect the feet from deformity if the infant is placed on his or her abdomen. Support the ankles with foam rubber pads so that the toes do not rest on the bed.

Good general nursing care and a caring attitude are vital for these infants. Special consideration should also be given to the parents to help them understand this disorder.

The alpha fetoprotein screen, which is performed on maternal serum between 15 and 20 weeks' gestation, can detect this neural tube defect. An ultrasound can confirm the diagnosis by enabling visualization of the defect. Early detection gives the parents a choice. They can continue the pregnancy, knowing that their newborn will need special attention at birth and may have permanent disabilities, or they can decide to terminate the pregnancy within the legal time restrictions. In either case, nursing support is needed to help a family understand the nature of a neural tube defect and all the possible outcomes.

DOWN SYNDROME

Down syndrome is a congenital disorder that involves irreparable brain and body damage, Figure 4–9. It is associated with chromosomal abnormalities, primarily a third chromosome 21, but the cause of these abnormalities is not clear. Among generalized syndromes caused by chromosomal anomalies, Down syndrome is the most common. Its occurrence is more likely with increasing maternal age, Figure 4–10.

Mental retardation is sometimes severe. Deformities are most often noticed in the skull and eyes. The eyes are set close together and slanted, the nose is flat, and the tongue is large and usually protrudes from an open mouth. The head is small, and the hands are short and

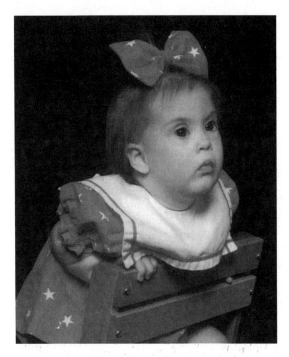

Figure 4–9   *Down syndrome infant*

thick. The skin may be mottled. Muscle tone may be weak. Some of these children die early in life because of infection, which their bodies cannot handle.

HYDROCEPHALUS

Hydrocephalus is due to a blockage or to an inadequate absorption of cerebrospinal fluid and an increase of fluid—and pressure—within the intracranial cavity, Figure 4–11. The accumulation of fluid in the ventricles generally enlarges the infant's skull since the bones are not yet closed and will yield to pressure.

Symptoms of hydrocephalus include an unusually large head at birth (or a rapidly enlarging head after birth), bulging fontanels, and the "setting-sun" sign (sclera visible above the iris). A CT scan or MRI may be done to confirm suspected hydrocephalus.

DOWN SYNDROME AND MATERNAL AGE	
Maternal Age	**Frequency of Down Syndrome**
30	1 in 885 births
31	1 in 826 births
32	1 in 725 births
33	1 in 592 births
34	1 in 465 births
35	1 in 365 births
36	1 in 287 births
37	1 in 225 births
38	1 in 176 births
39	1 in 139 births
40	1 in 109 births
41	1 in 85 births
42	1 in 67 births
43	1 in 53 births
44	1 in 41 births
45	1 in 32 births
46	1 in 25 births
47	1 in 20 births
48	1 in 16 births
49	1 in 12 births

Figure 4–10   *Risk of giving birth to a Down syndrome infant by maternal age*

Treatment should begin as soon as symptoms appear and before damage to the brain results. Several shunting procedures are now in use. Prognosis depends on the promptness of treatment and the operation performed.

FACIAL PARALYSIS

Pressure of the forceps on the facial nerve may cause a temporary paralysis of the muscles on one side of the face. The mouth may be drawn to the other side; this lopsidedness is most noticeable when the baby cries. The

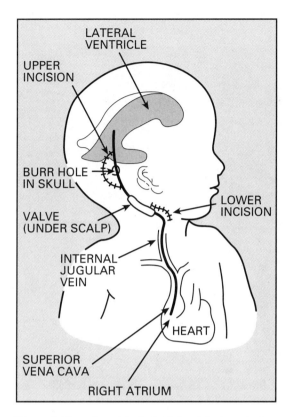

Figure 4–11 *A ventriculoatrial shunt drains spinal fluid in an infant with hydrocephalus.*

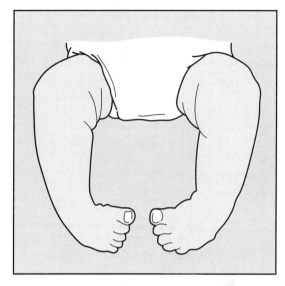

Figure 4–12 *Anterior view of bilateral talipes (clubfoot)*

condition usually disappears in a few days or even a few hours. The parents need reassurance that this is a temporary condition. During initial feedings, sucking may be difficult for the infant. The mother needs support and patience in feeding her baby.

MUSCULOSKELETAL SYSTEM OF THE NEWBORN

The bones provide support and protection. Skeletal muscles are attached to the bones. Body movements are due to the action of these muscles. Some disorders of the newborn affect this system.

TALIPES

Talipes (clubfoot), which may involve one or both feet, is the most common congenital foot abnormality, occurring twice as frequently in males as in females. The foot may turn inward, outward, downward, or upward, Figure 4–12. The cause of this disorder is not fully known but may have a hereditary component.

To treat talipes, a series of casts may be used. The cast usually covers the leg from the foot to mid-thigh and is changed regularly to correct the deformity gradually and gently. To maintain the correction, a Denis Browne splint may be worn for a period of at least 6 months. Then special shoes may be worn. If these treatments are unsuccessful, surgical correction may be necessary.

CONGENITAL HIP DYSPLASIA

Congenital hip dysplasia (congenital dislocation of the hip) is caused by improper embryonic development of the acetabulum (socket of the pelvis). Usually, the dislocation occurs when the head of the femur does not lie entirely within the shallow acetabulum. Dysplasia usually affects only one hip and occurs seven times more frequently in girls than it does in boys.

Dysplasia can be difficult to detect. However, signs may include:

- limited hip abduction (movement away from the body) on the affected side. Normally, when an infant is lying on his or her back with knees and hips flexed, the hip joint permits the femur to be abducted until the knee almost touches the table at a 90-degree angle. With dislocation, abduction on the affected side is 45 degrees or less.
- shortened leg on the affected side.
- asymmetrical thigh and gluteal folds that are more prominent on the affected side.
- Ortolani's click (palpable movement of the femur's head into the acetabulum as physician applies gentle pressure).

Treatment should be started as soon as the diagnosis is made. The objective of treatment is to create a normal joint by placing the head of the femur within the acetabulum and by enlarging and deepening the socket with constant pressure. This objective is usually accomplished by manipulating the femur into place and by applying a brace such as the Frejka pillow or the Pavlik harness, which is gradually adjusted to attain proper alignment of the femur, Figure 4–13. If the hip does not remain stable, a hip spica cast may be used for 3 to 6 months. If necessary, surgery is performed.

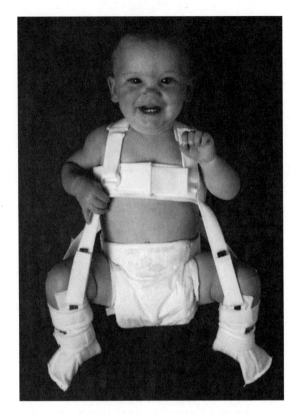

Figure 4–13 *Infant fitted with a Pavlik harness. (Courtesy Wheaton Brace Company, Carol Stream, IL)*

FRACTURES

Fractures may occur during delivery. The bones usually affected are the clavicle (collarbone), the humerus (upper arm), and the femur (thigh bone). The clavicle usually heals without treatment. Long bones need to be splinted, but these fractures typically heal quickly.

TORTICOLLIS

Torticollis is a condition caused by an abnormal shortening of the sternocleidomastoid muscle. The head is tilted to one side. Exercise or traction may be prescribed.

ERB'S PALSY

A newborn with **Erb's palsy** may suffer partial paralysis of the arm resulting from injury to the brachial plexus. The newborn cannot raise his or her arm. Usually, this injury is not permanent if it is caused during the delivery process.

URINARY SYSTEM OF THE NEWBORN

The kidneys, ureters, bladder, and urethra make up the urinary system. This system is responsible for waste excretion via urination and helps maintain fluid and electrolyte balance.

MALFORMATION OF THE URINARY TRACT

For every newborn, it is important to record the time, description, and kind of urine flow. Although little urine is voided in the first 2 days, ample water should be given to meet the newborn's needs for hydration and waste excretion. Malformations may lead to death if they are obstructive and renal failure occurs. Abnormalities of the ureters, double kidneys, and double pelves on one or both kidneys cause no harm in themselves but may lead to renal infection and problems of the urinary tract.

EXSTROPHY OF THE BLADDER

Exstrophy of the bladder results from failure of the abdominal wall and related structures to fuse in utero. This defect leaves the interior of the bladder completely exposed through an abdominal opening. The bladder's exposed mucosa appears reddened and is easily irritated. Because this defect exposes the bladder and lets urine flow directly onto the surrounding skin, the newborn is at high risk for infection and trauma. Because of inadequate drainage and infection, kidney damage is also a danger.

During the neonatal period, surgery should be done to close the bladder. However, the parents should be informed that surgery does not ensure normal voiding and that urinary diversion may be required. Final corrective surgery should be completed before the child begins school.

HYPOSPADIAS AND EPISPADIAS

In **hypospadias**, the urethra terminates on the underside of the penis. Although hypospadias does not prevent urination, it prevents the child from directing his urinary stream while standing. Usually, surgery is performed early to correct this defect. It is typically done before age 18 months to help prevent body image problems as well as the embarrassment and ridicule that an older child with this condition may experience.

In **epispadias**, the urethra opens on the upper surface of the penis. This condition is less common than hypospadias and is sometimes associated with exstrophy of the bladder. It, too, is correctable by surgery.

REPRODUCTIVE SYSTEM OF THE NEWBORN

The external sex organs and related inner structures comprise the reproductive system. This system is concerned with the production of new individuals.

CRYPTORCHIDISM

Cryptorchidism is a condition in which one or both of the testes fail to descend into the scrotum. The cause of this disorder is unknown. If uncorrected, it can lead to sterility.

In an infant with cryptorchidism, the testes usually descend spontaneously during the first year of life. If they do not descend by then, treatment should begin. Treatment sometimes starts with injections of human chorionic gonadotropic hormone. If this is not effective, surgery is performed. (For more information, see Chapter 26.)

SEXUAL AMBIGUITY

Abnormal sexual development in utero can lead to sexual ambiguity (ambiguous or inappropriate genitalia) at birth. The degree of ambiguity can vary greatly. For example, a newborn's genitalia may conform closely to those of one sex, or a newborn may have the genitalia of both sexes.

Two conditions that cause sexual ambiguity are **pseudohermaphroditism** and **hermaphroditism**. A newborn with pseudohermaphroditism has the external sex organs of one sex and the gonads (glands that produce gametes, or reproductive cells) of the other sex. This newborn is said to be intersexual. Female pseudohermaphrodites have female internal organs, but the enlarged clitoris and fused labia of the external organs resemble a penis and scrotum. Male pseudohermaphrodites have testes that usually do not descend from the abdomen and may have feminine external genitals. However, they have no ovaries. A hermaphrodite has the gonads and genitals of both sexes.

For a newborn with ambiguous genitalia, hasty sex determination based solely on appearance can ultimately be devastating. Therefore, various diagnostic tests may be done to establish the genetic sex and to help determine the gender choice. (Generally, the newborn's anatomy—not genetic sex—determines the gender choice.) Treatment consists of performing corrective surgery as needed; to treat hermaphroditism, the gonads of one sex are removed. Families will need the nurse's support and encouragement to deal with this emotionally charged condition.

INBORN ERRORS OF METABOLISM

In addition to disorders that affect specific body systems, newborns may have inborn errors of metabolism. Because metabolism includes all chemical processes in the body, it affects growth, energy generation, waste elimination, and the promotion of other bodily functions. Therefore, errors of metabolism can have systemic effects.

PHENYLKETONURIA

Normally, the liver produces an enzyme that acts on an amino acid called phenylalanine; the enzyme changes it to tyrosine. Phenylketonuria (PKU) is a metabolic disease caused by failure of the body to oxidize phenylalanine because of the missing or inadequate enzyme. Since the amino acid isn't broken down, it builds up in the blood and tissues, causing damage to the brain. Symptoms of PKU include vomiting, hyperactivity, eczema, and a musty urine odor. If the disease is left untreated, mental retardation usually results.

Blood and urine tests can detect PKU. A

blood test is done routinely on a newborn in the hospital nursery after the infant has ingested protein but before discharge. The test is repeated within 3 weeks if the specimen was collected within the first 24 hours after birth. Retardation can be prevented with early detection and prompt treatment.

Treatment consists of dietary management restricting phenylalanine intake. Because phenylalanine makes up 5% of the protein in all foods, a low-phenylalanine diet is very limited. The infant should receive a low-phenylalanine formula, such as Lofenalac or Phenexol. Through adolescence, the child must avoid meat, fish, nuts, legumes, dairy products, and bread. Best results are obtained if treatment begins by the third week of life and if the serum phenylalanine level remains between 2 and 8 mg/dL.

GALACTOSEMIA

In the rare disorder **galactosemia**, an enzyme is missing that normally converts galactose into glucose. Typically, the affected infant appears normal at birth but later experiences difficulties after consuming milk, which contains galactose.

The primary symptoms of galactosemia are jaundice, vomiting, and weight loss. If caregivers do not withhold milk, additional problems may develop, such as cataracts, brain damage, enlargement of the liver and spleen, and death. To detect galactosemia, many states now require blood testing as part of routine newborn screening.

Treatment for galactosemia focuses on removing all forms of lactose (galactose is derived from lactose) from the diet. This includes breast milk. For infants, galactose-free formula (such as various soy-protein formulas) should be substituted for milk. For older children, the diet must continue to be free of lactose. Basically, it omits all types of dairy products.

CONGENITAL HYPOTHYROIDISM

Congenital hypothyroidism is a deficiency of thyroid hormones at birth. It may be permanent or transient and may result from a congenital absence or inability of the thyroid gland to function, resulting in a lack of thyroid hormone.

At birth, a newborn with congenital hypothyroidism usually appears normal. About 6 weeks later, the newborn may begin to display characteristic facial features, such as a short forehead, puffy eyes, flattened bridge of the nose, and a large tongue. Other symptoms may include vomiting; feeding difficulties; a hoarse cry; thick, dry, mottled skin; poor feeding; abdominal distention; constipation; umbilical hernia; and slow bone development. The infant sleeps for long periods and seldom cries. Parents may comment that the newborn is an especially good baby.

To detect congenital hypothyroidism early, facilities in most states routinely assess levels of the thyroid hormones. Some perform the test when the newborn is 2 to 6 days old. Others perform it as part of screening for PKU and galactosemia—when the newborn is 24 to 48 hours old. Early detection and treatment are important to prevent physical and mental impairment.

When the disorder is confirmed, life-long thyroid hormone replacement should begin. The agent of choice is levothyroxine sodium (Synthroid), a synthetic thyroid hormone. During this therapy, blood levels of thyroid hormones should be monitored and the dosage adjusted as needed. Bone age surveys to assess bone growth should also be performed.

REVIEW QUESTIONS

A. Multiple choice. Select the best answer.

1. Asphyxia neonatorum could be caused by
   a. physiological jaundice
   b. placenta abruptio
   c. omentum
   d. cyanosis

2. Which of the following is a consideration when an infant who does not breathe spontaneously at birth is being treated?
   a. proper positioning
   b. stimulation of the infant's legs and arms
   c. application of Nystatin to the mouth
   d. phototherapy

3. Jaundice that appears before the third day after birth
   a. has little medical significance
   b. is called physiological jaundice
   c. may indicate a hemolytic disease
   d. is to be expected in all infants

4. Excessive gas accumulation in the newborn may predispose the infant to
   a. pyloric stenosis
   b. umbilical hernia
   c. colic
   d. imperforate anus

5. The normal stool color of a breast-fed infant is
   a. black
   b. yellow
   c. black and yellow
   d. greenish yellow

6. Meningomyelocele is a condition in which
   a. a vertebra is defective
   b. the meninges protrude through the opening of the spinal cavity
   c. the spinal cord and meninges protrude through the defect in the bony rings of the spinal canal
   d. the posterior portion of the laminae of the vertebrae fails to close

7. Which of the following is characteristic of an infant with Down syndrome?
   a. a rounded nasal bridge
   b. mental retardation
   c. rapid growth and development
   d. a large head

8. Temporary paralysis of the muscles on one side of the face can be caused by
   a. pressure of the forceps on the facial nerve
   b. severe uterine contractions
   c. analgesic drugs given to the mother during labor
   d. disproportionate sizes of the baby's head and the mother's pelvis

9. Erb's palsy is defined as
   a. an abnormal shortening of the sternocleidomastoid muscle
   b. partial paralysis of the arm due to injury to the brachial plexus
   c. temporary paralysis of the muscle on one side of the face
   d. the turning inward, outward, downward, or upward of one or both feet

10. A male newborn with an undescended testicle has
    a. cryptorchidism
    b. hypospadias
    c. epispadias
    d. hermaphroditism

11. A metabolic disease caused by failure of the body to oxidize a certain amino acid is
    a. erythroblastosis fetalis
    b. torticollis
    c. narcosis
    d. phenylketonuria

12. Mental retardation can be caused by
    a. phenylketonuria
    b. narcosis
    c. hypospadias
    d. pyloric stenosis

B. Match the term in column I to the correct description in column II.

Column I	Column II
1. anoxia	a. unconscious or stuporous state caused by drugs
2. asphyxia neonatorum	b. deprivation of oxygen
3. bilirubin	c. fissure in the roof of the mouth
4. cleft palate	d. product of red blood cell destruction
5. dyspnea	e. exposure to fluorescent blue light
6. cleft lip	f. vertical split in upper lip
7. hyaline membrane disease	g. an amino acid
8. narcosis	h. failure of the newborn to breathe spontaneously
9. phenylalanine	i. respiratory distress syndrome
10. phototherapy	j. difficult breathing

C. Briefly answer the following questions.

1. What are five signs of respiratory distress?
2. What is the treatment for erythroblastosis fetalis?

SUGGESTED ACTIVITIES

• Discuss the possible causes of birth defects. Talk about emotions a family of an infant with a birth defect would most likely experience. Draw on any personal knowledge.

• Write a report on how you think you would react when assisting in the birth of a severely deformed infant. Determine ways to overcome negative feelings you may have.

• Identify organizations that have birth defects as their focus. What services do they offer?

• Research the causes of mental retardation. Present a paper or a talk on one of the causes.

• Compare the clinical findings, diagnostic tests, and treatments associated with various inborn errors of metabolism.

BIBLIOGRAPHY

Betz, C., M. Hunsberger, and S. Wright. *Family-Centered Nursing Care of Children*, 2nd ed. Philadelphia: W. B. Saunders, 1994.

Cohen, S., C. Kenner, and A. Hollingsworth. *Maternal, Neonatal, and Women's Health Nursing*. Springhouse, PA: Springhouse, 1991.

Daberkow, E., and R. Washington. Cardiovascular diseases and surgical intervention. In G. Merenstein and S. Gardner, eds. *Handbook of Neonatal Intensive Care*, 2nd ed. St. Louis, MO: Mosby–Year Book, 1989.

Gellis, S., and B. Kagan, eds. *Current Pediatric Therapy*, 13th ed. Philadelphia: W. B. Saunders, 1990.

Hazinski, M. *Nursing Care of the Critically Ill Child*, 2nd ed. St. Louis, MO: Mosby–Year Book, 1992.

Jackson, D., and R. Saunders. *Child Health Nursing: A Comprehensive Approach to the Care of Children and Their Families.* Philadelphia: J. B. Lippincott, 1993.

Peterson, P. Spina bifida: Nursing challenge. *RN* 55, no. 3 (1992): 40–46.

Schaming, D., et al. When babies are born with orthopedic problems, *RN* 53, no. 4 (1990): 62–67.

Steele, S. Phenylketonuria: Counseling and teaching functions of the nurse on an interdisciplinarian team. *Issues in Comprehensive Pediatric Nursing*, 12, no. 5 (1989): 395–409.

Whitis, G., and P. Iyer. *Patient Outcomes in Pediatric Nursing.* Springhouse, PA: Springhouse, 1995.

Wong, D. L. *Whaley & Wong's Nursing Care of Infants and Children*, 5th ed. St. Louis, MO: Mosby–Year Book, 1995.

Growth and Development

CHAPTER

5

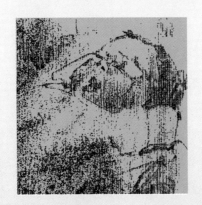

Principles of Growth and Development

Objectives

After studying this chapter, the student should be able to:

- Discuss principles of growth and development.

- Distinguish between cephalocaudal growth and proximodistal growth.

- Identify the variations in growth rate that occur as children mature.

- Describe the differences in growth rates for various parts of the body.

- Identify two factors that influence growth and development and give an example of each.

GROWTH

DEVELOPMENT

CEPHALOCAUDAL

PROXIMODISTAL

DIFFERENTIATION

INTEGRATION

rowth is the continuous and complex process in which the body and its parts increase in size. It can be evaluated numerically; for example, height, weight, arm length, leg length, and head circumference can be measured using numbers. **Development** is the qualitative, continuous process in which the child's level of functioning and progression of skills become more complex. For example, children babble before they use words and use two- or three-word phrases before they speak in sentences.

Several principles that govern how growth and development proceed are listed in Figure 5–1. This chapter discusses these principles and provides an overview of general patterns in growth and development. More detailed information on physical growth, cognitive development, and developmental milestones is provided in Chapters 6 and 7.

PATTERNS OF DEVELOPMENT

DIRECTIONAL PATTERNS

Growth and development proceed in a cephalocaudal and a proximodistal direction, Figure

PRINCIPLES OF GROWTH AND DEVELOPMENT

- Growth and development proceed in a cephalocaudal and proximodistal direction and follow an orderly, sequential pattern.

- The pace of growth and development varies, and different parts of the body grow and develop at different rates.

- Behavior becomes more versatile as development proceeds.

- Differentiation of skills occurs with maturation and practice.

- Development involves the ability to move from simple to more complex tasks.

- Growth and development are influenced by such factors as heredity and environment. Development cannot proceed without appropriate stimulation.

Figure 5–1

5–2. **Cephalocaudal** refers to the process in which maturation begins at the head and moves downward to the toes. For instance, infants are able to lift their heads before they can lift their chests, and they have control of their hands before they have control of their feet. **Proximodistal** refers to the process in which development proceeds from the center of the body outward toward the extremities. Again, infants control their shoulder movements before their hand movements, grasp objects with their whole hand before using their fingers, and gaze at items before they can reach out and grasp them.

PREDICTABLE PATTERNS

Throughout childhood and adolescence, other definite patterns in motor, physical, cognitive, and psychosocial growth and development can also be observed. Although the time and rate at which growth and development occur

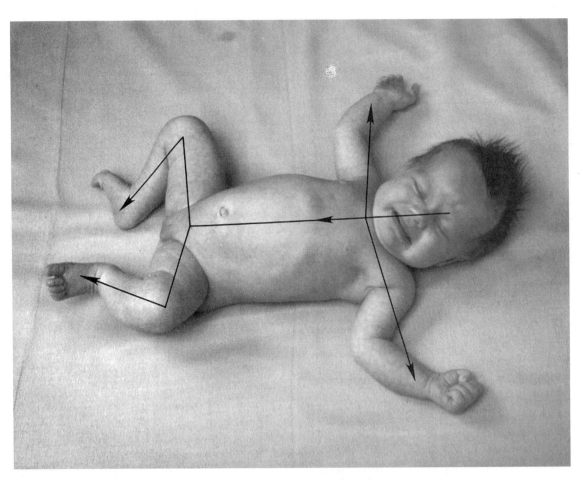

Figure 5–2   *Growth and development proceed in a cephalocaudal and a proximodistal direction.*

may vary from child to child, growth and development are predictable and follow an orderly sequence. Children achieve milestones in motor development at different ages but within an expected time frame. Although one child may walk at 10 months of age and another at 12 months, both children achieve this milestone at the expected point in their development. Furthermore, the sequence of motor development is fairly consistent; most children sit before they stand and stand before they walk.

Cognitive development also proceeds in an orderly and sequential pattern. For example, 2-year-olds use one word to describe several objects; thus, the word *ball* describes both apple and ball. Five-year-olds, on the other hand, use words that accurately represent the objects; an apple is called an apple and a ball is called a ball. In addition, children progress from literal interpretation of words to more complex associations in a predictable sequence (Erikson 1963).

DEVELOPMENTAL PACE

Although growth and development are orderly and sequential, the pace of these processes varies throughout childhood and adolescence. In the fetus and infant, the rate of growth is very rapid. After the age of 12 months, however, growth slows and progresses at a steady pace. The growth rate again increases dramatically during adolescence. The pace of maturation for different body systems also varies. For example, the cardiovascular system matures earlier than the respiratory system. In addition, when one area is developing, development of another area seems to slow down. Thus, while children are learning to walk they concentrate on this activity, and their speech development slows.

Rates of growth and development of the parts of the body also differ. Infants' heads are large compared with the rest of their bodies;

their arms and legs are relatively short. The feet and legs of toddlers and preschoolers grow more rapidly than the trunks of the body. This disproportion makes toddlers clumsy, and contributes to the number of falls they experience.

DIFFERENTIATION

Children progress from general and simple responses to more specific and complex responses as they mature. This process is termed **differentiation**. Differentiation can be seen in language development. In infancy, children only cry and babble, but by adolescence they can express complex thoughts and feelings (Gottlieb 1983). The same is true of gross motor skills. For example, 2-year-olds can jump in place, and 7-year-olds can jump rope. Differentiation also takes place throughout psychosocial development as children progress from concrete thinking to abstract thinking (Erikson 1963). Differentiation is influenced by maturation and practice. Thus, children are not able to ride a bicycle until their muscles are developmentally ready and until they have had the opportunity to learn how to ride the bicycle and practice the necessary skills.

INTEGRATION OF SKILLS

As they mature, children are able to combine simple movements or skills to achieve complex tasks (Dacey and Travers 1991). This pattern, referred to as **integration**, is seen in the progression from the simple movements of crawling to the more complex movements of walking, running, and hopping. Children learn to play catch long before they combine the skills of throwing, catching, fielding, and batting in the game of baseball. Integration is also demonstrated in cognitive development. For instance, children progress from performing simple addition and subtraction to using these abilities in the more complex calculations of higher mathematics.

Factors Influencing Growth and Development

Growth and development are influenced by many interacting factors such as heredity and environment.

Influence of Heredity (Genetic Factors)

Genetic factors influence the child's physical characteristics, such as bone structure and height and weight. Intellectual potential and personality type are also determined by inheritance. The sex of the child, which is randomly determined at conception, affects growth patterns and how others behave toward the child.

Certain physical or mental defects that affect the child's development may be inherited. For example, muscular dystrophy (of which there is more than one kind) is a chronic, hereditary, degenerative muscle disease that affects muscle development. Children with Duchenne muscular dystrophy, the most common and severe form of the disease, usually develop noticeable muscle weakness by the third year of life. Eventually they are confined to a wheelchair.

Influence of Environment

Although a child is born with certain potential features and capacities, interaction with the environment influences how and to what extent this potential is realized. If children are well nourished, growth is stimulated. If, however, children are malnourished, growth is retarded (Tanner 1978).

A stimulating environment is also important to fostering growth and development. The period of infancy and each developmental stage thereafter require stimulation by parents and caregivers. Parents can provide auditory and visual stimulation to their infants by simply talking to them while maintaining eye contact. Physical contact between parents and their young children is also important. Simple toys such as balls and wooden blocks encourage development and early exploration of the environment. Involvement in appropriate activities promotes and enhances growth and development.

Social, economic, and educational factors are part of the cultural environment that affects growth and development. Children learn how to act in certain situations by observing the people around them. Behavior that is acceptable in some families may be considered improper in other families from different ethnic backgrounds.

Nursing Care Related to Principles of Growth and Development

- Knowledge of the principles of growth and development is an important aspect of the care that nurses provide to children and adolescents.
- Nurses should anticipate the needs of parents in fostering optimal growth and development in their children.
- Nurses should act as advocates for children and adolescents so that people who work with children (teachers, coaches, and others) understand what the child is capable of accomplishing at various developmental stages.

REVIEW QUESTIONS

A. Multiple choice. Select the best answer.

1. Which of the following is most true about growth?
    a. It can be measured numerically.
    b. It refers to changes in behavior as well as size.
    c. It proceeds most rapidly in school-age children.
    d. It proceeds mainly in the limbs of newborns and infants.

2. Being able to sit before being able to stand is an example of
    a. cephalocaudal development
    b. developmental pace
    c. growth
    d. stimulation

3. Growth and development proceed
    a. from the feet to the head
    b. at a constant rate through infancy and childhood
    c. in predictable sequences
    d. without outside stimulation

4. Which of the following variations in the rate of growth and development would you most expect?
    a. rapid growth in the preschool years
    b. rapid growth in the school-age years
    c. rapid growth in adolescence
    d. steady growth in infancy

5. Which of the following are you most apt to see?
    a. toddlers with head and body well proportioned
    b. well-coordinated toddlers
    c. preschoolers that seem to be all legs
    d. infants with head and body well proportioned

6. Which of the following is true of differentiation?
    a. It is a progression from specific to general responses in a given area of ability.
    b. It applies primarily to psychosocial development.
    c. It is interrupted by practice.
    d. It increases as muscles develop.

7. Integration has occurred in which of the following examples?
    a. being able to use a fork to help cut food after learning to hold the fork
    b. being able to sit on a bicycle before being able to ride it
    c. being able to hold a bat before being able to swing it
    d. being able to hold knitting needles before being able to knit

8. Which of the following is not an example of environmental influences on growth and development?
    a. diet
    b. culturally defined ways of training children
    c. an inherited hip defect
    d. parental expectations

B. Match the term in column I to the correct definition in column II.

Column I	Column II
1. integration	a. head-to-toe direction
2. growth	b. from center to extremity
3. proximodistal	c. an increase in size
4. differentiation	d. increase in level of functioning
5. development	e. combining simple movements or skills to achieve complex tasks
6. cephalocaudal	f. general responses becoming more specific

Suggested Activities

- Research and report on one of the following:
  - the impact of the environment on growth and development
  - the impact of heredity on growth and development

- Prepare a teaching poster to demonstrate how parents or other caregivers can stimulate some aspect of childhood development.

- List three examples of:
  - cephalocaudal development
  - proximodistal development

- Interview the parent of one child to do a case history of growth and development for a period of a child's life.

- Work individually or in teams to find three examples of each of the following developmental concepts:
  - differentiation
  - integration

Bibliography

Dacey, J., and J. Travers. *Human Development across the Lifespan*. Dubuque, IA: Wm. C. Brown Publishers, 1991.

Erikson, E. H. *Childhood and Society*, 2nd ed. New York: W. W. Norton, 1963.

Gottlieb, G. The psychobiological approach to developmental issues. In P. Mussen, ed. *Handbook of Child Psychology*, 4th ed. New York: Wiley, 1983.

Tanner, J. M. *Foetus into Man: Physical Growth from Conception to Maturity*. Cambridge, MA: Harvard University Press, 1978.

CHAPTER

6

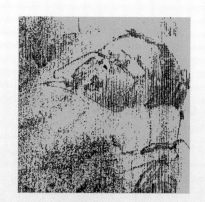

*P*hysical Growth

OBJECTIVES

AFTER STUDYING THIS CHAPTER, THE STUDENT SHOULD BE ABLE TO:

- IDENTIFY THE MOST RAPID PERIOD OF GROWTH OCCURRING DURING THE LIFESPAN.

- DESCRIBE THE CHANGES IN HEIGHT AND WEIGHT THAT OCCUR DURING INFANCY, TODDLERHOOD, AND THE PRESCHOOL YEARS.

- DESCRIBE THE CHANGES THAT OCCUR IN THE SCHOOL-AGE YEARS AND DURING ADOLESCENCE.

- IDENTIFY THE AVERAGE AGE OF SKELETAL MATURITY IN BOYS AND GIRLS.

- DESCRIBE THE PROCESS OF PRIMARY (DECIDUOUS) AND SECONDARY (PERMANENT) TOOTH ACQUISITION.

KEY TERMS

INFANCY	PREPUBERTAL GROWTH SPURT
TODDLERHOOD	ADOLESCENT GROWTH SPURT
PRESCHOOL	SEXUAL MATURITY
SCHOOL AGE	PRIMARY (DECIDUOUS) TEETH
ADOLESCENCE	SECONDARY (PERMANENT) TEETH

hysical growth is one of the most visible changes of childhood. The tiny newborn becomes a strong and sturdy toddler, a slender schoolchild, and finally a gangly adolescent. Parents and relatives are often astonished at the rapid changes that occur during infancy, early childhood, and adolescence. "I can't believe how big you've gotten," is a common refrain during this period.

This chapter describes patterns of height and weight gain, skeletal growth, and tooth eruption from infancy through adolescence. Growth patterns during this period can be summarized as follows:

Infancy: A period of very rapid growth and development occurring between birth and 1 year of age

Toddlerhood: A period of slower growth occurring between 1 and 3 years of age

Preschool: A period in which physical growth slows and stabilizes occurring between 3 and 6 years of age

School Age: A period of slow, steady growth occurring between 6 and 12 years of age

Adolescence: A period of increased physical growth and development, characterized by the development of primary and secondary sex characteristics, occurring between the ages of 12 and 19 years

Cross-sectional growth charts are used to plot a child's growth from infancy through adolescence. These charts provide a statistical definition of what is considered normal by comparing the child with others of similar age and sex. Normal variations in growth may reflect ethnic or individual genetic differences in both potential for growth and timing of growth spurts (Rudolph 1991). Chapter 12 provides a detailed discussion of the techniques

PHYSICAL GROWTH DURING INFANCY	
Age	**Physical Size**
1–6 months	Birth weight is regained by 10th–14th day; gains 1.5 pounds per month until 5 months.
	Birth weight doubles by 6 months.
	Grows 1 inch per month during the first 6 months.
6–12 months	Birth weight triples by 12 months.
	Birth length increases 50% by the end of the first year.

Figure 6–1

for measuring physical growth; refer to the appendixes at the back of this textbook for pediatric growth charts.

PHYSICAL GROWTH

In the first year, physical growth is faster than it will be in any other period of the lifespan. The newborn baby gains weight and length rapidly, maturing into a stronger and more active infant and toddler. Physical growth continues more slowly between toddlerhood and the school-age years, until another rapid growth spurt occurs at puberty.

INFANCY AND TODDLERHOOD

By the age of 6 months, the average infant has doubled his or her birth weight, attaining a weight of about 15 pounds. By one year, birth weight has tripled, to about 22 pounds. The infant's height increases during this period by about 10 to 12 inches, with the average 1-year-old attaining a height of about 30 inches, Figure 6–1.

This period of rapid growth decreases during the second and third years. The average child gains about 5 to 6 pounds and grows approximately 3½ to 5 inches by the second birthday. During the third year, the increase is less, about 3 to 5 pounds and 2 to 2½ inches, Figure 6–2.

As the child grows, body proportions change as well. The head, which is disproportionately large in the newborn baby and toddler, becomes smaller in proportion to the rest of the body until the individual reaches his or her full adult height, Figure 6–3. Most children also become leaner in this period. Thus, by age 3, the characteristically potbellied toddler has become a slender preschooler.

PHYSICAL GROWTH DURING TODDLERHOOD	
Age	**Physical Size**
1–2 years	Gains ½ pound or more per month. Grows 3½–5 inches during this year.
2–3 years	Gains 3–5 pounds per year. Grows 2–2½ inches per year.

Figure 6–2

PRESCHOOL AND SCHOOL-AGE YEARS

During the preschool (3–6) and school-age (6–12) years, the average child goes through a period of slow but steady growth, Figure 6–4. As the young child grows, body weight and

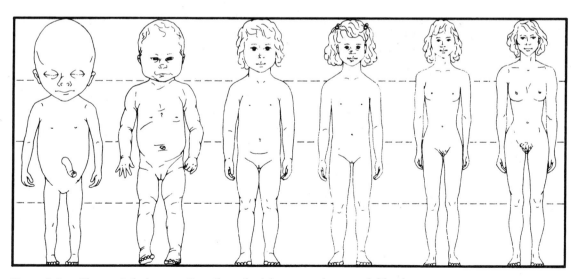

Figure 6–3   *Changes in body proportions through adolescence and young adulthood*

PHYSICAL GROWTH DURING PRESCHOOL AND SCHOOL-AGE YEARS	
Age	**Physical Size**
3–6 years (preschool)	Gains 3–5 pounds per year. Grows 1½–2½ inches per year. Birth length doubles by 4 years.
6–12 years (school-age)	Gains 3–5 pounds per year. Grows 1½–2½ inches per year.

Figure 6–4

PHYSICAL GROWTH DURING ADOLESCENCE	
Age	**Physical Size**
12–18 years	Weight gain peaks during growth spurts and accounts for over 40% of the ideal body weight. During growth spurt, girls gain approximately 20–25 pounds; boys approximately 15–20 pounds. Girls grow approximately 5–6 inches and boys 4½–5 inches. This secondary growth spurt accounts for approximately 25% of final adult height.

Figure 6–5

shape change as well. The legs are the fastest-growing part of the body during childhood. Fat tissue increases slowly until approximately age 7, when the **prepubertal growth spurt** begins. This phase precedes the true growth spurt of adolescence.

PUBERTY AND ADOLESCENCE

The trunk and legs continue to become proportionately longer during adolescence. Puberty is characterized by a rapid growth spurt, which generally begins in girls between the ages of 9 and 14½ (usually at about age 10) and in boys between the ages of 10½ and 16 (usually at about age 12 or 13). This period of accelerated growth typically lasts about 2 years.

In both sexes, the **adolescent growth spurt** affects practically all skeletal and muscular growth. During this period, the adolescent gains almost half of his or her final adult weight, and the skeleton and organ systems double in size. These changes are more pronounced in boys than in girls and follow their own timetables. Thus, parts of the body may be out of proportion for a time. The familiar awk-

wardness that characterizes the teenage years is a result of this unbalanced, rapid growth. During adolescence, boys also develop broader shoulders and greater muscle mass than girls, and girls develop a wider pelvis in preparation for childbearing. Growth in height is virtually complete by age 18, Figure 6–5.

Soon after the growth spurt ends, the adolescent reaches **sexual maturity**. Under the influence of the hypothalamus, pituitary, and gonadal hormones, the reproductive organs double in size during adolescence and mature to adult function. The principal sign of sexual maturity in girls is menstruation. The principal sign of sexual maturity in boys is the presence of sperm in the urine. Like that of the adolescent growth spurt, the timing of sexual maturity in boys and girls varies greatly, Figure 6–6.

Refer to the appendixes at the back of this textbook for growth charts from infancy through adolescence.

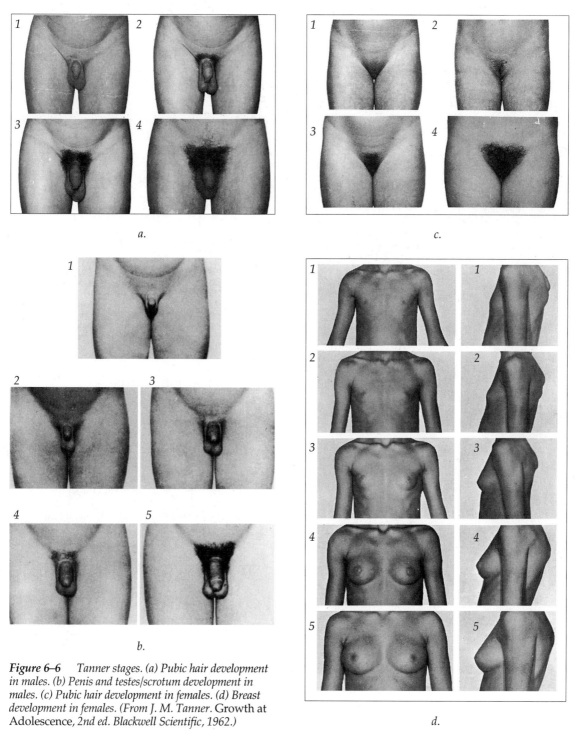

Figure 6–6   *Tanner stages. (a) Pubic hair development in males. (b) Penis and testes/scrotum development in males. (c) Pubic hair development in females. (d) Breast development in females. (From J. M. Tanner.* Growth at Adolescence, *2nd ed. Blackwell Scientific, 1962.)*

a.

c.

b.

d.

SKELETAL GROWTH

Changes in body proportion as the child grows from infancy to adulthood are related to the pattern of skeletal growth.

Skeletal growth is considered complete when the growth plates of the long bones of the arms and legs have completely fused. Completion of skeletal growth occurs, on average, in boys at 17½ years and in girls at 15½ years.

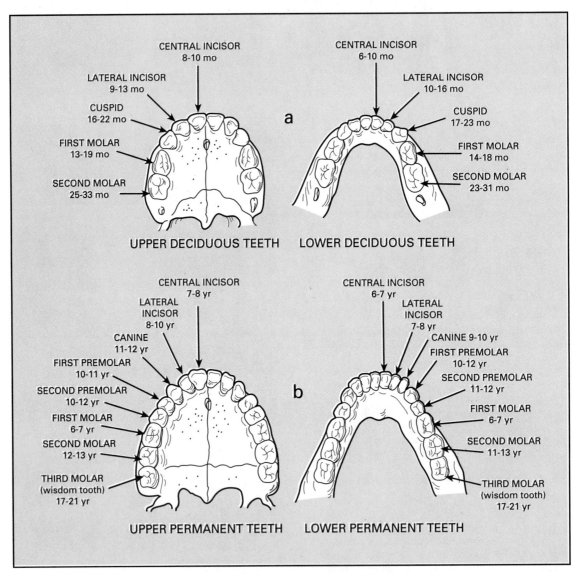

Figure 6–7   Tooth development. (a) Primary (deciduous) teeth. (b) Secondary (permanent) teeth.

Minor skeletal growth continues until approximately age 30, as additional bone is deposited to the upper and lower surfaces of the vertebrae. But this additional bone deposition accounts for only a 3- to 5-mm increase in height.

TOOTH DEVELOPMENT

PRIMARY (DECIDUOUS) TEETH

In most infants, the first tooth erupts between the ages of 5 and 9 months. By 1 year, 6 to 8 teeth usually are present. By the time a toddler reaches 33 months, approximately 20 **primary (deciduous) teeth** will have been acquired in a characteristic pattern, Figure 6–7a.

SECONDARY (PERMANENT) TEETH

The first **secondary (permanent) teeth** emerge at about 6 years, and the child continues to shed and replace teeth throughout childhood and early adulthood, see Figure 6–7b. The timing of the shedding of primary teeth and that of the eruption of secondary teeth vary widely among children.

REVIEW QUESTIONS

A. Multiple choice. Select the best answer.

1. The most rapid rate of growth during the lifespan occurs
    a. in the first year
    b. during adolescence
    c. between 3 and 6 years of age
    d. between 6 and 12 years of age

2. Which of the following is most true of first-year growth?
    a. Weight at the age of 6 months is about triple the birth weight.
    b. Birth weight triples by the end of the first year.
    c. Infant height doubles by the age of 6 months.
    d. Infant height at the end of the first year is about 40 inches.

3. You are likely to observe which of the following changes in body proportions as the child grows?
    a. The head of the toddler is well proportioned relative to the body.
    b. The legs of the growing child will be longer relative to the rest of the body than in infancy.
    c. The potbelly of the school-age child will flatten as adolescence approaches.
    d. The trunk of the adolescent looks smaller relative to the limbs than that of the school-age child.

4. After the age of 2, the number of pounds gained each year
   a. will increase until the age of 18
   b. will remain constant until the adolescent growth spurt
   c. will be about 10
   d. will be about 6

5. Which statement is true? Height increases
   a. about ½ inch per month during the first 6 months
   b. 2 to 2½ inches per year for the toddler
   c. are smaller each year from ages 3 to 12
   d. 5 to 6 inches per year for girls during the adolescent growth spurt

6. Which of the following statements is true of the adolescent growth spurt?
   a. The adolescent gains almost half of his or her final adult weight.
   b. It lasts approximately 4 years.
   c. It usually occurs between the ages of 10 and 12 years in boys.
   d. Organs triple in size.

7. Sexual maturity
   a. occurs immediately before the adolescent growth spurt
   b. occurs soon after the adolescent growth spurt ends
   c. is characterized primarily by the growth of breasts in girls
   d. is characterized primarily by the voice change in boys

8. Which of the following best describes skeletal growth?
   a. Skeletal growth is considered complete when the growth plates of the arms and legs have completely fused.
   b. The long bones of the arms and legs fuse during the school-age years.
   c. Minor skeletal growth continues throughout adult life.
   d. All skeletal growth stops after adolescence.

9. Tooth development shows which of the following patterns?
   a. The first tooth erupts between 2 and 4 months.
   b. The shedding and replacement of natural teeth continue throughout life.
   c. Before the toddler is 2 years old, 20 primary (deciduous) teeth will erupt.
   d. The first permanent teeth emerge at about 6 years of age.

10. Which of the following best describes the growth patterns of boys and girls?
    a. Growth patterns are similar during infancy and childhood.
    b. Growth patterns are markedly different in the preschool years.
    c. The rate of skeletal development differs throughout early childhood.
    d. Teeth erupt at different times in boys and girls.

SUGGESTED ACTIVITIES

- List the physical changes that you expect to occur in:
  - infancy
  - toddlerhood
  - preschool years
  - school-age years
  - adolescence

- Make color-coded charts to help you remember and compare changes in height and weight for each stage.

- List changes discussed in this chapter that you have observed in a growing infant, young child or adolescent. Discuss your findings in groups.

BIBLIOGRAPHY

Behrman, R. E. and V. C. Vaughn. *Nelson's Textbook of Pediatrics*, 13th ed. Philadelphia: W. B. Saunders, 1987.

Papalia, D. E. and S. W. Olds. *A Child's World: Infancy through Adolescence*, 6th ed. New York: McGraw-Hill, 1993.

Rudolph, A. M. *Rudolph's Pediatrics*, 19th ed. Norwalk, CT: Appleton & Lange, 1991.

Seidel, H. M., J. W. Ball, J. E. Dains, and G. W. Benedict. *Mosby's Guide to Physical Examination*, 2nd ed. St. Louis, MO: Mosby-Year Book, 1991.

Tanner, J. M. *Foetus into Man: Physical Growth from Conception to Maturity*. Cambridge, MA: Harvard University Press, 1978.

Wong, D. L. *Whaley & Wong's Essentials of Pediatric Nursing*, 4th ed. St. Louis, MO: Mosby-Year Book, 1993.

CHAPTER

7

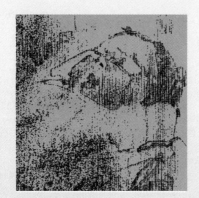

Developmental Stages

OBJECTIVES

AFTER STUDYING THIS CHAPTER, THE STUDENT SHOULD BE ABLE TO:

- IDENTIFY AND DESCRIBE THE STAGES OF FREUD'S THEORY OF PSYCHOSEXUAL DEVELOPMENT.

- IDENTIFY AND DESCRIBE THE STAGES OF ERIKSON'S THEORY OF PSYCHOSOCIAL DEVELOPMENT.

- IDENTIFY AND DESCRIBE THE STAGES OF PIAGET'S THEORY OF COGNITIVE DEVELOPMENT.

- IDENTIFY AND DESCRIBE THE LEVELS OF KOHLBERG'S THEORY OF MORAL DEVELOPMENT.

- DESCRIBE PHYSICAL CHARACTERISTICS OF CHILDREN AT VARIOUS STAGES OF DEVELOPMENT.

- IDENTIFY FINE MOTOR ABILITY AT VARIOUS STAGES OF DEVELOPMENT.

- IDENTIFY GROSS MOTOR ABILITY AT VARIOUS STAGES OF DEVELOPMENT.

- IDENTIFY LANGUAGE SKILLS AT VARIOUS STAGES OF DEVELOPMENT.

- IDENTIFY SENSORY ABILITY AT VARIOUS STAGES OF DEVELOPMENT.

*i*nfants and children act on their environment and in turn are stimulated by the responses they help to bring about. Through this interaction, motor, cognitive, language, and social skills are developed. This chapter introduces several theories of child development and identifies behaviors and skills that are characteristic of children at various stages of development. This information provides a useful guide for nurses who care for pediatric patients of various ages.

The following developmental stages are used in this chapter and throughout the text:

Infant: Birth through 1 year
Toddler: 1 through 3 years
Preschool Child: 3 through 6 years
School-Age Child: 6 through 12 years
Adolescent: 12 through 19 years

PERSONALITY AND TEMPERAMENT

Each child is a unique individual whose personality and temperament influence how the child deals with others and with the environment. **Personality** is the pattern of characteristic thoughts, feelings, and behaviors that distinguishes one person from another (Phares 1991). **Temperament** refers to a person's style of approaching other people and situations (Thomas and Chess, 1977). Early in life, children display identifiable differences in temperament. For example, parents of a new baby girl may tell the nurse, "She's such a fussy baby; she cries all the time. Our older child was so different; she was such an easy baby, laughing and smiling constantly." A child's temperament usually remains consistent as the child grows older.

THEORIES OF DEVELOPMENT

Many theorists have examined the process of child development. Among the most well known are Freud, Erikson, Piaget, and Kohlberg. These theorists identified stages of development common to all children as they mature. But because each child develops individually, he or she also demonstrates unique differences in achievement of developmental milestones.

FREUD'S THEORY OF PSYCHOSEXUAL DEVELOPMENT

According to Sigmund Freud, the personality consists of three aspects: the id, ego, and superego. The **id** represents one's desires. It is present at birth and seeks immediate gratification under the pleasure principle. The pleasure principle is the attempt to gratify needs immediately. The **ego** represents reason or common sense. The goal of the ego is to find a way to gratify the id. The **superego** represents one's conscience. It incorporates socially approved "shoulds" and "should nots" into the person's own value system.

Freud's theory of **psychosexual development** focuses on the shift of gratification from one body zone to another as the child matures. According to Freud, the developing child passes through five stages: *oral, anal, phallic, latent,* and *genital,* Figure 7–1.

ERIKSON'S THEORY OF PSYCHOSOCIAL DEVELOPMENT

Erik Erikson's theory of **psychosocial development** stresses societal and cultural influences on the ego at eight stages of the lifespan (Erikson 1963). Only the first five stages are related to childhood, Figure 7–2. Erikson identifies a conflict or problem — that is, a particular challenge — that must be resolved during critical periods of personality development in order for a healthy personality to develop.

PIAGET'S THEORY OF COGNITIVE DEVELOPMENT

Cognitive (or intellectual) **development** encompasses a wide variety of mental abilities, including learning, language, memory, reasoning, and thinking. Jean Piaget proposed that changes in children's thought processes result in a growing ability to acquire and use knowledge about their world (Piaget 1969). If the child is given nurturing experiences, his or her ability to think will unfold and mature naturally.

Piaget identified several stages and substages of cognitive development. The principal stages are the *sensorimotor stage*, from birth to 2 years; the *preoperational stage*, from 2 to 7 years; the *concrete operational thought stage*, from 7 to 11 years; and the *formal operational thought stage*, from 11 years through adulthood (Piaget 1969). Figure 7–3 summarizes the changes that occur during each stage.

KOHLBERG'S THEORY OF MORAL DEVELOPMENT

Lawrence Kohlberg's focus is on the aspect of cognitive development that deals with moral reasoning. He identifies three levels of **moral development**: preconventional, conventional, and postconventional (Kohlberg 1975). At the *preconventional level* (4–7 years), the young child's decisions are based on the desire to please others and avoid punishment. At the *conventional level* (7–11 years), conscience or an internal set of standards becomes increasingly important. At the *postconventional level* (12 years and older), the child uses internalized ethical standards in making decisions. The person

FREUD'S STAGES OF PSYCHOSEXUAL DEVELOPMENT		
Stage	**Age**	**Description**
Oral	Birth–1 year	Infant gains pleasure through the mouth, with sucking and eating the primary desires.
Anal	1–3 years	Pleasure is centered in the anal area, with control over excretion a primary force in behavior.
Phallic	3–6 years	Sexual energy becomes centered in the genitalia. During this stage the child shifts his or her identification from the parent of the same sex to the parent of the opposite sex.
Latent	6–12 years	Sexual energy is at rest. Children focus on skills and traits learned earlier. Energy is directed at learning and play.
Genital	12 years–adulthood	Focus is on mature sexual function and developing relationships with others.

Figure 7–1

who achieves this level is able to evaluate different moral approaches and make decisions on the basis of personal ethical standards.

Although Kohlberg provides age guidelines for the attainment of these levels, he emphasizes that they are approximate and that many individuals never reach the postconventional level of moral development.

DEVELOPMENTAL SCREENING

The **Denver II Developmental Screening Test** is given to children between 1 month and 6 years of age in order to assess normal development and identify potential developmental delays, Figure 7–4 (pages 96–97). The test assesses four areas: gross motor skills, fine motor skills, personal and social development, and language development.

Gross motor skills demonstrate the child's ability to control the large muscle groups of the body. Examples of gross motor skills are rolling over, crawling, and throwing a ball. **Fine motor skills** demonstrate the child's ability to coordinate the small muscle groups. Examples of fine motor skills are grasping an object, holding a crayon, and playing a musical instrument.

Development is difficult to assess because all children demonstrate individual variations in behavior and in their acquisition of skills.

ERIKSON'S STAGES OF PSYCHOSOCIAL DEVELOPMENT

Stage	Age	Description
Trust versus mistrust	Birth–1 year	The infant must develop trust in the people who provide care. Caregivers encourage this trust when they provide food, cleanliness, touch, warmth, comfort, and freedom from pain. From this basic sense of trust develops a sense of trust in the world, other people, and oneself, and feelings of faith and optimism. If these needs are not met, the infant will mistrust others.
Autonomy versus shame and doubt	1–3 years	The toddler demonstrates a sense of autonomy or independence through control over his or her body and environment and by saying "no" when asked to do something. From this sense of autonomy, the child develops self-control and willpower. Children who are consistently criticized for expressions of independence or for lack of control will develop a sense of shame about themselves and will doubt their abilities.
Initiative versus guilt	3–6 years	The child explores the world, tries out new activities, and considers new ideas. This period of exploration creates a child who is involved and busy, with a sense of purpose and direction. Conversely, consistent criticism during this period will lead to feelings of guilt and lack of purpose.
Industry versus inferiority	6–12 years	Characterized by involvement in many interests and activities. The older child takes pride in his or her accomplishments at school, home, and in the community and learns to compete and cooperate with others. The child who is free to exercise skill and intelligence in the completion of activities develops a sense of competence. A sense of inferiority can develop if the child cannot accomplish what is expected.
Identity versus role confusion	12–18 years	Characterized by examination and redefinition of the self or identity. The adolescent questions the self, family, peers, and the community. Successful completion of this stage results in devotion and fidelity, the ability to maintain allegiance to others and to values and ideologies that are accepted during this period. Conversely, the adolescent who is unable to establish a meaningful definition of self will experience role confusion later in life.

Figure 7–2

Stage	Age	Description
PIAGET'S STAGES OF COGNITIVE DEVELOPMENT		
Sensorimotor	Birth–2 years	The child learns about the world through input from the senses and by motor activity.
		During this period, the child begins to link cause with effect and to recognize object permanence (i.e., that an object continues to exist even when it cannot be seen).
		Language provides the child with a tool for understanding the world.
Preoperational	2–7 years	The child now thinks by using words as symbols, but logic is not well developed.
Concrete operational thought	7–11 years	The child develops a more accurate understanding of cause and effect, and reasons well if concrete objects are used.
Formal operational thought	11 years–adulthood	Mature intellectual thought is attained. The adolescent can reason abstractly and consider different alternatives or outcomes.

Figure 7–3

Overall Denver II test results are analyzed, and the child is classified as normal, suspect, or untestable. When results are not normal, retesting and referral should occur.

ANTICIPATORY GUIDANCE

Anticipatory guidance is an important form of teaching that provides parents with information to help them understand their children's behavior and improve their parenting skills. Anticipatory guidance about the range of normal behaviors characteristic of a particular developmental stage can increase parents' confidence in their parenting abilities by reinforcing that their expectations for their child are typical. Parents can benefit from information about the following topics:

- normal growth and development
- safety
- stimulation
- nutrition and feeding practices
- bathing
- immunizations
- sexual curiosity
- toilet training
- exercise
- vocational guidance (adolescents)
- common health problems

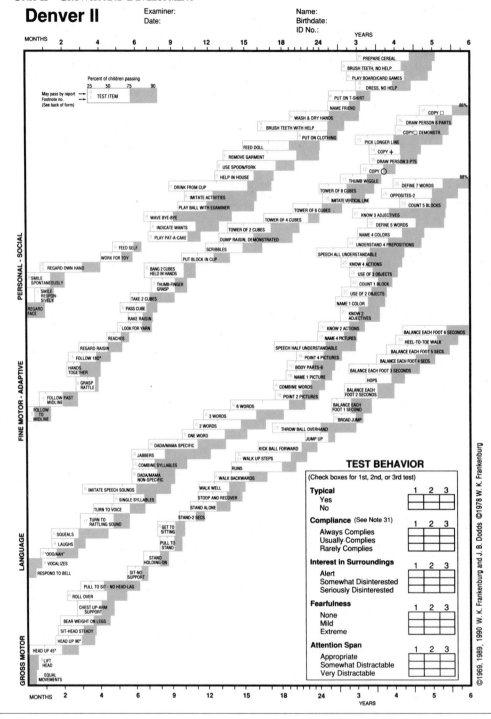

Figure 7-4 *Denver II — Revision and Restandardization of the Denver Developmental Screening Test. (From W. K. Frankenberg and J. B. Dodds, 1990)*

DIRECTIONS FOR ADMINISTRATION

1. Try to get child to smile by smiling, talking or waving. Do not touch him/her.
2. Child must stare at hand several seconds.
3. Parent may help guide toothbrush and put toothpaste on brush.
4. Child does not have to be able to tie shoes or button/zip in the back.
5. Move yarn slowly in an arc from one side to the other, about 8" above child's face.
6. Pass if child grasps rattle when it is touched to the backs or tips of fingers.
7. Pass if child tries to see where yarn went. Yarn should be dropped quickly from sight from tester's hand without arm movement.
8. Child must transfer cube from hand to hand without help of body, mouth, or table.
9. Pass if child picks up raisin with any part of thumb and finger.
10. Line can vary only 30 degrees or less from tester's line. /
11. Make a fist with thumb pointing upward and wiggle only the thumb. Pass if child imitates and does not move any fingers other than the thumb.

   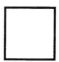

12. Pass any enclosed form. Fail continuous round motions.

13. Which line is longer? (Not bigger.) Turn paper upside down and repeat. (pass 3 of 3 or 5 of 6)

14. Pass any lines crossing near midpoint.

15. Have child copy first. If failed, demonstrate.

When giving items 12, 14, and 15, do not name the forms. Do not demonstrate 12 and 14.

16. When scoring, each pair (2 arms, 2 legs, etc.) counts as one part.
17. Place one cube in cup and shake gently near child's ear, but out of sight. Repeat for other ear.
18. Point to picture and have child name it. (No credit is given for sounds only.)
    If less than 4 pictures are named correctly, have child point to picture as each is named by tester.

 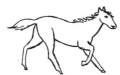   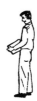

19. Using doll, tell child: Show me the nose, eyes, ears, mouth, hands, feet, tummy, hair. Pass 6 of 8.
20. Using pictures, ask child: Which one flies?... says meow?... talks?... barks?... gallops? Pass 2 of 5, 4 of 5.
21. Ask child: What do you do when you are cold?... tired?... hungry? Pass 2 of 3, 3 of 3.
22. Ask child: What do you do with a cup? What is a chair used for? What is a pencil used for? Action words must be included in answers.
23. Pass if child correctly places <u>and</u> says how many blocks are on paper. (1, 5).
24. Tell child: Put block **on** table; **under** table; **in front of** me, **behind** me. Pass 4 of 4. (Do not help child by pointing, moving head or eyes.)
25. Ask child: What is a ball?... lake?... desk?... house?... banana?... curtain?... fence?... ceiling? Pass if defined in terms of use, shape, what it is made of, or general category (such as banana is fruit, not just yellow). Pass 5 of 8, 7 of 8.
26. Ask child: If a horse is big, a mouse is __? If fire is hot, ice is __? If the sun shines during the day, the moon shines during the __? Pass 2 of 3.
27. Child may use wall or rail only, not person. May not crawl.
28. Child must throw ball overhand 3 feet to within arm's reach of tester.
29. Child must perform standing broad jump over width of test sheet (8 1/2 inches).
30. Tell child to walk forward, ⊂○⊂⊃⊂○⊃⊂○⊃► heel within 1 inch of toe. Tester may demonstrate. Child must walk 4 consecutive steps.
31. In the second year, half of normal children are non-compliant.

OBSERVATIONS:

Figure 7–4   *continued*

INFANT
(BIRTH THROUGH 1 YEAR)

GENERAL CHARACTERISTICS

Physical growth and development occur more rapidly during infancy than at any other period of life. During the first year, the infant triples his or her birth weight and by the year's end begins to walk and communicate with others.

MOTOR, LANGUAGE, AND SENSORY DEVELOPMENT

Over the course of the first year, the infant develops greater motor control, following a cephalocaudal and proximodistal pattern of development (see Chapter 5). The infant participates actively in learning through the senses and through motor activities, progressing from reflexive behaviors such as sucking and grasping to purposeful activities, such as the manipulation of objects.

Communication skills also progress rapidly during this period. Within the first few weeks of life, two-way interaction is occurring between the infant and parents or caregivers. The infant expresses comfort by cooing, cuddling, and eye contact. Discomfort is displayed by kicking the legs, arching the back, and vigorous crying. By the end of the first year, the infant has refined these communication skills and is able to speak several words.

Changes in motor, language, and sensory development during infancy are summarized in Figure 7–5.

TODDLER
(1 THROUGH 3 YEARS)

GENERAL CHARACTERISTICS

The term *toddler* aptly describes children from 1 to 3 years old, who toddle from side to side as they walk, holding out their arms for balance. The ability to walk increases the toddler's independence from parents. For this reason, the toddler period has been called the first adolescence. An infant only months before, the toddler now demonstrates increasing autonomy and negativism, responding with an emphatic "No!" to parents' instructions.

MOTOR, LANGUAGE, AND SENSORY DEVELOPMENT

During the toddler period, motor skills continue to develop. The eyes now work well together, and hearing is well developed. Sometime between the end of the second and third years, toddlers learn bowel and bladder control.

The rapid growth of language skills during this period emphasizes the importance of communication with toddlers. The 12- to 15-month-old child may use four to six words in addition to "mama" and "dada." By the end of this period, the 3-year-old has a vocabulary of more than 500 words and uses short sentences.

Changes in motor, language, and sensory development during toddlerhood are summarized in Figure 7–5.

PRESCHOOL CHILD
(3 THROUGH 6 YEARS)

GENERAL CHARACTERISTICS

The preschool years are characterized by increasing initiative and independence. Preschoolers have mastered many gross motor and some fine motor skills, and they can communicate both verbally and nonverbally. During the preschool period, these skills are refined, and children learn the social skills that will prepare them to function in the school environment.

Developmental Stage — Infancy

Age

Birth–
1 month

Gross Motor

- Assumes tonic neck posture

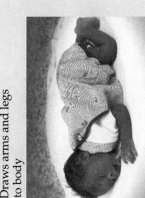

- When prone lifts and turns head

Fine Motor

- Holds hands in fist
- Draws arms and legs to body

Language

- Cries

Sensory

- Comforts with holding and touch
- Looks at faces
- Follows objects when in line of vision
- Alert to high-pitched voices
- Smiles

2–4
months

- Can raise head and shoulders when prone to 45°–90°; supports self on forearms
- Rolls from back to side

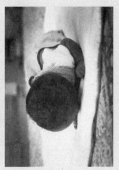

- Hands mostly open
- Looks at and plays with fingers
- Grasps and tries to reach objects

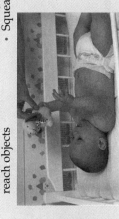

- Vocalizes when talked to; coos, babbles
- Laughs aloud
- Squeals

- Smiles
- Follows objects 180 degrees
- Turns head when hears voices or sounds

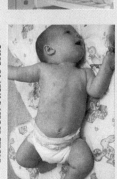
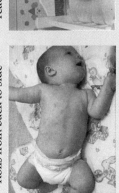

Figure 7–5   Stages of development; infancy through adolescence (Developed by Barbara Ellen Norvitz, BSN, RN, PNP)

Developmental Stage — Infancy

Age	Gross Motor	Fine Motor	Language	Sensory
4–6 months	• Turns from stomach to back and then back to stomach • When pulled to sitting almost no head lag • By 6 months can sit on floor with hands forward for support	• Can hold feet and put in mouth • Can hold bottle • Can grasp rattle and other small objects • Puts objects in mouth	• Squeals	• Watches a falling object • Responds to sounds

Figure 7–5   continued

DEVELOPMENTAL STAGE — INFANCY

Age	Gross Motor	Fine Motor	Language	Sensory
6–8 months	• Puts full weight on legs when held in standing position	• Transfers objects from one hand to the other • Can feed self a cookie • Can bang two objects together	• Babbles vowel like-sounds, ooh or aah • Imitation of speech sounds, (mama, dada) beginning • Laughs aloud	• Responds by looking and smiling • Recognizes own name

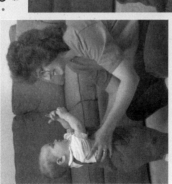

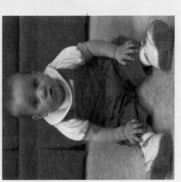

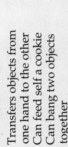

• Can sit without support
• Bounces when held in a standing position

Figure 7–5   continued

DEVELOPMENTAL STAGE — INFANCY

Age	Gross Motor	Fine Motor	Language	Sensory
8–10 months	• Crawls on all fours or uses arms to pull body along floor	• Beginning to use thumb-finger grasp • Dominant hand use • Has good hand-mouth coordination	• Responds to verbal commands • May say one word in addition to "mama" and "dada"	• Recognizes sounds
	• Can pull self to sitting • Can pull self to standing			

Figure 7-5   continued

DEVELOPMENTAL STAGE — INFANCY

Age	Gross Motor	Fine Motor	Language	Sensory
10–12 months	• Can sit down from standing • Walks around room holding onto objects • Can stand alone	• Picks up and drops objects • Can put small objects into toys or containers through holes	• Understands "no" and other simple commands • Learns 1–2 other words • Imitates speech sounds • Speaks gibberish	• Follows fast-moving objects • Indicates wants

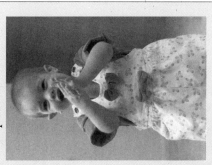
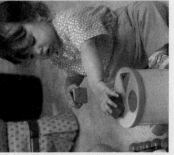
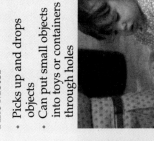
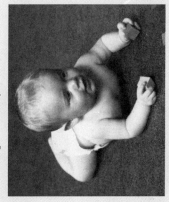

• Turns many pages in a book at one time
• Picks up small objects

• Likes to play imitative games such as patty cake and peek-a-boo

Figure 7–5   continued

DEVELOPMENTAL STAGE — TODDLERHOOD

Age	Gross Motor	Fine Motor	Language	Sensory
12–15 months	• Can walk alone well • Can crawl up stairs	• Can feed self with cup and spoon • Puts raisins into a bottle • May hold crayon or pencil and scribble • Builds a tower of two cubes	• Says four to six words	• Binocular vision developed

Figure 7–5   continued

DEVELOPMENTAL STAGE — TODDLERHOOD

Age	Gross Motor	Fine Motor	Language	Sensory
18 months	• Runs, falling often • Can jump in place • Can walk up stairs holding on	• Can build a tower of 3–4 cubes • Can use a spoon	• Says 10 or more words • Points to objects or body parts when asked	• Visual acuity 20/40

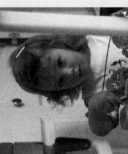

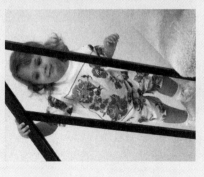

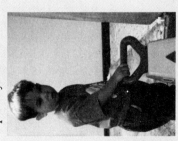

• Plays with push and pull toys

Figure 7–5   *continued*

DEVELOPMENTAL STAGE — TODDLERHOOD

Age	Gross Motor	Fine Motor	Language	Sensory
24 months	• Can walk up and down stairs • Can kick a ball • Can ride a tricycle	• Can draw a circle • Tries to dress self	• Talks a lot • Approximately 300-word vocabulary • Understands commands • Knows first name, refers to self • Verbalizes toilet needs	
30 months	• Throws a ball • Jumps with both feet • Can stand on one foot for a few minutes	• Can build a tower of 8 blocks • Can use crayons • Learning to use scissors	• Knows first and last name • Knows the name of 1 color • Can sing • Expresses needs • Uses pronouns appropriately	

Figure 7–5   *continued*

Developmental Stage — Preschool Age

Age	Gross Motor	Fine Motor	Language	Sensory
3–6 years	• Can ride a bike with training wheels • Can throw a ball overhand • Skips and hops on one foot • Can climb well • Can jump rope	• Can draw a six-part person • Can use a scissors • Can draw circle, square or cross • Likes art projects, likes to paste and string beads • Can button • Learns to tie and buckle shoes • Can brush teeth	• Language skills are well developed with the child able to understand and speak clearly • Vocabulary grows to over 2,000 words • Talks endlessly and asks questions	• Visual acuity well-developed • Focused on learning letters and numbers

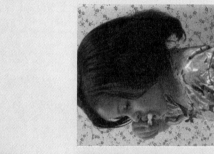
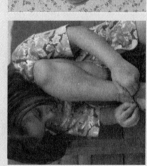
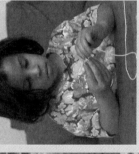
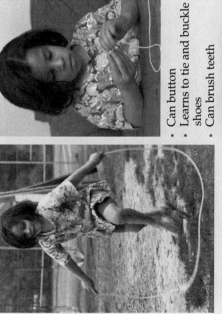

Figure 7–5   continued

Developmental Stage — School Age

Age	Gross Motor	Fine Motor	Language	Sensory
6–12 years	• Can use rollerblades or ice skates • Able to ride two-wheeler • Plays baseball	• Can put models together • Likes crafts • Enjoys board games, plays cards	• Vocabulary increases • Language abilities continue to develop	• Reading • Able to concentrate on activities for longer periods

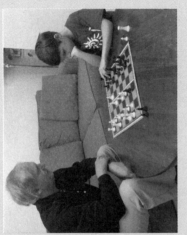
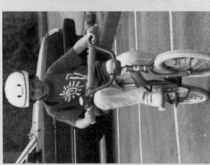
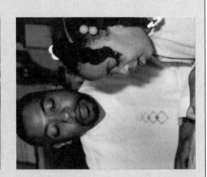

Figure 7-5   *continued*

DEVELOPMENTAL STAGE — ADOLESCENCE

Age	Gross Motor	Fine Motor	Language	Sensory
12–19 years	• Muscles continue to develop • At times awkward, with some lack of coordination	• Well-developed skills	• Vocabulary fully developed	• Development complete

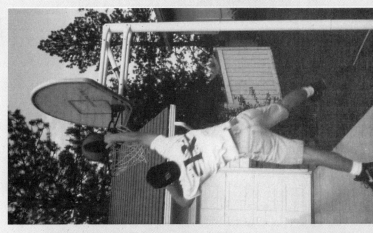

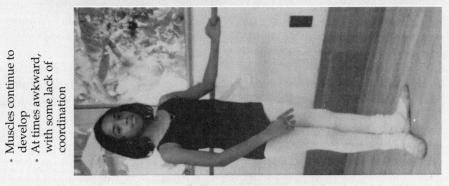

Figure 7–5 *continued*

MOTOR, LANGUAGE, AND SENSORY DEVELOPMENT

Most preschool children display more precisely controlled movements than they demonstrated as toddlers. The ability to participate successfully in games and other physical activities enhances preschoolers' self-esteem. Interaction with others during play, in turn, encourages the growth of social skills.

Language skills continue to expand during the preschool years. The preschooler has a vocabulary of more than 2,000 words and uses complete sentences of several words. Although many words are used, the preschooler's grasp of their meaning is usually quite literal. For example, children may interpret a statement such as "you're going to cough your head off" to mean that their head is going to fall off.

Figure 7–5 summarizes changes in motor, language, and sensory development during the preschool years.

SCHOOL-AGE CHILD (6 THROUGH 12 YEARS)

GENERAL CHARACTERISTICS

Interactions with peers, growth of intellectual skills, and continued refinement of fine motor and gross motor skills characterize children in the school-age period. Activities such as playing an instrument or helping with chores help the school-age child to develop a sense of self-worth.

MOTOR, LANGUAGE, AND SENSORY DEVELOPMENT

School-age children have the fine motor skills necessary to color, draw, write, and play a musical instrument or board game, and they have the physical and social skills needed for team sports and group activities. Vocabulary continues to increase, and the child's reading and writing skills expand rapidly. Children in this period also learn to apply rules for interacting with people outside their families.

Refer to Figure 7–5 for a summary of changes in motor, language, and sensory development during the school-age years.

ADOLESCENT (12 THROUGH 19 YEARS)

GENERAL CHARACTERISTICS

Adolescence is generally thought of as a time of transition into adulthood. Adolescents are trying to establish an identity of their own by experimenting with adult roles and behaviors.

MOTOR, LANGUAGE, AND SOCIAL DEVELOPMENT

Although some awkwardness and lack of coordination may accompany the adolescent growth spurt, increased dexterity, strength, and endurance are characteristic of the teenage years. Language skills are well developed. The adolescent increasingly demonstrates independence from parents, establishing close ties with peers. These relationships form the basis of an adult identity. Traditional values that were accepted during childhood are often questioned. But the adolescent must also develop the emotional maturity and motivation to make wise choices. Encouragement from family and significant others and practice in dealing with difficult decisions can help adolescents to become less impulsive and self-centered when solving problems.

Refer to Figure 7–5 for a summary of changes in motor, language, and sensory development during adolescence.

NURSING CARE RELATED TO DEVELOPMENTAL STAGES

- When caring for or teaching pediatric patients, always keep in mind the age and developmental stage of the child.
- Review with parents realistic expectations for their child's stage of development, and caution them not to expect skills that are beyond the developmental level of their child.
- Provide infants with touch, comfort, and security.
- Anticipate the infant's need to suck by providing a pacifier.
- Anticipate the preschool child's concerns about sexuality by providing privacy and clear explanations about any procedures involving the genital area.
- When speaking to preschoolers, remember that they interpret your words literally.
- Allow children to manipulate medical equipment safely in order to see for themselves how it works.
- Anticipate the adolescent's focus on relationships by asking about friends and family.
- Provide adolescents with information and allow them, when possible, to choose among alternative treatments.

REVIEW QUESTIONS

A. Multiple choice. Select the best answer.

1. The theory of cognitive (intellectual) development was proposed by
   a. Freud
   b. Piaget
   c. Erikson
   d. Kohlberg

2. The final stage of development in Freud's theory is
   a. oral
   b. anal
   c. phallic
   d. genital

3. According to Erikson, a child between the ages of 3 and 6 years is in the stage of
   a. trust versus mistrust
   b. autonomy versus shame and doubt
   c. initiative versus guilt
   d. identity versus industry

4. The final stage of cognitive development according to Piaget is
   a. formal operational thought
   b. sensorimotor
   c. concrete operational thought
   d. preoperational

5. The highest level of moral development according to Kohlberg is the
   a. conventional
   b. preconventional
   c. postconventional
   d. nonconventional

6. Which of the following statements is true according to Kohlberg's theory?
    a. The young child's moral decisions are based on the desire to please others or to avoid being punished.
    b. The young child earns approval by following rules.
    c. The school-age child begins to internalize ethical standards for forming his or her own decisions and weighing the value of differing moral approaches.
    d. Most people reach the postconventional level before age 20.

7. Erikson's theory holds that
    a. trust develops first in children between 3 and 6 years of age
    b. the toddler must learn to obey others
    c. the adolescent is mainly concerned with building a sense of competence
    d. a particular social or psychological challenge has to be met at each stage for a healthy personality to develop

8. Freud's stages focus on
    a. shifts in gratification from one body area to another as development unfolds
    b. how a child learns right from wrong
    c. how children think as they develop
    d. developmental tasks

9. The Denver II Developmental Screening Test assesses
    a. cognitive development
    b. intelligence quotient
    c. personal and social development
    d. sexual development

10. The infant stage of development is typically characterized by
    a. the infant's active participation in sensory and motor learning
    b. one-way interaction until the second week of life
    c. lack of purposeful activities
    d. a vocabulary of more than 100 words

11. During the toddler stage, you can observe
    a. the ability to coordinate games with other toddlers
    b. well-developed fine motor skills
    c. a precisely controlled gait
    d. the use of short sentences

12. The preschool child
    a. has mastered all fine motor skills
    b. cannot yet participate in games with other children
    c. uses complete sentences of several words
    d. has mastered few gross motor skills

13. When working with preschoolers, you ought to
    a. joke about their literal interpretation of words
    b. acknowledge concerns about sexuality by maintaining privacy and giving clear explanations about procedures involving the genital area
    c. avoid explaining procedures in order to lessen anxiety
    d. discourage parents from participating in care in order to promote independence

14. When dealing with adolescents, you will want to
    a. avoid focusing on the importance of relationships in their lives
    b. prevent them from making choices about their own care
    c. help them become less impulsive when solving problems
    d. encourage self-centeredness

SUGGESTED ACTIVITIES

- Interview a parent about his or her child's behavior patterns. Find two examples of each of the four theories discussed in this chapter.

- Try to write a history of your own development to see how many examples of developmental changes you can recall.

- Identify three personality patterns in yourself or someone you are close to.

- Visit a day-care center or early childhood learning center and observe children's skills and activities at various ages.

- Prepare an anticipatory guidance poster for teaching parents. You choose the age group and topic to be presented.

- List the five stages of development and three characteristics unique to each one.

- Compare several children of the same age in one of the following areas:
  - fine motor ability
  - gross motor ability
  - sensory ability
  - language skills

BIBLIOGRAPHY

Erikson, E. H. *Childhood and Society*, 2nd ed. New York: W. W. Norton, 1963.

Kohlberg, L. The cognitive-developmental approach to moral education. *Phi Delta Kappa* 56, (1975): 670–677.

Papalia, D. E., and S. W. Olds. *A Child's World: Infancy through Adolescence*, 6th ed. New York: McGraw-Hill, 1993.

Phares, E. J. *Introduction to Personality*, 3rd ed. Glenview, IL: Scott, Foresman, 1991.

Piaget, J. *The Theory of Stages in Cognitive Development*. New York: McGraw-Hill, 1969.

Thomas, A. and S. Chess. *Temperament and Development*. New York: Brunner/Mazel, 1977.

Thompson, J. M., and A. C. Bowers. *Health Assessment: An Illustrated Pocket Guide*, 3rd ed. St. Louis, MO: Mosby-Year Book, 1992.

Wong, D. L. *Whaley & Wong's Essentials of Pediatric Nursing*, 4th ed. St. Louis, MO: Mosby-Year Book, 1993.

Pediatric Health Promotion

CHAPTER

8

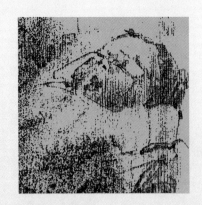

$\mathcal{B}$asic Nutrition

OBJECTIVES

AFTER STUDYING THIS CHAPTER, THE STUDENT SHOULD BE ABLE TO:

- LIST ESSENTIAL NUTRIENTS OF A WELL-BALANCED DIET AND DESCRIBE THEIR FUNCTIONS.

- IDENTIFY SEVERAL SOURCES OF EACH ESSENTIAL NUTRIENT.

- IDENTIFY AGE-RELATED NUTRITIONAL NEEDS OF CHILDREN.

- EXPLAIN CHARACTERISTIC EATING PATTERNS OF CHILDREN OF DIFFERENT DEVELOPMENTAL STAGES.

- PROVIDE NUTRITIONAL TEACHING TO ASSIST PARENTS IN PLANNING A HEALTHY DIET FOR CHILDREN FROM INFANCY THROUGH ADOLESCENCE.

KEY TERMS

NUTRIENTS

MALNUTRITION

LACTOSE

NONESSENTIAL AMINO ACIDS

ESSENTIAL AMINO ACIDS

LIPIDS

TRIGLYCERIDES

FATTY ACIDS

FOOD PYRAMID

RECOMMENDED DIETARY ALLOWANCES

RITUALISTIC BEHAVIOR

*N*utrition is essential to the health and well-being of children. Adequate nutrition is especially important during periods of rapid growth and development, such as infancy and early childhood (Marotz et al. 1993). Life-long eating habits are formed in early childhood, and a healthy diet can lay the foundation for healthy eating habits in adulthood.

THE ROLE OF THE NURSE

Nurses are frequently involved in counseling children and families about diet and the importance of good nutrition. Nutritional counseling can be challenging as well as rewarding. It is important to emphasize positive eating habits that already exist in the child's diet. To be effective in counseling families and children, the nurse needs to be able to:

1. Recognize outward signs of good and poor nutrition.
2. Assess a family's nutritional intake.
3. Modify existing dietary habits to meet the goals of a prescribed treatment plan.
4. Plan meals that incorporate the child's food preferences, where possible.

Culture and religion influence the selection of food. Because there are many different cultural and religious groups in the United States, nurses must also have a knowledge of cultural food habits and preferences that affect diet, Figure 8–1.

ESSENTIAL NUTRIENTS AND THEIR FUNCTIONS

Five major **nutrients** are essential for proper body function: carbohydrates, protein, fats,

minerals, and vitamins. Water, which is essential to life, is sometimes included in the category of essential nutrients. A daily intake of essential nutrients depends on eating a variety of foods in adequate amounts. Inadequate intake of essential nutrients results in **malnutrition**, Figure 8–2 (page 120).

CARBOHYDRATES

The primary function of carbohydrates is to meet the body's need for energy. Carbohydrates are the most readily available and easily converted source of energy for body metabolism. There are two categories of carbohydrates: simple and complex.

Simple carbohydrates include monosaccharides, such as glucose, fructose, and galactose, and disaccharides, such as sucrose (table sugar) and **lactose** (found in milk). Complex carbohydrates include starch and dietary fiber. The dietary fiber in carbohydrates passes through the intestinal tract unchanged because the body lacks the enzymes to digest it. There are many sources of carbohydrates, including grains and grain products, fruits, root vegetables, sugars, and syrups.

The nurse needs to use a sensible approach when teaching parents guidelines for a child's intake of sugar. Many "scare tactics" have been used to discourage sugar ingestion, leading some parents to give honey to infants and sugar substitutes to children. Parents should be warned that honey has been linked to cases of botulism in infants and that the long-term effects of many sugar substitutes are yet to be determined. A moderate approach to the intake of sugars in childhood is therefore advised.

A carbohydrate deficiency is manifested by weight loss, because protein and fat sources are being used for energy. Prolonged carbohydrate deficiency can lead to liver damage.

ETHNIC AND REGIONAL FOOD PATTERNS

Ethnic Group	Bread and Cereal	Eggs, Meat, Fish, Poultry	Dairy Products	Fruits and Vegetables	Seasonings and Fats
Italian	Northern Italy Crusty white bread, cornmeal, and rice Southern Italy Pasta	Beef, chicken, eggs, fish	Milk in coffee, cheese	Broccoli, zucchini, other squash, eggplant, artichokes, string beans, tomatoes, peppers, asparagus, fresh fruit	Olive oil, vinegar, salt, pepper, garlic
Puerto Rican	Rice, noodles, spaghetti, oatmeal, cornmeal	Dry salted codfish, meat, salt pork, sausage, chicken, beef	Coffee with hot milk	Starchy root vegetables, green bananas, plantain, legumes, tomatoes, green pepper, onion, pineapple, papaya, citrus fruits	Lard, herbs, oil, vinegar
Near Eastern	Bulgur (wheat)	Lamb, mutton, chicken, fish, eggs	Fermented milk, sour cream, yogurt, cheese	Nuts, grape leaves	Sheep's butter, olive oil
Greek	Plain wheat bread	Lamb, pork, poultry, eggs, organ meats	Yogurt, cheese, butter	Onions, fresh fruit, tomatoes, legumes	Olive oil, parsley, lemon, vinegar

Figure 8–1   (Compiled from Mahan, L. K. and M. Arlin. Krause's Food, Nutrition, and Diet Therapy, 8th ed. Philadelphia: W. B. Saunders, 1992).

ETHNIC AND REGIONAL FOOD PATTERNS

Ethnic Group	Bread and Cereal	Eggs, Meat, Fish, Poultry	Dairy Products	Fruits and Vegetables	Seasonings and Fats
Mexican	Lime-treated corn	Little meat (ground beef or pork), poultry, fish	Cheese, evaporated milk as beverage for infants	Pinto beans, tomatoes, potatoes, onions, lettuce	Chili pepper, salt, garlic
Chinese	Rice, wheat, millet, corn, noodles	Little meat and no beef, fish (including raw fish), eggs of hen, duck, and pigeon	Water buffalo milk occasionally, soybean milk, cheese	Soybeans, soybean sprouts, bamboo sprouts, soy curd cooked in lime water, radish leaves, legumes, vegetables, fruits	Sesame seeds, ginger, almonds, soy sauce
American Black	Hot breads, cookies, pastries, cakes, cereals, white rice	Chicken, salt, pork, ham, bacon, sausage	Milk and milk products	Kale, mustard, turnip greens, cabbage, hominy grits, sweet potatoes	Molasses
Jewish	Noodles, crusty white seed rolls, rye bread, pumpernickel bread	Kosher meat (from fore-quarters and organs from beef, lamb, veal), milk not eaten at same meal, fish	Milk and milk products	Vegetables — usually cooked with meat (kosher), fruits	

Figure 8–1   continued

SIGNS OF HEALTH AND MALNUTRITION

	Normal/Healthy	Malnourished
Hair	Shiny and firm in scalp	Dull, brittle, dry and loose
Eyes	Clear pink membranes; adjust easily to darkness	Pale membranes, spots, redness; adjust slowly to darkness
Skin	Smooth, hydrated skin	Pale, sallow, ashen, scaly, and cracked skin
Tongue	Red, bumpy, rough	Smooth, sore, purplish, swollen
Nails	Smooth and pink	Spoon-shaped, brittle, ridged
Behavior	Alert and attentive	Irritable and inattentive, apathetic or hyperactive

Figure 8–2 (*Adapted from E. Whitney and S. Rolfes.* Understanding Nutrition. *Minneapolis/St. Paul: West Publishing, 1993*).

Excess ingestion of simple carbohydrates can result in obesity and dental caries.

It is now recommended that approximately 55% to 60% of daily caloric intake be in the form of carbohydrates, with no more than 10% of these in the form of simple sugars (Marotz et al. 1993).

PROTEIN

The primary function of protein is to promote cellular and tissue growth and repair. Protein is used as an energy source only when other sources (carbohydrates and fats) are lacking. Proteins are made up of hundreds of individual units called amino acids. **Nonessential amino acids** can be manufactured by the body and, therefore, do not need to be obtained from the diet. **Essential amino acids** cannot be manufactured and must be provided in food.

Proteins are classified as complete or incomplete depending on whether they supply all of the essential amino acids needed by the body in adequate amounts. Complete proteins are generally found in animal sources such as meat, fish, poultry, and dairy products, which also tend to be high in fat and cholesterol. Plant sources, such as nuts, seeds, vegetables, and legumes, individually supply incomplete proteins. These sources, however, can be combined to provide the equivalent of a complete protein.

The child who lacks protein appears weak and apathetic, with edema and muscle wasting. The child's skin may appear patchy and scaly, and the hair dull and colorless.

FATS

Fats are stored in the body and serve an important role in the diet as a reserve of energy. Too much fat, however, can be harmful. Fats, oils, and fatlike substances called sterols are classified as **lipids**. Chemically, fats are made up of **triglycerides**, which consist of three fatty acids combined with glycerol.

Fatty acids are classified as saturated or unsaturated. All animal products — including milk, butter, egg yolks, and red meat — contain some amounts of saturated fat. Polyunsaturated or monounsaturated fat is found in vegetable fats and oils (with the exception of coconut oil and palm oil). Saturated fats have been linked with high levels of cholesterol and low-density lipoproteins (LDLs) and with an incidence of hypertension in children.

When excess kilocalories are ingested, they are turned into fat and stored for later use. Fat functions to maintain body temperature, cushion vital organs, and facilitate the absorption of the fat-soluble vitamins (A, D, E, and K). It is also the source of the one essential fatty acid, linoleic acid. Excess ingestion of fat, however, can lead to obesity and atherosclerosis.

No more than 30% of daily calories should come from fat.

Minerals

Minerals help to regulate body functions and build body tissue. Calcium, phosphorus, potassium, and sodium are four minerals that are essential to proper body functioning. Milk products, meats, whole grains, legumes, and green leafy vegetables are good sources of many minerals. A well-balanced diet supplies necessary quantities of these and other minerals, such as iron, iodine, magnesium, and zinc.

Children need calcium and phosphorus for normal bone and tooth development. Fluoride is an important mineral that makes teeth harder and more resistant to decay. Fluoride supplementation of drinking water and the use of fluoride-containing toothpastes is therefore recommended during childhood to help prevent dental caries (Marotz et al. 1993). Iron supplements are usually recommended for infants after the age of 6 months to prevent deficiency (see later discussion). Other mineral supplements are usually unnecessary for children who consume a variety of foods.

Vitamins

Vitamins are essential for the regulation of normal body functions. For example, vitamins regulate energy metabolism, cellular reproduction and growth, bone growth, neuromuscular activities, and blood formation (Marotz et al. 1993). Vitamins are classified as either fat-soluble or water-soluble.

The fat-soluble vitamins are A, D, E, and K. These vitamins are stored in the body, mainly in the liver. Vitamin A helps the eyes to accommodate to dim light and also maintains the skin and mucous membranes. Vitamin D aids in the formation of bones and teeth. Food sources high in vitamins A and D include yellow fruits and vegetables and green leafy vegetables. Other sources include fish liver oil, animal liver, and sunlight.

Water-soluble vitamins are the B-complex vitamins and vitamin C. Once the body has absorbed a maximum concentration of these vitamins, the excess is excreted in the urine. Because water-soluble vitamins are not stored in the body, children need a daily intake of these vitamins to maintain health.

The B-complex vitamins include thiamin, riboflavin, niacin, B_{12}, folacin, pantothenic acid, and biotin. These vitamins aid in energy metabolism. Wheat germ, whole grains, legumes, organ meats, and eggs are good sources of B-complex vitamins. Deficiencies of these vitamins can result in symptoms of anorexia, muscle weakness, anemia, diarrhea, nausea, irritability, or depression.

Vitamin C, also known as ascorbic acid, has a significant role in the formation of collagen. It also functions in the metabolism of amino acids, the absorption of iron, and the synthesis of collagen. Vitamin C is found in citrus fruits (such as oranges, strawberries, and grapefruit) and dark green leafy vegetables. A deficiency of vitamin C can result in easy bruising, scurvy, sore mouth and gums, and joint tenderness due to disruption of cartilage.

GUIDELINES FOR NUTRITIONAL INTAKE DURING CHILDHOOD

Growth rate, body size, and physical activity influence a child's nutritional requirements. Several guidelines are available to help in planning nutritionally sound diets for children from infancy through adolescence.

Most nutritional recommendations until 1992 were based on the four basic food groups (milk and milk products, meat and meat alternatives, fruits and vegetables, and bread and cereal). In 1992, however, the U.S. Department of Agriculture (USDA) published a new guide for daily food planning, the **food pyramid**, Figure 8–3. This revised planning guide encourages limited intake of fats, increased intake of fiber (fruits, vegetables), and increased intake of carbohydrates (grains and grain products).

The U.S. **Recommended Dietary Allowances**

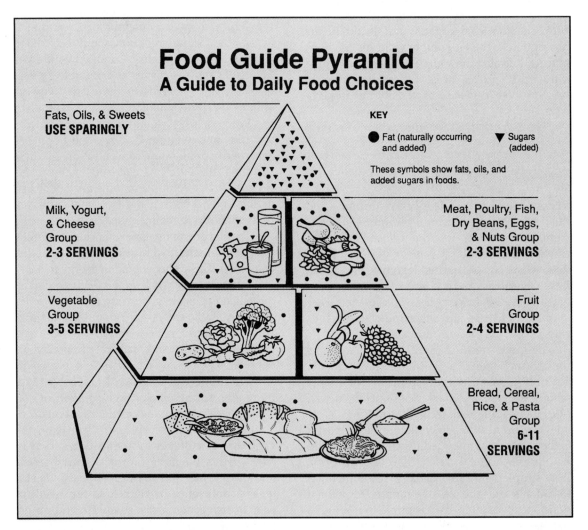

Figure 8–3   *(Courtesy of the U.S. Department of Agriculture)*

(RDAs), developed and updated periodically by the Food and Nutrition Board of the National Academy of Sciences, is a guide to intake of essential nutrients from infancy through adulthood, Figure 8–4. The committee on Nutrition of the American Academy of Pediatrics has also published several guidelines related to infant feeding, composition of formulas, and recommended dietary intake for children.

INFANT

During the first year of life, breast milk or infant formula is the infant's major source of food. Breast milk has certain advantages over formula. Breast milk contains easily digested protein and carbohydrate (in the form of lactose), fat (including linoleic acid), and minerals and vitamins. It is less likely to cause food allergies and also contains maternal antibodies, which help protect the infant from infection in the first months of life. Cow's milk or soy-based formulas closely parallel the nutritional content of breast milk. Cow's milk alone, however, is insufficient as a source of food for infants (American Academy of Pediatrics 1983). It lacks sufficient quantities of vitamin C and iron, contains excess sodium and less-digestible forms of protein, is higher in fat, and contains less sugar than breast milk.

The addition of solid foods in pureed form to the infant's diet is not recommended for the first 4 to 6 months of life (American Academy of Pediatrics 1984). Although the infant's stomach and intestines are able to digest the components of breast milk and formula, they cannot digest the starches found in many other foods. By the time an infant is 4 to 6 months of age, he or she is producing enzymes capable of digesting complex carbohydrates and proteins.

Neonatal iron stores are exhausted between 4 and 6 months of age, and this deficit becomes a significant factor when considering the infant's diet. Iron recommendations for infants are 10 mg per day by 6 months of age. An iron supplement or iron-fortified cereal is usually recommended after the age of 6 months to decrease the risk of iron deficiency and associated developmental delays.

New foods should be introduced one at a time at intervals of about one week in order to observe for symptoms of allergy or sensitivity. Iron-fortified rice cereal is usually the first solid food introduced, followed by pureed fruits, vegetables, and meats. Rice cereal, pears, yellow vegetables, and lamb usually are introduced first because they are the least likely to cause reactions. Another factor influencing introduction of foods is the need to select foods high in vitamin C to enhance iron absorption.

By 12 months of age, the normal infant has tripled his or her birth weight and is nearing a three-meal-per-day pattern. Explain to parents that experimentation with foods and feeding is a normal part of the infant's growth and development. Allow the older infant to begin self-feeding at 7 to 8 months of age.

Nursing Considerations. Teach parents the following points about the infant's diet and nutritional intake:

- Breast milk or formula provides a complete diet for the infant during the first 6 months of life.
- Self-feeding should be encouraged when the infant reaches about 7 months of age.
- Solids in pureed form may be added one at a time to the infant's diet after the age of 4 months.
- When new foods are introduced, observe for signs of food allergy or sensitivity (vomiting, diarrhea, abdominal pain, hives, and eczema).
- Because iron stores normally will be low after 6 months, iron-fortified food or iron supplementation may be required.
- Never prop bottles or allow the infant to take a bottle to bed. Juice, sweetened water, and formula can pool in the infant's mouth, causing tooth decay (nursing bottle-mouth syndrome). A propped bottle may cause choking and aspiration.

TODDLER

After the age of 1 year, the rapid growth and development of infancy begins to slow and the toddler's body begins to change proportions (see Chapter 7). The toddler's nutritional needs are directly related to these physical changes.

During this period, the child's appetite and the need for calories decrease. Adequate protein intake is necessary, however, to main-

RECOMMENDED DIETARY ALLOWANCES

Recommended dietary allowances[a] designed for the maintenance of good nutrition of practically all healthy people in the United States

Category	Age (years) or condition	Weight[b] (kg)	Weight[b] (lb)	Height[b] (cm)	Height[b] (in)	Protein (g)	Fat-soluble vitamins			
							Vitamin A (µg RE)[c]	Vitamin D (µg)[d]	Vitamin E (mg/α-TE)[e]	Vitamin K (µg)
Infants	0.0–0.5	6	13	60	24	13	375	7.5	3	5
	0.5–1.0	9	20	71	28	14	375	10	4	10
Children	1–3	13	29	90	35	16	400	10	6	15
	4–6	20	44	112	44	24	500	10	7	20
	7–10	28	62	132	52	28	700	10	7	30
Males	11–14	45	99	157	62	45	1000	10	10	45
	15–18	66	145	176	69	59	1000	10	10	65
	19–24	72	160	177	70	58	1000	10	10	70
	25–50	79	174	176	70	63	1000	5	10	80
	51+	77	170	173	68	63	1000	5	10	80
Females	11–14	46	101	157	62	46	800	10	8	45
	15–18	55	120	163	64	44	800	10	8	55
	19–24	58	128	164	65	46	800	10	8	60
	25–50	63	138	163	64	50	800	5	8	65
	51+	65	143	160	63	50	800	5	8	65
Pregnant						60	800	10	10	65
Lactating	1st 6 months					65	1300	10	12	65
	2nd 6 months					62	1200	10	11	65

From Food and Nutrition Board, National Research Council: *Recommended dietary allowances*, ed 10, Washington, DC, 1989. National Academy of Sciences.

[a]The allowances, expressed as average daily intakes over time, are intended to provide for individual variations among most normal persons as they live in the United States under usual environmental stresses. Diets should be based on a variety of common foods in order to provide other nutrients for which human requirements have been less well defined.

[b]Weights and heights of reference adults are actual medians for the U.S. population of the designated age, as reported by National Health and Nutrition Examination Survey (NHANES) II. The median weights and heights of those under 19 years of age were taken from Hamill PV and others: Physical growth: National Center for Health Statistics percentiles. *Am J Clin Nutr* 32:607–629, 1979. The use of these figures does not imply that the height-to-weight ratios are ideal.

Figure 8–4   *(Reprinted with permission from* Recommended Dietary Allowances, *10th ed. Copyright 1989 by The National Academy of Sciences. Courtesy of the National Academy Press, Washington, D.C.)*

tain optimal growth. Milk is an excellent source of protein for children, and from 16 to 24 ounces of milk per day is recommended. No more than 24 ounces is desirable, however, as milk contains little iron and excess intake can result in inadequate intake of other foods containing this mineral. Toddlers from 1 to 3 years of age remain at high risk for iron-deficiency anemia because of the rapid growth and depletion of iron stores during infancy

Water-soluble vitamins							Minerals						
Vita-min C (mg)	Thiamin (mg)	Ribo-flavin (mg)	Niacin (mg NE)[f]	Vita-min B$_6$ (mg)	Folate (µg)	Vita-min B$_{12}$ (µg)	Calcium (mg)	Phos-phorus (mg)	Mag-nesium (mg)	Iron (mg)	Zinc (mg)	Iodine (µg)	Sele-nium (µg)
30	0.3	0.4	5	0.3	25	0.3	400	300	40	6	5	40	10
35	0.4	0.5	6	0.6	35	0.5	600	500	60	10	5	50	15
40	0.7	0.8	9	1.0	50	0.7	800	800	80	10	10	70	20
45	0.9	1.1	12	1.1	75	1.0	800	800	120	10	10	90	20
45	1.0	1.2	13	1.4	100	1.4	800	800	170	10	10	120	30
50	1.3	1.5	17	1.7	150	2.0	1200	1200	270	12	15	150	40
60	1.5	1.8	20	2.0	200	2.0	1200	1200	400	12	15	150	50
60	1.5	1.7	19	2.0	200	2.0	1200	1200	350	10	15	150	70
60	1.5	1.7	19	2.0	200	2.0	800	800	350	10	15	150	70
60	1.2	1.4	15	2.0	200	2.0	800	800	350	10	15	150	70
50	1.1	1.3	15	1.4	150	2.0	1200	1200	280	15	12	150	45
60	1.1	1.3	15	1.5	180	2.0	1200	1200	300	15	12	150	50
60	1.1	1.3	15	1.6	180	2.0	1200	1200	280	15	12	150	55
60	1.1	1.3	15	1.6	180	2.0	800	800	280	15	12	150	55
60	1.0	1.2	13	1.6	180	2.0	800	800	280	10	12	150	55
70	1.5	1.6	17	2.2	400	2.2	1200	1200	320	30	15	175	65
95	1.6	1.8	20	2.1	280	2.6	1200	1200	355	15	19	200	75
90	1.6	1.7	20	2.1	260	2.6	1200	1200	340	15	16	200	75

[c]Retinol equivalent. 1 retinol equivalent = 1 mg retinol or 6 mg b-carotene.

[d]As cholecalciferol. 10 µg cholecalciferol = 400 IU vitamin D.

[e]α-Tocopherol equivalents. 1 mg d-α-tocopherol = 1 α-TE.

[f]1 NE (niacin equivalent) is equal to 1 mg of niacin or 60 mg of dietary tryptophan.

Figure 8–4 continued

(Mahan 1992). Thus, intake of foods rich in iron is advised.

Toddlers have fluctuating appetites with strong food likes and dislikes. Serving size is important. Toddlers tend to like colorful dishes with foods cut into bite-size pieces. **Ritualistic behavior** at mealtime is common. For example, toddlers like to use a special plate, fork, or spoon; they may want to eat one food first at each meal or follow a sequence in eating.

Nursing Considerations. Teach parents the following points about the toddler's diet, nutritional needs, and eating patterns:

. Limit milk to no more than 24 ounces per day.
. Toddlers can feed themselves and want to do so, Figure 8–5.
. Toddlers demonstrate definite food likes and dislikes. Be flexible but consistent in presenting food. Serve small portions.
. Toddlers are easily distracted during meals. Avoid interruptions.
• Insufficient iron intake during infancy can leave toddlers vulnerable to iron-deficiency anemia.

PRESCHOOL CHILD

Nutritional requirements for preschool children are similar to those for toddlers. Caloric requirements continue to decrease slightly between 3 and 6 years of age. Fluid requirements also decrease slightly, and protein requirements remain much the same. Preschool children, like toddlers, have definite food likes and dislikes and occasionally display ritualistic behavior By 5 years of age, however, most preschoolers become more agreeable to trying new foods, especially if they are allowed to help in food preparation.

The quantity of food a preschooler eats is not as important as the quality. The American Academy of Pediatrics' Committee on Nutrition

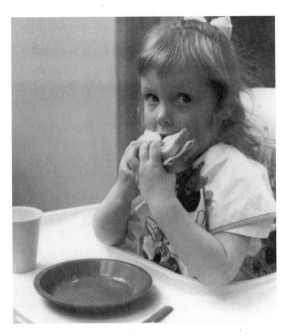

Figure 8–5 *A toddler enjoys self-feeding and demonstrates definite food likes and dislikes.*

(1984) recommends a moderate intake of fat (30% to 40% of total energy-source intake), but cautions against extremes in dietary restrictions.

During the preschool period children should be screened for nutritional deficiencies. A healthy diet during this period can lay the foundation for healthy eating patterns as an adult.

Nursing Considerations. Teach parents the following points about the preschool child's diet, nutritional needs, and eating patterns:

. The preschool child has definite food preferences.
. Preschool children are vulnerable to communicable diseases. Illness and fever increase metabolic rate, and therefore caloric needs.
. As ritualistic behavior diminishes, the preschooler becomes more flexible in eating habits.

SCHOOL-AGE CHILD

Because the young school-age child (age 6 to 7 years) chooses which foods to eat when at school or away from parental supervision, deficiencies in iron, vitamin A, and riboflavin are common during this period. Uneven growth patterns and lack of interest in eating contribute to the extreme fluctuations in the appetite of school-age children. In addition, peer pressure related to eating habits begins to appear.

Unless the diet of an 8- or 9-year-old child is well planned, it may be deficient in calcium, iron, and thiamin. Meats, legumes, and milk in sufficient quantities are needed to assure adequate amounts of these minerals and vitamins.

In the late school-age period (8 to 10 years) and in preadolescence (11 to 12 years), caloric requirements increase and nutritious snacks are required to meet dietary requirements. As the child reaches 11 to 12 years of age, protein requirements diminish. Growth of new bone and muscle slows; however, energy needs to maintain the child's additional tissue mass are high.

The manner in which food is offered to the school-age child is important. Encourage nutritious meals by presenting food in an appealing manner. Children can be encouraged to choose nutritious foods by labeling them "food to make us grow." Similarly, holiday foods such as dried fruit in Christmas stockings, peanuts in Easter baskets, and fresh fruit at Halloween promote good nutrition. One mother's approach exemplifies this philosophy: "When they were good I gave them a vegetable as a reward. Now they ask for vegetables and other nutritious snacks."

Nursing Considerations. Teach parents the following points about the school-age child's diet, nutritional needs, and eating patterns:

• During the school-age years, children's food choices begin to be influenced by peers, fads, and "junk food" advertising.

• School-age children are vulnerable to deficiencies in iron, calcium, and B-complex vitamins.
• The child's activities may interfere with mealtime routines and good eating habits.

ADOLESCENT

Caloric needs during adolescence are high because of the accelerated growth and development characteristic of this developmental stage. Individual variation is the single most significant feature of adolescent growth. Girls usually begin pubertal growth at about 10 years and complete their growth spurt by 16 years of age. Boys tend to start their pubertal growth two years later than girls (refer to Chapter 6).

Stress, fatigue, and peer pressure influence the adolescent's appetite and dietary intake. Most adolescent boys have a fairly adequate dietary intake because they eat massive quantities of food. This diet, however, is often high in fat. The diet of adolescent girls is often lacking in essential nutrients. Low-calorie diets and poor food choices contribute to nutrient deficiencies, particularly of calcium, protein, B vitamins, and iron. Eating disorders such as anorexia nervosa and bulimia nervosa often manifest during adolescence (refer to Chapter 30).

Although the adolescent's diet should be similar to the ideal diet recommended for adults, teenagers frequently model their eating patterns after adults who have poor diets. The nurse needs to understand the factors influencing adolescents' dietary intake when helping them plan meals. Creative approaches can help to promote a healthy diet. Teenagers who eat fast foods can be encouraged to eat pizza instead of high-salt, high-fat hamburgers and french fries from fast-food outlets, Figure 8–6.

Teenagers are concerned about their body image and a diet that enables them to maintain a healthy, physically fit body will be followed more readily than one that does not. Adolescents are also more likely to comply with a planned diet if they are involved in the decision-making process regarding food choices.

Nursing Considerations. Teach parents the following points regarding adolescent diet, nutritional needs, and eating patterns:

- The adolescent has an increased appetite and an increased need for calories.
- Requirements for calcium, iron, and protein are increased during adolescence.
- Diet during this period is greatly influenced by peer groups.
- Adolescents are vulnerable to eating disorders and food fads.

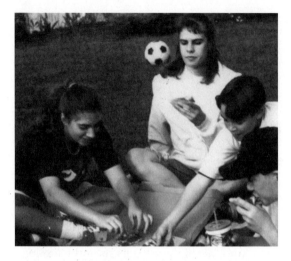

Figure 8–6 *Adolescents should be encouraged to eat healthy alternatives such as pizza, rather than high-fat, high-salt, low-nutrient fast foods.*

REVIEW QUESTIONS

A. Multiple choice. Select the best answer.

1. In counseling a mother whose 10-month-old infant is overweight, what advice should be given first?
   a. Recommend reducing the quantity of food given at each meal and allow one bottle feeding.
   b. Recommend the use of skim milk instead of whole milk in infant's formula.
   c. Ask the mother to keep a log of feedings and bring it to the clinic next week.
   d. Tell the mother that the baby needs to be more active.

2. Which of the following practices may help prevent the development of obesity?
   a. Encourage eating animal protein rather than plant protein.
   b. Avoid fats.
   c. Eat saturated fats, not polyunsaturated fats.
   d. Ingest caloric requirements for maintenance and growth.

3. Which of the following foods is the least likely to cause an infant to have an allergic reaction?
   a. apples
   b. green vegetables
   c. pears
   d. oatmeal

4. How does human milk differ from cow's milk? Human milk
   a. is more easily digested
   b. supplies more protein
   c. provides fewer calories
   d. contains less lactose

5. A 3-year-old boy is encouraged to drink a cup of orange juice to promote
   a. tissue regeneration
   b. iron absorption
   c. carbohydrate metabolism
   d. an acidic urine

6. Most normal infants who weigh 7 pounds (3.175 kg) at birth can be expected at 12 months of age to weigh
   a. 14 pounds (6.35 kg)
   b. 21 pounds (9.325 kg)
   c. 28 pounds (12.5 kg)
   d. 35 pounds (15.675 kg)

7. A mother at the well-baby clinic says she is worried because her 2-year-old daughter's appetite is decreasing. Which is the best response?
   a. Advise supplementing her meals with nutritious snacks several times a day.
   b. Suggest restricting her play activities until she eats all of the food at each meal.
   c. Emphasize that her caloric needs are lower now and her appetite reflects these reduced needs.
   d. Advise adding high-calorie foods to her diet to improve caloric intake.

8. The 6-year-old child who is at the expected developmental level will most likely have which of the following characteristic attitudes about food and eating?
   a. food likes and dislikes that fluctuate from day to day
   b. an eagerness to try new foods
   c. a dislike of fruits and vegetables
   d. a preference for familiar foods that are simply prepared

9. The infant should be weaned from only breast or bottle feeding to eating some solid foods at approximately 6 months of age because
   a. the infant should learn new tastes and textures
   b. extended breast and bottle feeding promote tooth decay
   c. the infant requires dietary fiber for proper growth and development
   d. the child's iron stores begin to diminish at 6 months of age

10. The adolescent's diet often lacks which of the following nutrients?
    a. carbohydrates and vitamin D
    b. fats and zinc
    c. proteins and iron
    d. fluids and calcium

SUGGESTED ACTIVITIES

- Identify four suggestions that you can give parents to encourage preschoolers to eat new or different foods. Be specific.

- Describe key differences in nutritional requirements and diet from infancy through adolescence.

BIBLIOGRAPHY

American Academy of Pediatrics, Committee on Nutrition. The use of whole cow's milk in infancy. *Pediatrics* (1993): 253–255.

American Academy of Pediatrics, Committee on Nutrition. Toward a prudent diet for children. *Pediatrics* 73 (1984): 876.

Anderson, J. B. The status of adolescent nutrition. *Nutrition Today* (March/April, 1991): 7–10.

Laquatra, I., and M. J. Gerlach. *Nutrition in Clinical Nursing.* Albany, NY: Delmar Publishers, 1990.

Mahan, L. K. and M. Arlin *Krause's Food, Nutrition and Diet Therapy*, 8th ed. Philadelphia: W. B. Saunders, 1992.

Marotz, L. R., M. Z. Cross, and J. M. Rush. *Health, Safety, and Nutrition for the Young Child*, 3rd ed. Albany, NY: Delmar Publishers, 1993.

Pipes, P., and C. Trahms. *Nutrition in Infancy and Childhood*, 5th ed. St. Louis, MO: Mosby-Year Book, 1993.

Whitney, E., and S. Rolfes. *Understanding Nutrition*. Minneapolis/St. Paul: West Publishing, 1993.

CHAPTER

9

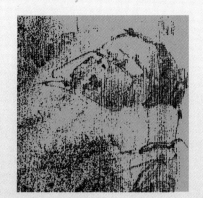

*P*reventive Health Care

OBJECTIVES

AFTER STUDYING THIS CHAPTER, THE STUDENT SHOULD BE ABLE TO:

- DISCUSS THE RECOMMENDED PHYSICAL EXAMINATIONS AND SCREENINGS FOR HEALTHY CHILDREN.
- DESCRIBE THE COMPONENTS OF THE HEALTH HISTORY.
- DISTINGUISH BETWEEN PASSIVE AND ACTIVE IMMUNITY.
- DISCUSS THE RECOMMENDED IMMUNIZATION SCHEDULE FOR HEALTHY CHILDREN.
- DESCRIBE THE CURRENT ACTIVE IMMUNIZATIONS AVAILABLE TO CHILDREN AND POSSIBLE REACTIONS TO THESE IMMUNIZATIONS.
- DESCRIBE GENERAL CONCERNS AND NURSING RESPONSIBILITIES WHEN ADMINISTERING VACCINES TO CHILDREN.
- DISCUSS THE IMPORTANCE OF DENTAL CARE.
- IDENTIFY THREE WAYS TO PREVENT DENTAL CARIES.

131

KEY TERMS

IMMUNE RESPONSE	LIVE ATTENUATED VIRUS
ACTIVE IMMUNITY	KILLED INACTIVATED VIRUS
PASSIVE IMMUNITY	TEETHING
VACCINE	DENTAL CARIES
TOXOID	SEALANTS

reventive health care is an important part of nursing care. Even before the baby is born, monitoring the health of an expectant mother and instilling good health care habits can prevent illness and help ensure good health during childhood and throughout life. Regular physical examinations, screenings, immunizations, dental care, and health care counseling to promote good health care habits are the keys to preventive health care.

SCHEDULED PHYSICAL EXAMINATIONS AND SCREENINGS

Regularly scheduled physical examinations and screenings are vital to a child's preventive health care. Their scheduling is based on individual needs. For the healthy child with adequate parenting, however, the American Academy of Pediatrics recommends regular examinations, including screenings and immunizations, at specific scheduled intervals from birth through adolescence, Figure 9–1. Laboratory tests, immunizations, and screenings may be a routine part of the examination or may be indicated as a result of the examina-

tion. Screenings are examinations or tests, such as a tuberculin test for tuberculosis or blood pressure measurement for hypertension, to detect a particular disease, disorder, or risk factors for a disease.

THE HEALTH HISTORY

The health history serves as a guide to the physical examination and includes background information for laboratory findings, nursing diagnoses, and planning. It is a record of the child's past health history, growth and development, nutritional status, and mental or psychosocial health as well as present health. The complete health history is taken at the child's initial health care visit and is updated with each examination. The child's past health history includes a prenatal, birth, and neonatal history; immunization records; and any illnesses, accidents, hospitalizations, surgery, and allergies. A history of the child's growth and development reveals how the child is progressing compared to other children of the same age, sex, and culture. The family history provides information about any chronic illness or communicable disease in the immediate family that may predispose the child to illness, and any activities among

RECOMMENDATIONS FOR PREVENTIVE PEDIATRIC HEALTH CARE

Committee on Practice and Ambulatory Medicine

Each child and family is unique; therefore, these **Recommendations for Preventive Pediatric Health Care** are designed for the care of children who are receiving competent parenting, have no manifestations of any important health problems, and are growing and developing in satisfactory fashion. **Additional visits may become necessary** if circumstances suggest variations from normal.

These guidelines represent a consensus by the Committee on Practice and Ambulatory Medicine in consultation with national committees and sections of the American Academy of Pediatrics. The Committee emphasizes the great importance of **continuity of care** in comprehensive health supervision and the need to avoid **fragmentation of care.**

A **prenatal visit** is recommended for parents who are at high risk, for first-time parents, and for those who request a conference. The prenatal visit should include anticipatory guidance and pertinent medical history. Every infant should have a newborn evaluation after birth.

	INFANCY[3]								EARLY CHILDHOOD[3]					MIDDLE CHILDHOOD[3]				ADOLESCENCE[3]										
AGE[4]	NEWBORN[1]	2-4d[2]	By 1mo	2mo	4mo	6mo	9mo	12mo	15mo	18mo	24mo	3y	4y	5y	6y	8y	10y	11y	12y	13y	14y	15y	16y	17y	18y	19y	20y	21y
HISTORY																												
Initial/Interval	•	•	•	•	•	•	•	•	•	•	•	•	•	•	•	•	•	•	•	•	•	•	•	•	•	•	•	•
MEASUREMENTS																												
Height and Weight	•	•	•	•	•	•	•	•	•	•	•	•	•	•	•	•	•	•	•	•	•	•	•	•	•	•	•	•
Head Circumference	•	•	•	•	•	•	•	•	•	•	•																	
Blood Pressure												•	•	•	•	•	•	•	•	•	•	•	•	•	•	•	•	•
SENSORY SCREENING																												
Vision	S	S	S	S	S	S	S	S	S	S	S	O[5]	O	O	S	S	O	S	O	S	S	O	S	S	O	S	S	S
Hearing[6]	S/O	S	S	S	S	S	S	S	S	S	S	O	O	O	S	S	O	S	O	S	S	O	S	S	O	S	S	S
DEVELOPMENTAL/ BEHAVIORAL ASSESSMENT[7]	•	•	•	•	•	•	•	•	•	•	•	•	•	•	•	•	•	•	•	•	•	•	•	•	•	•	•	•
PHYSICAL EXAMINATION[8]	•	•	•	•	•	•	•	•	•	•	•	•	•	•	•	•	•	•	•	•	•	•	•	•	•	•	•	•
PROCEDURES – GENERAL[9]																												
Hereditary/Metabolic Screening[10]	←	—	•																									
Immunization[11]	•—	—	→	•	•	•		←	•	→			←	•	→			• —	—	—	—	—	→					
Lead Screening[12]							• —	→			•																	
Hematocrit or Hemoglobin			←	—	—	—	•											←	—	—	—	•[13]	—	—	—	—	—	→
Urinalysis														•				←	—	—	—	•[14]	—	—	—	—	—	→
PROCEDURES – PATIENTS AT RISK																												
Tuberculin Test[15]								*	*	*	*	*	*	*	*	*	*	*	*	*	*	*	*	*	*	*	*	*
Cholesterol Screening[16]											*	*	*	*	*	*	*	*	*	*	*	*	*	*	*	*	*	*
STD Screening[17]																		*	*	*	*	*	*	*	*	*	*	*
Pelvic Exam[18]																		*	*	*	*	*	*	← *	*	*[18]	*	* →
ANTICIPATORY GUIDANCE[19]	•	•	•	•	•	•	•	•	•	•	•	•	•	•	•	•	•	•	•	•	•	•	•	•	•	•	•	•
Injury Prevention[20]	•	•	•	•	•	•	•	•	•	•	•	•	•	•	•	•	•	•	•	•	•	•	•	•	•	•	•	•
INITIAL DENTAL REFERRAL[21]								←	—	—	—	•																

1. Breastfeeding encouraged and instruction and support offered.
2. For newborns discharged in less than 48 hours after delivery.
3. Developmental, psychosocial, and chronic disease issues for children and adolescents may require frequent counseling and treatment visits separate from preventive care visits.
4. If a child comes under care for the first time at any point on the schedule, or if any items are not accomplished at the suggested age, the schedule should be brought up to date at the earliest possible time.
5. If the patient is uncooperative, rescreen within six months.
6. Some experts recommend objective appraisal of hearing in the newborn period. The Joint Committee on Infant Hearing has identified patients at significant risk for hearing loss. All children meeting these criteria should be objectively screened. See the Joint Committee on Infant Hearing 1994 Position Statement.
7. By history and appropriate physical examination: if suspicious, by specific objective developmental testing.
8. At each visit, a complete physical examination is essential, with infant totally unclothed, older child undressed and suitably draped.
9. These may be modified, depending upon entry point into schedule and individual need.
10. Metabolic screening (eg, thyroid, hemoglobinopathies, PKU, galactosemia) should be done according to state law.
11. Schedule(s) per the Committee on Infectious Diseases, published periodically in *Pediatrics*. Every visit should be an opportunity to update and complete a child's immunizations.
12. Blood lead screen per AAP statement "Lead Poisoning: From Screening to Primary Prevention" (1993).
13. All menstruating adolescents should be screened.
14. Conduct dipstick urinalysis for leukocytes for male and female adolescents.
15. TB testing per AAP statement "Screening for Tuberculosis in Infants and Children" (1994). Testing should be done upon recognition of high risk factors. If results are negative but high risk situation continues, testing should be repeated on an annual basis.
16. Cholesterol screening for high risk patients per AAP "Statement on Cholesterol" (1992). If family history cannot be ascertained and other risk factors are present, screening should be at the discretion of the physician.
17. All sexually active patients should be screened for sexually transmitted diseases (STDs).
18. All sexually active females should have a pelvic examination. A pelvic examination and routine pap smear should be offered as part of preventive health maintenance between the ages of 18 and 21 years.
19. Appropriate discussion and counseling should be an integral part of each visit for care.
20. From birth to age 12, refer to AAP's injury prevention program (TIPP®) as described in "A Guide to Safety Counseling in Office Practice" (1994).
21. Earlier initial dental evaluations may be appropriate for some children. Subsequent examinations as prescribed by dentist.

Key: • = to be performed * = to be performed for patients at risk S = subjective, by history O = objective, by a standard testing method ←•→ = the range during which a service may be provided, with the dot indicating the preferred age.
NB: Special chemical, immunologic, and endocrine testing is usually carried out upon specific indications. Testing other than newborn (eg, inborn errors of metabolism, sickle disease, etc.) is discretionary with the physician.
The recommendations in this publication do not indicate an exclusive course of treatment or serve as a standard of medical care. Variations, taking into account individual circumstances, may be appropriate.

Figure 9–1 *From the American Academy of Pediatrics. Recommendations for preventive pediatric health care.* Pediatrics *vol. 96, 2. August 1995. Used with permission.*

family members, such as smoking, that can affect the child's health. Information about the child's eating habits, and any weight gain or loss, food allergies, or gastrointestinal problems help identify nutritional problems or concerns. Questions about the child's interactions at school as well as with family and friends provide data concerning the child's mental and psychosocial health. A review of systems involves questions relating to the status of each system. Information about present health covers health habits and focuses on any current illness, complaints, or concerns.

Communication is vital during the interview and health history, as well as throughout the examination. The nurse should speak with the child as much as possible. Asking about school, family, and friends as well as any symptoms or concerns can elicit important information about the child's physical health, development, and mental health. Developing cooperation and trust can help the nurse to obtain information crucial to detecting potential as well as existing health problems and to determine areas in which counseling or education is needed.

THE PHYSICAL EXAMINATION

The physical examination begins with a general inspection, physical measurements, and vital sign assessment (see Chapter 12). An examination of systems follows (see Chapters 20–28). The sequence and extent of the examination of systems depends on the age of the child, the child's health, and any anxiety. Those areas of immediate concern will need the most attention. Only those areas to be examined should be exposed.

For the infant or toddler who is quiet, auscultation of the heart, lungs, and abdomen is generally performed first. It is important to keep the infant warm. The parent can assist in holding or comforting the child. The most distressing procedures, such as the examination of the ears, nose, and throat, are generally performed last. Talking calmly to the infant and toddler will encourage cooperation and help make the child feel comfortable. Allow the child to examine instruments such as stethoscopes and otoscopes. Toys or stuffed animals help provide a pleasant atmosphere.

Reassure the preschool age child about procedures. Allow the child to voice concerns and encourage any questions. The child may want to examine and play with instruments. Portions of the examination that are likely to cause discomfort are usually performed last. Include health education. Engaging the child as much as possible during the examination will help the child feel at ease.

Provide privacy for the school-age child who is dressing or undressing. Examinations of the ear, nose, and throat and the genitalia are usually performed last. An explanation of the procedures will help the child feel comfortable. Provide education about health care and sexual development. Encourage the child to ask questions.

Privacy and confidentiality are important for the adolescent. The adolescent may be interviewed with or without the parent or guardian present. Encourage trust and discussion by being direct, honest, and nonjudgmental. Provide educational counseling on sexuality, sexually transmitted diseases (STDs), contraception, substance abuse, and mental health, if needed. Boys should receive instruction on testicular self-examination, Figure 9–2. Girls should have a breast examination with instruction on breast self-examination (BSE), Figure 9–3. Sexually active girls should have a pelvic examination and Pap smear. All sexually active adolescents should be screened for STDs. The genitalia are usually examined last.

IMMUNIZATIONS

The routine immunization of children against specific infectious diseases is one of the most significant advances in health care worldwide. The occurrence of childhood diseases that were once considered major public health problems has been dramatically reduced because of the development of immunizing agents that prevent specific diseases.

In 1977 the U.S. Department of Health and Human Services initiated a childhood immunization program. Many children were immunized against childhood diseases because of this initiative and the enactment of laws by all 50 states requiring documentation of immunization as a condition of a child's enrollment into school.

Many children still remain underimmunized today, however. In some cities in the United States, as many as 50% of children under the age of 2 have not received the recommended immunizations. Nurses can be important advocates of childhood immunizations and should become familiar with the immunizations available to children, as well as the immune responses that these immunizations produce to specific childhood diseases.

THE IMMUNE RESPONSE

Immunity is a state in which an individual is resistant to a particular disease. Individuals become immune to specific diseases through exposure to the disease or vaccination against the disease. An **immune response** occurs when the body's lymphocytes are stimulated to produce antibodies that react with antigens (protein substances found on the surface of microorganisms). These disease-specific antibodies destroy or neutralize antigens and remain in the blood plasma to prevent reinfection by the specific infectious agent.

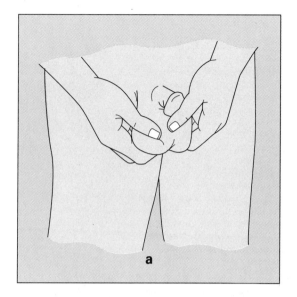

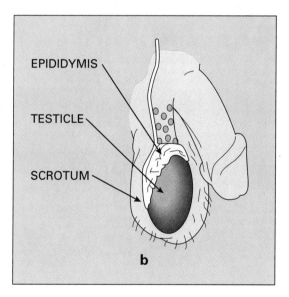

EPIDIDYMIS

TESTICLE

SCROTUM

b

Figure 9–2   *Testicular self-examination (a) Examine testicles once a month, preferably after a shower. Roll each testicle between the thumb and fingers of each hand. Do not mistake the cordlike structure, or epididymis, for an abnormality. Notify your doctor if you feel any lumps or changes. (b) Male reproductive organs. (Adapted from* Testicular Self-Examination, National Cancer Institute, *NIH Publication No. 94-2636, Reprinted February 1994)*

Here's what you should do to check for changes in your breasts.

1 Stand in front of a mirror that is large enough for you to see your breasts clearly. Check each breast for anything unusual. Check the skin for puckering, dimpling, or scaliness. Look for a discharge from the nipples.

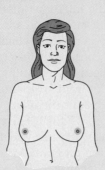

Do steps 2 and 3 to check for any change in the shape or contour of your breasts. As you do these steps, you should feel your chest muscles tighten.

2 Watching closely in the mirror, clasp hands behind your head and press your hands forward.

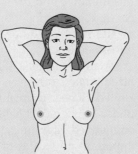

3 Next, press your hands firmly on your hips and bend slightly toward your mirror as you pull your shoulders and elbows forward.

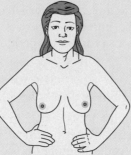

4 Gently squeeze each nipple and look for a discharge.

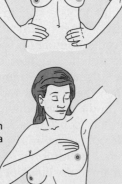

5 Raise one arm. Use the pads of the fingers of your other hand to check the breast and the surrounding area–firmly, carefully, and thoroughly. Some women like to use lotion or powder to help their fingers glide easily over the skin. Feel for any unusual lump or mass under the skin. Feel the tissue by pressing your fingers in small, overlapping areas about the size of a dime. To be sure you cover your whole breast, take your time and follow a definte pattern.

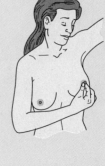

Some research suggests that many women do BSE more thoroughly when they use a pattern of up-and-down lines or strips. The important thing is to cover the whole breast and to pay special attention to the area between the breast and the underarm, including the underarm itself. Check the area above the breast, up to the collarbone and all the way over to your shoulder.

LINES: Start in the underarm area and move your fingers downward little by little until they are below the breast. Then move your fingers slightly toward the middle and slowly move back up. Go up and down until you cover the whole area.

6 It's important to repeat step 5 while you are lying down. Lie flat on your back, with one arm over your head and a pillow or folded towel under the shoulder. This position flattens the breast and makes it easier to check. Check each breast and the area around it very carefully using one of the patterns.

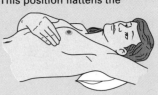

7 Some women repeat step 5 in the shower. Your fingers will glide easily over soapy skin, so you can concentrate on feeling for changes underneath.

If you notice a lump, a discharge, or any other change during the month–whether or not it is during BSE–contact your doctor.

Figure 9–3   *Breast self-examination. (Adapted from* What you Need to Know about Breast Cancer, *National Cancer Institute, NIH Publication No. 94-1556, Revised July 1993)*

Active immunity (or humoral immunity) occurs when individuals form antibodies or antitoxins against specific antigens, either by exposure to the infectious agent or by introduction of the antigen. For example, a child develops active immunity to the measles virus when he or she develops the disease or is vaccinated against the virus. In each instance, the child responds to the measles antigen by forming antibodies against it. If the child is exposed to measles again, reinfection will not occur because active immunity against the disease has been developed.

Passive immunity occurs when an individual receives ready-made antibodies from a human or animal that has been actively immunized against the disease. An example of passive immunity is the transfer of antibodies from a mother to her fetus. A newborn baby who has received measles antibodies from his or her mother in utero will be immune from measles for as long as 6 months to 1 year of age. Passive immunity provides only temporary immunity because the recipient has not developed his or her own antibodies against the disease.

VACCINES

Active immunity is achieved through the introduction of a **vaccine**, an active immunizing agent that incorporates an infectious antigen. The vaccine can be given in the form of a **toxoid**, an agent that has been treated to destroy its toxic qualities; a **live attenuated virus**, a weakened virus; or a **killed inactivated virus**.

Vaccines stimulate the body to produce antitoxins or antibodies against the specific disease. Some immunizing agents provide lifetime protection against a disease, some provide partial protection, and some must be readministered at intervals in the form of booster immunizations to maintain the antibodies at protective levels (American Academy of Pediatrics 1991).

RECOMMENDED IMMUNIZATION SCHEDULE

There are currently ten infectious diseases for which routine immunizations in childhood are recommended: diphtheria, tetanus, pertussis, infections caused by *Hemophilus influenzae*, polio, measles (rubeola), rubella (German measles), mumps, hepatitis B, and varicella.

The American Academy of Pediatrics' Committee on Infectious Diseases recommends that immunization for children begin at 2 months of age, with the exception of the hepatitis B vaccine, which can be given initially at birth (American Academy of Pediatrics 1991). Figure 9–4 gives the recommended schedule for active immunization of healthy infants and children.

DIPHTHERIA, TETANUS, AND PERTUSSIS VACCINES

Diphtheria-Tetanus-Pertussis. The diphtheria-tetanus-pertussis (DTP) immunization is usually given in one injection of combined diphtheria and tetanus toxoids, and a suspension of killed whole-cell pertussis organisms. For primary immunization of children, DTP is given in a series of four doses. The first three doses of 0.5 mL each are given intramuscularly at four- to eight-week intervals (usually at 2 months, 4 months, and 6 months of age). A booster dose of DTP is given to children at least 6 months after the third dose (between 12 and 18 months of age). At 4 to 6 years, or before entering school, children who have received the fourth dose of DTP at ages younger than 4 years should receive a fifth dose of DTP. An interruption in the recommended schedule does not affect immunity. It is not necessary to begin the series again if an immunization is delayed.

Forty to seventy percent of children will experience mild reactions following administration of the DTP immunization. These mild reactions include redness and tenderness at the injection site, fever, drowsiness, fretfulness,

RECOMMENDED CHILDHOOD IMMUNIZATION SCHEDULE
UNITED STATES, JANUARY – JUNE 1996

Vaccines are listed under the routinely recommended ages. Bars *indicate range of acceptable ages for vaccination.* Shaded bars *indicate catch-up vaccination: at 11-12 years of age, hepatitis B vaccine should be administered to children not previously vaccinated, and Varicella Zoster Virus vaccine should be administered to children not previously vaccinated who lack a reliable history of chickenpox.*

Age ▲ ▶ Vaccine	Birth	1 mo	2 mos	4 mos	6 mos	12 mos	15 mos	18 mos	4–6 yrs	11–12 yrs	14–16 yrs
Hepatitis B[1,2]	Hep B-1		Hep B-2			Hep B-3				Hep B[2]	
Diphtheria, Tetanus, Pertussis[3]			DTP	DTP	DTP		DTP[3] (DTaP at 15+ m)		DTP or DTaP	Td	Td
H. influenzae type b[4]			Hib	Hib	Hib[4]	Hib[4]					
Polio[5]			OPV[5]	OPV	OPV	OPV			OPV		
Measles, Mumps, Rubella[6]						MMR			MMR[6]	MMR[6] or MMR[6]	
Varicella Zoster Virus Vaccine[7]						Var	Var			Var[7]	

Approved by the Advisory Committee on Immunization Practices (ACIP), the American Academy of Pediatrics (AAP), and the American Academy of Family Physicians (AAFP).

Figure 9–4 *Recommended schedule of vaccinations for all children (From American Academy of Pediatrics, Report of the Committee on Infectious Diseases, 22nd ed. 1991)*

RECOMMENDED CHILDHOOD IMMUNIZATION SCHEDULE
UNITED STATES, JANUARY – JUNE 1996

[1]**Infants born to HBsAg-negative mothers** should receive 2.5 μg of Merck vaccine (Recombivax HB) or 10 μg of SmithKline Beecham (SB) vaccine (Engerix-B). The 2nd dose should be administered ≥ 1 mo after the 1st dose.

Infants born to HBsAg-positive mothers shouldreceive 0.5 mL Hepatitis B Immune Globulin (HBIG) within 12 hr of birth, and either 5 μg of Merck vaccine (Recombivax HB) or 10μg of SB vaccine (Engerix-B) at a separate site. The 2nd dose is recommended at 1–2 mos of age and the 3rd dose at 6 mos of age.

Infants born to mothers whose HBsAg status is unknown should receive either 5 μg of Merck vaccine (Recombivax HB) or 10 μg of SB vaccine (Engerix-B) within 12 hr of birth. The 2nd dose of vaccine is recommended at 1 mo of age and the 3rd dose at 6 mos of age.

[2]Adolescents who have not previously received 3 doses of hepatitis B vaccine should initiate or complete the series at the 11–12 year-old visit. The 2nd dose should be administered at least 1 mo after the 1st dose, and the 3rd dose should be administered at least 4 mos after the 1st dose and at least 2 mos after the 2nd dose.

[3]DTP4 may be administered at 12 mos of age, if at least 6 mos have elapsed since DTP3. DTaP (diphtheria and tetanus toxoids and acellular pertussis vaccine) is licensed for the 4th and/or 5th vaccine dose(s) for children ≥ 15 mos and may be preferred for these doses in this age group. Td (tetanus and diphtheria toxoids, absorbed, for adult use) is recommended at 11–12 years of age if at least 5 years have elapsed since the last dose of DTP, DTaP, or DT.

[4]Three *H. influenzae* type b (Hib) conjugate vaccines are licensed for infant use. If PRP-OMP (PedvaxHIB [Merck]) is administered at 2 and 4 mos of age, a dose at 6 mos is not required. After completing the primary series, any Hib conjugate vaccine may be used as a booster.

[5]Oral poliovirus vaccine (OPV) is recommended for routine infant vaccination. Inactivated poliovirus vaccine (IPV) is recommended for persons with a congenital or acquired immune deficiency disease or an altered immune status as a result of disease or immunosuppressive therapy, as well as their household contacts, and is an acceptable alternative for other persons. The primary 3-dose series for IPV should be given with a minimum interval of 4 wks between the 1st and 2nd doses and 6 mos between the 2nd and 3rd doses.

[6]The 2nd dose of MMR is routinely recommended at 4–6 yrs of age or at 11–12 yrs of age, but may be administered at any visit, provided at least 1 mo has elapsed since receipt of the 1st dose.

[7]Varicella zoster virus vaccine (Var) can be administered to susceptible children any time after 12 months of age. Unvaccinated children who lack a reliable history of chickenpox should be vaccinated at the 11–12 year-old visit.

Figure 9-4   Continued

and loss of appetite. Rarely children have more severe reactions; these include fever of 40.5°C (104.9°F) or higher, persistent crying for three or more hours, unusual high-pitched crying, and convulsions. If a severe reaction occurs, further immunization with pertussis is contraindicated (DHHS 1991a). Other contraindications to administration of pertussis vaccine are listed in Figure 9–5.

DTaP. In December 1991, the U.S. Food and Drug Administration (FDA) licensed a new pertussis vaccine. Instead of being made from killed whole-cell pertussis organisms, the new vaccine is made of a few parts of the pertussis cell (Edwards et al. 1991). Combined with the diphtheria and tetanus vaccines (DTaP) for administration, it can be used as the fourth and fifth dose for children only if they have been immunized previously with at least three doses of the DTP vaccine (DHHS 1992).

Diphtheria-Tetanus Pediatric. Diphtheria-tetanus (DT) pediatric vaccine is administered instead of DPT to children for whom the pertussis vaccine is contraindicated. DT con-

tains full amounts of the diphtheria and tetanus toxoids. This preparation is not given to children over the age of 7 because adverse reactions can occur from the administration of the full-strength diphtheria toxoid.

Diphtheria-Tetanus Adult. Diphtheria-tetanus (Td) adult vaccine is administered to children over the age of 11 and adults. It contains less diphtheria toxoid than the DPT or DT vaccines.

Poliovirus Vaccines. There are two types of polio vaccine available in the United States: live oral poliovirus vaccine (OPV) and inactivated polio vaccine (IPV).

OPV. OPV is the vaccine of choice for immunizing children against the poliovirus in the United States. This vaccine is given orally at the same time that the DTP immunization is administered. The primary series of three doses is usually given at 2 months, 4 months, and 6 to 18 months of age. A booster dose of OPV is given at 4 to 6 years of age.

OPV is a live attenuated virus that is

CONTRAINDICATIONS TO VACCINATIONS	
Vaccine	**Contraindications**
Pertussis	Progressive neurologic disorder
	Any of the following reactions after receiving the vaccine: convulsion, persistent uncontrollable cry, fever of 104°F or more
Live attenuated polio (OPV)	Immunosuppressed children or children who share a household with individuals who are immunosuppressed (e.g., those with HIV infection or those receiving steroids, chemotherapy, or radiation therapy)
Measles, mumps, rubella	Egg sensitivity (vaccine contains egg antigens), which may lead to an anaphylactic reaction
	Anaphylactic reaction to neomycin

Figure 9–5

excreted in the stool for about a month after administration. It should not be given to children if they or their household contacts are immunosuppressed from such conditions as cancer, HIV infection, or because of radiation or drug therapy that would make it difficult for the body to fight infection (DHHS 1991b), see Figure 9–5. Very rarely OPV will cause vaccine-related paralysis.

IPV. IPV is a killed virus that is given subcutaneously. It is recommended for children in whom OPV is contraindicated (American Academy of Pediatrics 1991).

Haemophilus Influenzae Type B Conjugate. *Haemophilus influenzae* type b infection is a major cause of meningitis, epiglottitis, septic arthritis, and bacteremia in infants and children under the age of 5. Current recommendations require all children be immunized by intramuscular injection with H. influenzae type b conjugate (Hib) beginning at approximately 2 months of age in a three-dose series at two-month intervals. A fourth dose is recommended at 12 to 15 months of age. Hib may be given simultaneously with DTP, polio, and measles, mumps, rubella (MMR) immunizations. A different injection site and separate syringes should be used (American Academy of Pediatrics 1991). Recently the FDA approved a combined Hib and DTP vaccine.

Hib is a very safe vaccine. About 2% of children receiving the vaccine develop redness and soreness at the injection site and mild fever.

Measles, Mumps, and Rubella Vaccines. Measles, mumps, rubella (MMR) is a live attenuated vaccine that is usually administered in one subcutaneous injection at 12 to 15 months of age. It is recommended that a second immunization be given to children 4 to 6 years or 11 to 12 years of age unless state law requires administration at 4 to 6 years.

Contraindications to the MMR vaccine are listed in Figure 9–5. Reactions may occur 5 to 12 days after administration of the measles, mumps, and rubella vaccines because they are live attenuated virus vaccines.

Measles. Measles (rubeola) is a serious disease that is easily prevented by the administration of the measles vaccine to all children. The vaccine is available in measles-only form (M), in combination with rubella (MR), and in combination with mumps and rubella (MMR). The initial measles immunization should be given at 12 to 15 months of age. If the vaccine is given earlier than 12 months, many children fail to become immune because of the presence of maternal antibodies to measles that were passed to the infant through the placenta during pregnancy. Any child vaccinated with MMR before 12 months of age should have a repeat vaccination at 15 months and a third dose at 4 to 6 years or 11 to 12 years (Merenstein et al. 1991).

Because of the increase in measles cases in vaccinated children, a two-dose schedule for administration of MMR is recommended (*Vaccine Bulletin* 1993). Some experts recommend that the second dose be given before entry into school (at 4 to 6 years), while others recommend that the second dose be given before entry into middle school (at 11 to 12 years) (*MMWR* 1989a).

The measles vaccine may sometimes cause a rash and fever.

Mumps. The mumps vaccine is a live attenuated virus that is usually combined with measles and rubella vaccines (MMR) for administration.

Rarely after receiving the mumps vaccine, the child may develop swelling of the parotid glands.

Rubella (German Measles). Rubella is usually a mild infection in children. When a pregnant woman develops the disease, however, serious consequences may occur. Babies born to mothers who have had rubella in pregnancy may be blind, deaf, or have heart disease (*MMWR* 1989b). Rubella vaccine is administered in a single subcutaneous dose of 0.5 mL in combination with measles and mumps (MMR), with measles (MR), or alone.

The current recommendation is to vaccinate all children 12 months of age or older. The vaccine usually is given combined with the measles and mumps vaccines (MMR), starting at 12 to 15 months of age. In addition, all postpubertal adolescent girls who are not known to be immune to rubella should be immunized (American Academy of Pediatrics 1991). Pregnancy, if a possibility, should be ruled out before immunization.

The rubella vaccine may cause swelling of the lymph glands or a rash. Mild pain or stiffness may also occur after one to three weeks.

Hepatitis B Vaccine. Hepatitis B virus infection is a major health problem in the United States. Both adolescents and adults are at high risk. Currently the hepatitis B vaccine is not required for entry into school (*MMWR* 1991).

Hepatitis B vaccine is recommended in a series of three intramuscular doses. The first dose is administered at birth. The second dose is given at 1 to 4 months of age and the third dose at 6 to 18 months of age, depending on the HBsAg status of the mother, see Figure 9–4.

Few reactions have been reported with hepatitis B vaccination. Those reported include soreness and redness at the injection site.

Varicella Virus Vaccine. The varicella virus vaccine, also known as the varicella zoster vaccine (VZV), is a live, attenuated vaccine used to prevent chickenpox. It is usually administered subcutaneously in a single 0.5 ml dose at 12 to 18 months or at 11 to 12 years. Children 13 years of age or older who have never had chickenpox should receive two doses, the second dose 4 to 8 weeks after the first.

GENERAL CONSIDERATIONS IN IMMUNIZATION

Informed Consent. The benefits and risks of the immunizations should be explained to parents before administering the vaccine. Religious beliefs may be a factor. For example, Christian Scientists may not permit their children to have immunizations.

Several documents developed by the Centers for Disease Control and Prevention (CDC) can be used for securing informed consent. These forms are frequently updated as new developments in immunization occur.

Record Keeping. Standard immunization records have been developed for parents' use, Figure 9–6. The child's health record should contain the following information about immunizations:

1. date of immunization (day, month, year)
2. vaccine
3. manufacturer
4. batch or lot number
5. site and route of administration
6. name and title of person administering immunization

The National Childhood Vaccine Injury Act (*MMWR* 1988) requires that any adverse reactions to the vaccine be reported to the state health department, which notifies the CDC.

Scheduling. Vaccinations should be postponed if the child has a febrile illness. An upper respiratory infection without fever does not necessitate postponing the immunization. A lapse in the routine schedule does not interfere with the immune response, so it is unnecessary to reinitiate the series if such a lapse occurs. If the child's immunization status is unknown, he or she should be considered susceptible (Derschewitz 1988).

Vaccine Administration Record

Patient Name _____

Birthdate _____

Record # _____

Clinic Name/Address

"I have been provided a copy, and have read or have had explained to me, information about the diseases and the vaccines listed below. I have had a chance to ask questions that were answered to my satisfaction. I believe I understand the benefits and risks of the vaccines cited, and ask that the vaccine(s) listed below be given to me or to the person named above (for whom I am authorized to make this request)."

Vaccine	Date Given m/d/y	Age	*Site	Vaccine Manufacturer	Vaccine Lot Number	**Handout Publ. Date	***Initials	Signature of Parent or Guardian
DTP1								
DTP2								
DTP3								
DTP/DTaP4								
DTP/DTaP5								
DT								
DTP/Hib1								
DTP/Hib2								
DTP/Hib3								
DTP/Hib4								
Td								
OPV/IPV1								
OPV/IPV2								
OPV/IPV3								
OPV/IPV4								
MMR1								
MMR2								
Hib1								
Hib2								
Hib3								
Hib4								
Hep B1								
Hep B2								
Hep B3								

*** Initials   Signature of Vaccine Administrator

_____
_____
_____
(Use reverse side if more signatures are needed)

*Site Given Legend
RA = Right Arm
LA = Left Arm
RT = Right Thigh
LT = Left Thigh
O = Oral

** If required by state law

American Academy of Pediatrics

Copyright©1992
Rev 7/93

HE0116

Figure 9–6   (Used with permission of the American Academy of Pediatrics, Elk Grove Village, IL)

NURSING CONSIDERATIONS WHEN ADMINISTERING VACCINES

- Refer to the manufacturer's insert for the proper storage and route of administration for the vaccine.

- Obtain informed consent from parents before administering the vaccine.

- Minimize minor, local reactions to intramuscular injection (for example, DTP) by:
  - using a 1-inch long, 22-gauge, needle
  - injecting the vaccine into the anterolateral thigh muscle in children 18 months old or younger (the deltoid muscle can be used in older children)

- Use a ⅝-inch long, 25–gauge needle for subcutaneous injections.

- Give each vaccine at a separate site.

- Adequately restrain the child when administering the vaccine.

- Know that multiple vaccines may be given in a single visit without adverse effects.

- Accurately document the administration of immunizations for parents and on the child's health record.

DENTAL CARE

The nurse plays an important role in a child's dental care through the education of both the child and the parent or guardian. Maintaining good health, including eating a balanced diet, and practicing good dental habits are vital to the development of healthy teeth. A child's dental health affects overall health. Healthy teeth are important to a child's self-esteem. They affect the child's appearance and aid in speech. They also affect the child's ability to chew in order to obtain needed nutrients.

Dental care of a child's teeth should begin even before the baby is born. Because teeth begin developing in the fetus, a balanced diet and a healthy expectant mother help ensure the development of healthy teeth in the newborn.

INFANT AND TODDLER

The parent can begin good dental health habits from the beginning of the child's life by wiping the baby's gums with a damp wash cloth or gauze pad after each feeding. The first teeth, which arrive when the infant is six or seven months old, can be brushed with a soft bristle toothbrush after each meal. The eruption of teeth, or **teething**, may cause red, swollen, and sensitive gums. The baby's discomfort can be alleviated with acetaminophen, by lightly rubbing gums with a cool wash cloth, wet gauze, or a clean finger, or a hard rubber teething ring or teething pretzel.

Babies who nurse or are bottle fed at naptime, at bedtime, or throughout the night can develop bottle mouth caries, also known as nursing bottle caries or baby bottle tooth decay. Bottle mouth caries are extensive **dental caries**, or tooth decay, in children from 12 months to 4 years of age caused by exposing the child's teeth to formula, milk, including breast milk, or sugary liquids such as juice or sweetened liquids for long periods of time. Dental decay is caused when bacteria and sugar form plaque, which destroys tooth enamel. The nurse should educate the mother to avoid feeding the child milk, formula, or juices at naptime and at bedtime; if the mother wishes to give the baby the bottle at those times, she should use water.

PROFESSIONAL DENTAL CARE

The child's first dental appointment should be scheduled when the first teeth appear. The child may see a regular dentist or a pedodontist, a dentist who specializes in the dental care of children. The purpose of the first dental visit is to acquaint the child with the dentist, the hygienist, the dental office, and the procedures of an examination and cleaning. X-rays may be taken to ensure that the teeth are developing properly. The dentist will also educate the parent and the child, depending on the age of the child, about dental care, including proper brushing, flossing, nutrition, and the use of fluoride in preventing dental caries. If the child does not have adequate fluoride in drinking water, the dentist may suggest fluoride supplements or fluoride treatments. Dental visits every six months should be part of the child's regular dental care; dental problems may necessitate more frequent visits.

PRESCHOOL CHILD

The preschool child will need the help of an adult with brushing and flossing activities. The child should use a children's soft bristle toothbrush of his own, which should be replaced when bristles are worn—about every 3 to 4 months. A small amount of fluoride toothpaste should be used; parents should make sure that children do not swallow the toothpaste.

The child should eat a well-balanced diet, high in calcium and phosphorus. Snacks should include high-protein foods, fruits, and vegetables, rather than sugary foods. When brushing after meals is not feasible, the child should be taught to rinse with water.

Deciduous, or primary, teeth affect the position of the permanent teeth and, like permanent teeth, the child's appearance and the ability to chew and to speak.

SCHOOL-AGE CHILD

At approximately age 6, the child begins to lose his deciduous teeth and the first permanent teeth, the 6-year-old molars, appear. The dentist may recommend the use of **sealants**, or thin, plastic coatings, to protect the molars, which may be susceptible to dental caries because of grooves in the tooth. Sealants prevent dental caries by prohibiting bacteria from penetrating the tooth. The school-age child should participate in his own dental care by brushing after meals and flossing at least once a day. He should avoid sugary snacks and instead eat foods such as meat, cheese, plain yogurt, nuts, and vegetables.

ADOLESCENT

Adolescents are largely responsible for their own dental care. Good oral hygiene habits learned during the preschool and school-age years will help to prevent dental caries. Adolescents, however, may eat in-between meals and may not have the opportunity to brush after all meals. The nurse needs to stress the importance of avoiding sugary snacks, eating well-balanced meals, and maintaining good oral hygiene because poor dental health can affect appearance and overall health. Adolescents also need to be careful to eat a well-balanced diet to promote overall health and healthy teeth. Children with braces need to practice diligent and careful dental care. Children who play sports and are especially susceptible to injury should wear a mouthguard, preferably fitted by a dentist. By practicing good dental health care, adolescents can help ensure that they will have healthy permanent teeth for a lifetime.

REVIEW QUESTIONS

A. Multiple choice. Select the best answer.

1. Preventive health care should begin
   a. at birth
   b. at 1 month of age
   c. before birth
   d. at the first doctor's visit

2. The health history serves as a
   a. record of nursing care plans
   b. laboratory finding
   c. guide to the physical examination
   d. screening to detect risk factors

3. When examining an infant, which of the following procedures is usually performed first?
   a. vision and hearing screening
   b. auscultation of the heart, lungs, and abdomen
   c. examination of the ears, nose, and throat
   d. examination of the genitalia

4. Vaccines can be given in which of the following forms?
   a. toxoid
   b. live active virus
   c. topical
   d. live enhanced virus

5. DTP immunizes against which of the following diseases?
   a. diphtheria, tetanus, polio
   b. diphtheria, toxoid, polio
   c. diphtheria, toxoid, pertussis
   d. diphtheria, tetanus, pertussis

6. Measles, mumps, and rubella vaccines are usually given
   a. if the child has a neomycin or egg sensitivity
   b. before 12 months of age
   c. while maternal antibodies are still present
   d. initially at about 12 to 15 months of age

7. The child's health record must contain the following information about immunizations
   a. the day and hour of immunization
   b. a family history of communicable diseases
   c. immunizations of brothers and sisters
   d. the site and route of administration

8. Vaccinations should be postponed
   a. if the child has an upper respiratory infection with no fever
   b. if the child has a febrile illness
   c. if a lapse in the routine immunization schedule has occurred
   d. if a nurse cannot determine the child's immunization status

9. When administering vaccines, the nurse's responsibilities include
   a. administering vaccines over the religious objections of parents
   b. giving each vaccine at the same site
   c. limiting administration to one vaccine per visit
   d. giving each vaccine at a separate site

10. The child's first professional dental examination should occur
    a. at 3 years of age
    b. just before the child begins school
    c. at 2 years of age
    d. when the first teeth erupt

SUGGESTED ACTIVITIES

- Identify actions that may help a fearful preschool child feel comfortable during a physical examination.

- Make a chart to teach parents when immunizations are given, what they protect against, and possible side effects or reactions.

- Make your own drug cards indicating the various forms of each vaccine, when indicated and contraindicated, and possible reactions.

- Plan a day at the office of a pedodontist. Make note of dental care problems among children and any preventive education given to children and parents.

BIBLIOGRAPHY

American Academy of Pediatrics. *Chickenpox and the New Vaccine.* Elk Grove Village, IL: American Academy of Pediatrics, 1995.

American Academy of Pediatrics. *Report of the Committee on Infectious Diseases,* 22nd ed. Elk Grove Village, IL: American Academy of Pediatrics, 1991.

American Cancer Society. *Facts on Testicular Cancer.* Atlanta, GA: American Cancer Society, 88-500M, 1988, Rev. 11/93.

American Cancer Society. *For Men Only.* Atlanta, GA: American Cancer Society, 91-500M, No. 2028, 1991.

American Dental Association. *Diet & Dental Health.* Chicago, IL: Bureau of Health Education and Audiovisual Services, 1983.

American Dental Association. *Nursing Bottle Mouth.* Chicago, IL: Bureau of Health Education and Audiovisual Services.

American Dental Association. *Your Child's Teeth.* Chicago, IL: Bureau of Health Education and Audiovisual Services, 1983.

Brunner, L. S., and D. S. Suddarth. *The Lippincott Manual of Nursing Practice.* Philadelphia: J. B. Lippincott, 1986.

Cada, D. J. *Drug Facts and Comparisons.* St. Louis, MO: Facts and Comparisons, 1995.

Center for Dental Information. *Preparing for a Lifetime of Smiles.* Princeton, NJ: Center for Dental Information.

Department of Health and Human Services (DHHS). *Diphtheria, Tetanus, Pertussis.* Atlanta, GA: Centers for Disease Control, October 15, 1991a.

Department of Health and Human Services (DHHS). *Polio.* Atlanta, GA: Centers for Disease Control, October 15, 1991b.

Department of Health and Human Services (DHHS). *DTaP.* Atlanta, GA: Centers for Disease Control, March 25, 1992.

Derschewitz, R. A. *Ambulatory Pediatrics.* Philadelphia: J. B. Lippincott, 1988.

Edwards, K. M., N. A. Halsey, T. Townsend, and D. T. Karson. Differences in antibody response to whole-cell pertussis vaccines. *Pediatrics* 88, no. 5 (1991): 1019–1023.

Johnson & Johnson Consumer Products. *Now, your child can grow up without a single cavity.* Skillman, NJ: Johnson & Johnson Consumer Products, 1990.

Julian, T. W. *Health Assessment and Physical Examination.* Albany, NY: Delmar Publishers, 1995.

Marks, M. G. *Broadribb's Introductory Pediatric Nursing,* 4th ed. Philadelphia: J. B. Lippincott, 1994.

Merenstein, G., W. Kaplan, and A. Rosenberg. *Handbook of Pediatrics.* Norwalk, CT: Appleton & Lange, 1991.

MMWR. National Childhood Vaccine Injury Act: Requirements for permanent vaccination records and for reporting of selected events after vaccination. *MMWR* 37, no. 13, (1988): 197–200.

MMWR. Measles prevention: Recommendations of the Immunization Practices Advisory Committee. *MMWR* 38 (S-9) (1989a).

MMWR. Rubella vaccine during pregnancy — United States, 1971–1988. *MMWR* 38, no. 17 (1989b): 289–293.

MMWR. Hepatitis B virus: A comprehensive strategy for eliminating transmission in the United States through universal childhood immunization. *MMWR* 40 (RR 13) (November, 1991).

Mott, S. R., S. R. James, and A. M. Sperhac. *Nursing Care of Children and Families*. Redwood City, CA: Addison-Wesley, 1990.

Pillitteri, A. *Maternal and Child Health Nursing*. Philadelphia: J. B. Lippincott, 1992.

Thompson, E. D., and J. W. Ashwill. *Pediatric Nursing: An Introductory Text*, 6th ed. Philadelphia: W. B. Saunders, 1992.

Vaccine Bulletin. Measles and herd immunity: The association of attack rates with immunization rates in preschool children. *Vaccine Bulletin* 61 (January, 1993).

Wong, D. L. *Whaley & Wong's Nursing Care of Infants and Children*, 5th ed. St. Louis, MO: Mosby–Year Book, 1995.

CHAPTER

10

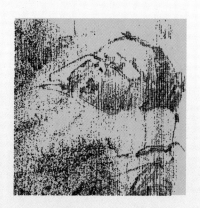

*C*hild Safety

OBJECTIVES

AFTER STUDYING THIS CHAPTER, THE STUDENT SHOULD BE ABLE TO:

- IDENTIFY THE LEADING CAUSE OF DEATH AND PERMANENT INJURY IN CHILDREN.

- IDENTIFY SPECIFIC FEDERAL REGULATIONS DESIGNED TO REDUCE THE INCIDENCE OF UNINTENTIONAL INJURY AMONG CHILDREN.

- DISCUSS MEASURES FOR PREVENTING UNINTENTIONAL INJURIES IN CHILDREN FROM INFANCY THROUGH ADOLESCENCE.

- IDENTIFY POISONS COMMONLY FOUND IN THE HOME.

- DEFINE CHILD ABUSE AND DIFFERENTIATE AMONG PHYSICAL ABUSE, EMOTIONAL ABUSE, SEXUAL ABUSE, AND NEGLECT.

- DESCRIBE SIGNS OF PHYSICAL ABUSE, SEXUAL ABUSE, AND NEGLECT.

- IDENTIFY THE ABCs OF CARDIOPULMONARY RESUSCITATION.

- DESCRIBE VARIATIONS FOR PERFORMING CARDIOPULMONARY RESUSCITATION ON AN INFANT OR CHILD VICTIM.

- DESCRIBE VARIATIONS FOR REMOVING A FOREIGN BODY OBSTRUCTION IN AN INFANT OR CHILD VICTIM.

KEY TERMS

GASTRIC LAVAGE

CHILD ABUSE

PHYSICAL ABUSE

EMOTIONAL ABUSE

SEXUAL ABUSE

NEGLECT

CARDIOPULMONARY RESUSCITATION (CPR)

RESCUE BREATHING

STRIDOR

HEIMLICH MANEUVER

*i*nfants and children depend on others to maintain a safe environment in which they can develop and grow. Providing a safe environment requires knowledge of behaviors that characterize children at different stages of their development. An essential part of the nurse's role involves educating parents about behaviors that place children at risk for unintentional injury or death.

Children who grow up in an abusive home environment are especially at risk for injury or death. Nurses must therefore be alert to the signs of physical or emotional abuse and ready to intervene promptly to protect the child from further harm. The nurse has a legal responsibility to report suspected abuse.

Emergency measures are, at times, necessary to help children who have sustained injury. Nurses and other health care providers must be able to perform techniques for cardiopulmonary resuscitation and removal of an object causing airway obstruction. Nurses should encourage parents and others in the community to become familiar with these lifesaving techniques.

ACCIDENTS

Accidents kill and permanently injure more children than any disease and are the leading cause of death in childhood. Most accidents occur in or near the home. Statistics also indicate that certain injuries are more common among specific age groups. Burns, for example, are a common occurrence in children. Toddlers are especially at risk, Figure 10–1. For

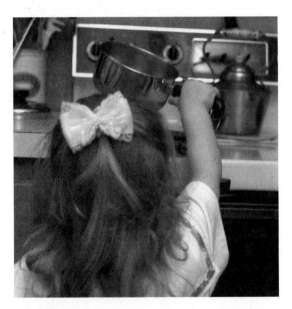

Figure 10–1   *Burns are a common cause of unintentional injury among toddlers, who can reach stove tops. Teach parents to place pots on back burners and turn pot handles toward the back of the stove, away from inquisitive hands.*

these reasons, a primary focus of nurses and other health care providers is educating parents about accident prevention through age-appropriate precautions, Figure 10–2.

The federal government and various private agencies have attempted to provide regulations for certain factors that influence some accidents. For example, regulations mandate the use of nonflammable fabric for children's sleepwear. Laws also require proper restraints for infants and small children while riding in automobiles, Figure 10–3. These restraints must meet standards set by the federal government.

ACCIDENT PREVENTION IN CHILDREN	
Injury	**Anticipatory Guidance**
Falls	• Secure infant in infant seat. • Do not leave infant unattended on tables or beds. • Use gates to block doorways and stairs. • Move chairs and ladders away from counters and cabinets.
Burns	• Be sure bath water and foods are not too hot. • Use safety covers on electrical outlets. • Keep fireplace screens closed. • Do not leave barbecue grills unattended. • Turn pot handles toward back of stove.
Poisoning	• Lock cabinets that contain medicines and cleaning products. • Keep all house plants out of child's reach. • Keep syrup of ipecac in the home. • Have poison control center number by the telephone.
Motor vehicle, pedestrian, biking accidents	• Be sure that car seats have approved infant/toddler restraint systems. • Use seat belts at all times. • Do not leave small children unattended out of doors. • Keep small children in a fenced-in yard if possible. • Have children use bicycle helmets at all times. • Teach children bicycle safety. • Have teenagers take driver education classes before getting their driver's license. • Discuss the importance of not drinking and using drugs while driving.
Drowning	• Do not leave children unsupervised near water or on a boat. • Use life jackets approved for children. • Keep home swimming pools covered when not in use. • Remember that a child can drown in a bath tub or a bucket of water.
Firearms	• Keep guns unloaded, out of reach, and locked away.

Figure 10–2

ALWAYS READ AND FOLLOW MANUFACTURER'S INSTRUCTIONS. If you do not have them, write to the company's consumer relations department, identifying the model number, name of seat, and date of manufacture. The manufacturer's address is on the label on the seat.

USING CAR SEATS CORRECTLY

After installing your car seat, be sure to check the following:

Is the seat facing the right way?
• **Never use an infant seat facing forward.** Infant car seats must always face toward the back of the car to support both the body and the head during a crash.

• **Use a convertible seat facing the rear for babies up to at least 20 pounds and at least 1 year of age.** The reclined, rear-facing position provides the best protection for your baby's neck.

• **Turn the convertible seat around to face forward for children who are over 20 pounds and at least 1 year of age.** When you face the seat forward, make three adjustments: move the seat into the upright position; move the shoulder straps to the set of harness slots indicated by the manufacturer's instructions (usually the highest slots); and route the seat belt through the proper belt path for this position.

Is your baby buckled into the car seat correctly?
• **Keep the harnesses snug,** and readjust them as your child grows. Use the plastic harness clip, if provided, at armpit level to hold shoulder straps in place.

• Make sure the straps lie flat and are not twisted. Keep the shoulder straps in the slots at or just below your baby's shoulders.

• Dress your baby in clothes that allow the straps to go between his or her legs. Keep the straps snug by adjusting them to allow for the thickness of your child's clothes.

• To keep a newborn from slouching, pad the sides of the seat and between the crotch with rolled up diapers or receiving blankets. If your infant's head flops forward, tilt the seat back until it is level by wedging firm padding, such as a rolled towel, under the front of the base of the seat.

Is the car seat installed in your vehicle correctly?
• **Check instructions to make sure the belt is in the correct path.** These are usually in different places in a convertible seat when the seat faces forward or rearward.

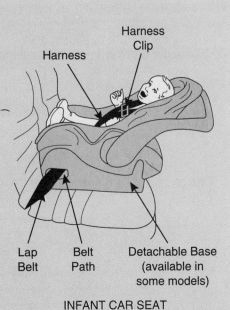

INFANT CAR SEAT

A

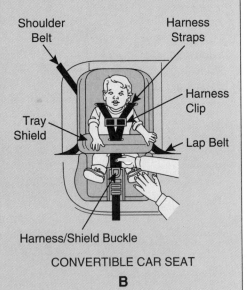

CONVERTIBLE CAR SEAT

B

Figure 10–3   *Proper use of a car seat for infants and small children is key to preventing or reducing injury in motor vehicle crashes. (Reproduced with permission of the American Academy of Pediatrics, Elk Grove Village, IL)*

• Route the seat belt through the correct path on the car seat and pull it tight.

• Before each trip, check to **make sure the belt that is holding the car seat in place is tight enough** by pushing on the car seat. It should not move easily from side to side or toward the front of the car. If it does:

• In a convertible seat, tighten the belt more while pressing the car seat firmly into the auto seat cushion with your knee.

• Feed the seat belt back into the wind-up reel to take up all the slack.

• Check the placement of the buckle. Make sure the buckle does not lie just at the point where the belt must bend around the frame of the car seat or through the slot of the car seat. If so, you will not be able to tighten the belt properly.

• If you are not able to tighten the belt, look for another set of belts in the car that can be tightened properly.

• Check your vehicle owner's manual to make sure your belts can be used to install car seats and for special instructions.

• Many lap/shoulder belts allow the passenger to move freely even when they are buckled. If your car has this type of seat belt, you will need to use a locking clip to secure the car seat. Locking clips are provided with all new car seats. **See the instructions that come with the car seat for information on how to use the locking clip.**

• Some vehicle lap belts (especially in front seats with automatic shoulder belts) need a special, heavy-duty locking clip. Check your car owner's manual or call the Hotline for help.

• Some car seats require the use of a tether strap. A tether strap is a belt that is attached to the car seat and bolted to the car. They are designed to give extra protection and keep the seat from being thrown forward in a crash. If you have a seat that requires or recommends a top tether strap when facing forward, be sure to install it according to instructions. A correctly used tether can offer improved protection and, in some cases, a safer, snug fit.

Remember: For current information about child safety seat recalls, safety notices, and replacement parts call the **Auto Safety Hotline at 800/424-9393** or the car seat manufacturer.

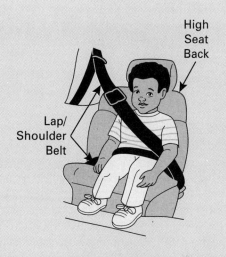

High Seat Back

Lap/ Shoulder Belt

SHIELD BOOSTER
C

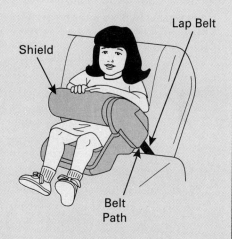

Lap Belt

Shield

Belt Path

SHIELD BOOSTER
D

Figure 10–3   *Continued*

The Child Protection and Toy Safety Act, passed in 1970, has helped to stop the distribution of unsafe toys. Nurses, however, should caution parents to inspect any toy purchased for small or loose parts that might cause injury.

POISONING

Poisoning — by the ingestion, inhalation, absorption, or injection of a toxic substance requiring intervention — is the most common pediatric emergency. Over 2 million poisoning cases involving children are reported to poison control centers in the United States each year; 5,000 of these cases result in death (Budassi Sheehy 1990). Poisoning is a major cause of preventable death in children under 5 years of age, with a peak incidence in children between 2 and 3 years of age. Children in this age group are at greater risk for poisoning because of their characteristic behaviors that involve exploration and testing of the environment (Eichelberger et al. 1992), Figure 10–4.

More than 90% of poisonings occur in the home and are usually caused by common household products, Figure 10–5. Poisonous substances that are commonly ingested by young children are listed in Figure 10–6. The Poison Prevention Packaging Act of 1970 requires that child safety caps be put on all potentially toxic substances and drugs. These caps are not, in fact, "child-proof," but rather are designed to delay access to the substance by a child under 4 years of age.

NURSING CONSIDERATIONS REGARDING CHILD SAFETY

- Teach parents accident prevention techniques regarding falls, burns, choking.
- Emphasize to parents the importance of keeping household plants out of the reach of children and locking up medications and household toxins.
- Stress to parents the proper use of car seats.
- Suggest that parents buy toys that are developmentally appropriate for their child.

DEVELOPMENTAL FACTORS THAT INCREASE POISONING RISK

- Child puts everything in the mouth as a means of exploring the environment.

- Child's sense of taste is not well developed, so he or she will drink or eat many liquids and substances that older children and adults would find distasteful.

- Child is becoming more independent, mobile, and curious.

- Child is now able to open drawers, closets, and most containers.

- Child cannot read labels.

Figure 10–4 *Developmental factors that place toddlers and small children at risk for poisoning (From Eichelberger, Ball, Pratsch, and Runion,* Pediatric Emergencies: A Manual for Prehospital Care Providers, *1992. Adapted by permission of Prentice-Hall, Englewood Cliffs, NJ)*

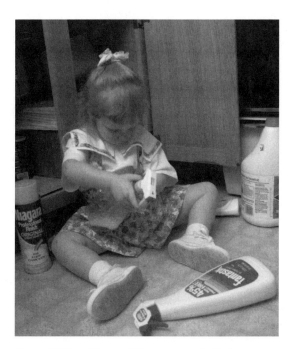

Figure 10–5 *Many substances found in the home present hazards to small children and should be kept in locked cabinets.*

In order to assess a situation and provide appropriate emergency instructions and care, the health care professional must obtain specific information from the parent or caregiver regarding the poison and the child's condition (Budassi Sheehy 1990), Figure 10–7. Because most substances are absorbed within two to four hours, it is important to act quickly.

Further absorption of a poison may be prevented by chemical removal, mechanical removal, or antidotes. Examples of each method are (1) syrup of ipecac, (2) gastric lavage, and (3) activated charcoal, respectively. The approach used will depend on the substance ingested.

Administer syrup of ipecac to stimulate vomiting. If a parent has syrup of ipecac at home, the recommended dose (Rosenstein and Fosarelli 1989) is

- *9 months:* 5 cc or 1 teaspoon (tsp)
- *9–12 months:* 10 cc or 2 tsp
- *1–12 years:* 15 cc or 1 tablespoon (Tbsp)
- *over 12 years:* 30 cc or 2 Tbsp

POISONOUS SUBSTANCES COMMONLY INGESTED BY CHILDREN

- Over-the-counter medications such as aspirin, acetaminophen, vitamins with iron, skin care preparations, and diaper care products

- Prescription drugs and sedatives

- House and garden plants, such as poinsettias, Boston ivy, elephant ear, ivy (leaves), mistletoe (berries), philodendron, daffodil (bulbs), azalea (foliage and flowers), and rhubarb (leaves)

- Household cleaners
- Petroleum products, such as heavy greases, oils, turpentine, furniture polish, gasoline, and lighter fluid
- Alcohol in alcoholic beverages, cold remedies, mouthwash, perfume, and alcohol-based paints and thinners
- Lead in lead-based paint, unglazed pottery, lead water pipes, and acid juices in leaded pottery

Figure 10–6   *(From Eichelberger, Ball, Pratsch, and Runion,* Pediatric Emergencies: A Manual for Prehospital Care Providers, *1992. Adapted by permission of Prentice-Hall, Englewood Cliffs, NJ)*

WHEN POISONING IS SUSPECTED

- What drug or product did the child take?

- How much did the child take?

- Is the child having any symptoms?

- Is the child having difficulty breathing?

- Has the child ever done this before?

- Tell parents or caregivers to transport the child to the nearest emergency department for evaluation and treatment if needed.

- Tell them to bring the product and product container — including empty containers — to the emergency department.

- Instruct them to save all emesis.

Figure 10–7 *Information to be obtained in suspected cases of pediatric poisoning (Adapted from Budassi Sheehy,* Mosby's Manual of Emergency Care, *3rd ed. Mosby-Year Book, St. Louis, 1990)*

NURSING CONSIDERATIONS REGARDING TOXIC SUBSTANCES

- Emphasize to parents the importance of keeping the poison control center number next to the telephone.

- Teach parents how to use syrup of ipecac, and stress the importance of keeping it in the home.

- Help parents express feelings of fear, anger, and guilt accompanying a child's unintentional injury or poisoning.

Ipecac usually takes effect in 15 to 20 minutes. Do not give ipecac if the child has ingested a caustic or hydrocarbon, is having a seizure, or is comatose. If there is no response to ipecac or vomiting is contraindicated, gastric lavage is ordered. **Gastric lavage** involves instilling large amounts of warm normal saline through a nasogastric tube into the child's stomach until the return is clear. Lavage is contraindicated for the ingestion of corrosives (lye, strong acids), strychnine, or hydrocarbons (kerosene, gasoline, paint thinner, cleaning fluid).

Ingestions are also treated with the administration of activated charcoal. Activated charcoal prevents absorption of the poison and promotes excretion from the body. There are no known contraindications or side effects. Charcoal has an ugly appearance and can be mixed with water, fruit juice, or syrup to make it easier for the child to drink. Charcoal can also be given by nasogastric or orogastric tube.

Ingestion of a poison may not, in fact, be accidental. Sometimes a child is abused by the administration of drugs. Often, the abuse continues while the child is in the hospital. Be suspicious if the child is less than 1 or more than 5 years of age; if more than one ingestion episode has occurred; if the clinical findings are inconsistent; and if risk factors for abuse are present (Rosenstein and Fosarelli 1989).

CHILD ABUSE

Child abuse — the intentional physical or emotional maltreatment or neglect of children — is a growing social problem. Physical abuse, physical neglect, emotional abuse, emotional neglect, verbal assault, or sexual assault are all forms of child abuse (Harris 1993).

In the United States, it is estimated that there are 50,000 to 70,000 child abuse cases each year (Budassi Sheehy 1990). After sudden infant death syndrome, child abuse is the leading cause of death in infants under 6 months of age (Eichelberger et al. 1992). Many children die each year as a result of child abuse injuries. The child should be removed from the abusive situation as soon as possible to prevent further injury.

It is the nurse's duty to report suspected cases of child abuse to the appropriate legal authorities. Every state has laws that protect children from abuse. Although coming to the realization that a child has been abused is difficult, it is a moral and legal responsibility to report such findings.

PSYCHOSOCIAL FACTORS CONTRIBUTING TO ABUSE

Abuse usually occurs because the abuser is having difficulty coping. Many factors can contribute to the abuse of a child, including economic stressors (poverty, unemployment, too many children), marital problems, single parenthood, inadequate or lack of support systems, and drug or alcohol abuse (Eichelberger et al. 1992). In addition, a child's personality, chronic illness, or physical disabilities can place him or her at high risk for abuse.

TYPES OF ABUSE

Physical Abuse. **Physical abuse** is defined as deliberate physical maltreatment that causes injury to the body. The injuries may be caused by beatings, burns, shaking, or throwing the

child. Characteristic signs of physical abuse are listed in Figure 10–8.

Emotional Abuse. Any interaction over a period of time that causes a child unnecessary psychological pain is **emotional abuse**, including excessive demands, verbal harassment, excessive yelling, belittling, teasing, or rejection. Because the signs of emotional abuse are often subtle, this is one of the most difficult types of abuse to identify and prevent.

Sexual Abuse. **Sexual abuse** entails sexual contact between a child, 16 years of age or younger, and a person in a position of authority, no matter what the age, in which the child's participation was obtained through force, threats, bribes, or gifts. Sexual contact can include intercourse, masturbation, fondling, exhibitionism, sodomy, or prostitution (Eichelberger et al. 1992, Rosenstein and Fosarelli 1989).

Physical signs of sexual abuse include bruises on the genitals; a small tear or laceration of the vagina, penis, or anus; semen on the body; and discharge from the urethra, vagina, or penis.

Neglect. **Neglect** refers to the deliberate or unintentional lack of care for a child's basic needs that places the child's life or health in danger (Eichelberger et al. 1992). Neglect can include poor nutrition, inadequate medical care, lack of psychosocial support systems, or lack of education. The absence of daily care and abandonment of the child are also considered neglect.

NURSING CONSIDERATIONS REGARDING CHILD ABUSE

- Become familiar with state laws for the prevention of child abuse and neglect.
- Develop skills to recognize the signs of abuse in children.

Signs of Physical Abuse in Children

- Small round burns or scars.

- Glove or stocking burns from immersion of the hands or feet in hot water. These burns have a characteristic lack of splash marks.

- Burns to buttocks, legs, and feet, often with creases behind the knees and lack of involvement of the upper thighs.

- Clearly defined burns showing the shape of the object used — for example, an iron, stove burner, oven rack, or radiator.

- Slap marks resembling the shape of a hand.

- Welts showing the shape of the object used — for example, a belt, buckle, hanger, electrical cord.

- Suspicious bruises in various stages of healing. Active children often have bruises over bony prominences such as the shins, hips, spine, lower arms, forehead, and under the chin. These are caused by falling and bumping into objects during play. Suspicious sites for bruises are on the upper arms, trunk, upper thighs, sides of the face, ears and neck, genitalia, and buttocks.

- Human bite marks indicating the pattern of teeth and size of an adult's mouth.

Figure 10–8 (From Eichelberger, Ball, Pratsch, and Runion, Pediatric Emergencies: A Manual for Prehospital Care Providers, 1992. *Adapted by permission of Prentice-Hall, Englewood Cliffs, NJ)*

Pediatric Basic Life Support: The ABCs of CPR

Cardiopulmonary Resuscitation

Cardiopulmonary resuscitation (CPR) provides basic life support to a victim who, unable to breathe or pump sufficient blood through the body, would otherwise die. There are three basic skill groups known as the ABCs of CPR: *Airway, Breathing,* and *Circulation.*

Airway — Determine Responsiveness. The nurse must first determine whether the infant or child is conscious and breathing. To determine the level of responsiveness, tap the child and speak loudly. When the child is unconscious, the muscles in the mouth and throat relax, allowing the tongue to fall back into the throat and obstruct the airway. The airway should be opened immediately using the head tilt–chin lift maneuver, Figure 10–9a, b. If neck injury is sus-

pected, the head tilt should be avoided and the airway opened using a jaw thrust, instead, keeping the cervical spine completely immobilized.

Breathing — Assessment. Once the airway is opened, check for breathing. Look for a rise and fall of the chest and abdomen, listen for exhaled air, and feel for exhaled air flow at the mouth. If no movement is observed, **rescue breathing** is begun, Figure 10–9c, d.

If the victim is an infant (under 1 year of age), place your mouth over the infant's nose and mouth, creating a seal. If the victim is a large infant or child (1–8 years of age), make a mouth-to-mouth seal, pinching the victim's nose tightly with your thumb and forefinger and maintaining the head tilt with your other hand. Provide two slow breaths to the victim, pausing in between to take a breath. If a mask with a one-way valve or other infection-control barrier is available, it should be used when performing rescue breathing.

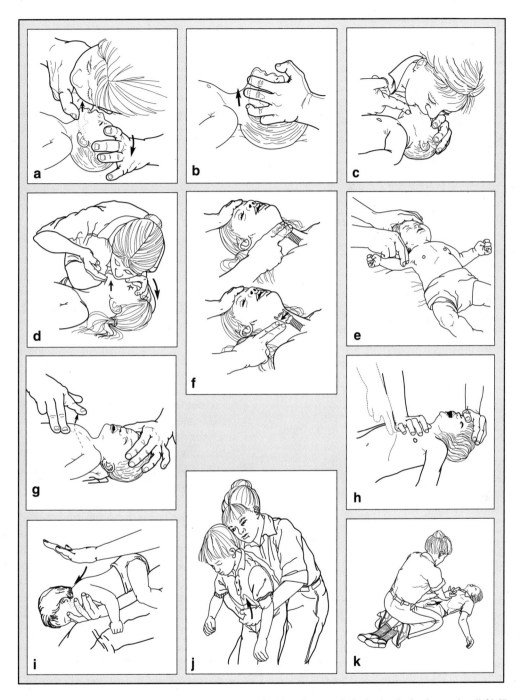

Figure 10–9 *Procedures for cardiopulmonary resuscitation (a–h) and removal of a foreign body obstruction (i–k) (From Emergency Cardiac Care Committee and Subcommittees, American Heart Association, 1992. Guidelines for cardiopulmonary resuscitation and emergency cardiac care. V. Pediatric basic life support.* Journal of the American Medical Association, *vol. 268, no. 16)*

If the chest does not rise after the initial breaths, airway obstruction may be the cause. Reposition the victim's head by performing the head tilt–chin lift or jaw thrust maneuver. If the chest still does not rise, the obstruction may be from a foreign body. Once the airway is opened and two rescue breaths have been provided, determine whether chest compression is needed.

Circulation — Assessment (Pulse Check). Assess the pulse in a large central artery. The short, chubby neck of children under 1 year of age makes rapid location of the carotid artery difficult, so palpation of the brachial artery is recommended, Figure 10–9e. In children over 1 year of age, the carotid artery on the side of the neck is used, Figure 10–9f.

If a pulse is present but the infant or child is not breathing, rescue breathing alone should be provided at a rate of 20 breaths per minute (once every 3 seconds) until spontaneous breathing resumes. If a pulse is not palpable, external chest compressions are begun.

Chest Compressions

Chest compressions must always be accompanied by ventilations. To achieve optimal compressions place the infant or child in a supine position on a hard, flat surface.

The area of compression for infants is the lower third of the sternum, Figure 10–9g. Landmarks and technique for chest compression in an infant are as follows:

1. Draw an imaginary line (intermammary line) between the nipples, over the breastbone.
2. Place your index finger on the sternum just below the intermammary line. Place your middle and ring fingers approximately a fingerwidth below the line where it intersects the sternum. Avoid compression of the xiphoid process.
3. Compress the chest ½ to 1 inch at the rate of at least 100 times per minute. Pause for ventilation.

4. At the end of each compression, pressure is released without removing the fingers from the surface of the chest.

Landmarks and technique for chest compression in a child are as follows:

1. Using the middle and index fingers of the hand nearer the victim's feet, trace the lower margin of the victim's rib cage, on the side of the chest next to you.
2. Using the middle finger, follow the margin of the rib cage to the notch where the ribs and sternum meet.
3. With the middle finger on this notch, place the index finger next to the middle finger.
4. Place the heel of the same hand next to the point where the index finger was located, with the long axis of the heel parallel to that of the sternum, Figure 10–9h. The fingers should be held up off the ribs while the heel of the hand remains in contact with the sternum.
5. Use your other hand to maintain the child's head position.
6. Compress the chest 1–1½ inches at the rate of 100 times per minute. Pause for ventilation.
7. Compressions should be smooth. Allow the chest to return to its resting position after each compression, but do not lift your hand off of the chest.

Coordination of Compressions and Rescue Breathing. External chest compressions must always be accompanied by rescue breathing. At the end of every five compressions, a pause of 1–1½ seconds should be allowed for a ventilation. The infant and small child should be reassessed after 20 cycles of compressions and ventilations (approximately 1 minute) and every few minutes thereafter for any sign of resumption of spontaneous breathing or pulses.

If you are alone, call for help after 1 minute of rescue support (20 breaths including chest compressions, if necessary). If the victim is small and no trauma is suspected, it may be possible to carry the child (supporting the head and neck carefully) to a telephone while CPR is provided so that you can call for help.

FOREIGN BODY AIRWAY OBSTRUCTION

The most common cause of respiratory distress in children is airway obstruction. Aspiration of a foreign body can result in airway obstruction and death. Foreign body aspiration is the second leading cause of unintentional injury deaths in infants between 1 month and 1 year of age and the fifth leading cause in children 1 to 4 years of age. Commonly aspirated foods include hot dogs, uncooked vegetables, peanuts, grapes, beans, candy, and seeds. The size, shape, and consistency of the object contribute to the severity of the symptoms.

The Infant. If an infant or child experiences the sudden onset of respiratory distress associated with coughing, gagging, or **stridor** (a high-pitched, noisy sound or wheezing), suspect foreign body aspiration. Relief of the obstruction should be attempted only if the cough is or becomes ineffective (loss of sound) or the child is having increasing respiratory difficulty, accompanied by stridor.

The Child: The Heimlich Maneuver. In children under 1 year of age, a combination of five back blows and five chest thrusts is used to try to remove the obstruction, Figure 10–9i. Back blows are delivered while the infant is supported in the prone position along the arm; chest thrusts are delivered while the infant is supine. Remove the foreign body if it can be seen.

In older children, subdiaphragmatic abdominal thrusts are performed with the child either sitting, standing, or lying (**Heimlich maneuver**), Figure 10–9j, k.

When the child is conscious and is either standing or sitting, perform the following steps.

1. Stand behind the child with your arms directly under the child's axillae and encircling the child's chest.
2. Make a fist with one hand, placing the thumb side against the midline of the child's abdomen, slightly above the navel and below the tip of the xiphoid process.
3. Grasp the fist with the other hand and exert a series of up to five quick upward thrusts. Take care not to press on the xiphoid or the rib cage because of the potential for damage to internal organs.

When the child is unconscious and lying on the floor, perform these steps.

1. Place the child supine and kneel beside the child or straddle the child's hips.
2. Place the heel of one hand in the midline of the child's abdomen above the navel and below the rib cage and xiphoid process. Place the other hand on top of the first.
3. Press both hands into the abdomen with a quick upward thrust. Each thrust is directed upward in the midline and should not be directed to either side of the abdomen.

Individual thrusts should continue until the foreign body is expelled or until five abdominal thrusts have been delivered. If the foreign body can be seen, remove it.

NURSING CONSIDERATIONS REGARDING CPR	
• Promote classes in CPR for the general public.	• Encourage new parents to learn CPR and to recertify periodically to maintain these skills.

REVIEW QUESTIONS

A. Multiple choice. Select the best answer.

1. Most deaths among children are caused by
   a. child abuse
   b. accidents
   c. burns
   d. drowning

2. The recommended dose of syrup of ipecac for a 3-year-old toddler is
   a. 5 cc (1 tsp)
   b. 10 cc (2 tsp)
   c. 15 cc (1 Tbsp)
   d. 30 cc (2 Tbsp)

3. Syrup of ipecac may be used
   a. to stimulate vomiting when some poisons have been ingested
   b. when the child is in a coma from poisoning
   c. to stop convulsions from poisoning
   d. as an antidote for caustics

4. Gastric lavage is indicated when
   a. a corrosive, such as lye or strong acid, has been ingested
   b. there is no response to ipecac or when vomiting is contraindicated
   c. strychnine poisoning occurs
   d. a child drinks a hydrocarbon such as kerosene

5. The incidence of child abuse in the United States each year is approximately
   a. 10,000–15,000 cases
   b. 20,000–30,000 cases
   c. 50,000–70,000 cases
   d. 100,000–150,000 cases

6. Which of the following is a form of neglect?
   a. excessive yelling
   b. rejection
   c. teasing
   d. poor nutrition

7. Which of the following is *not* true of sexual abuse?
   a. Sexual contact is not limited to intercourse.
   b. Most of the signs of sexual abuse are easily spotted.
   c. Overt signs of sexual abuse include bruising on the genitals, lacerations of the vagina or anus, semen on the body, discharge from the vagina or penis.
   d. It involves a child, 16 years or younger, with another person in a position of authority.

8. The rate of chest compressions used when performing CPR on a 10-year-old child should be
   a. 60 times/minute
   b. 80 times/minute
   c. 100 times/minute
   d. 120 times/minute

9. When performing CPR on an unconscious child, one should not
   a. shake the child gently to determine the level of response
   b. open the airway manually using the head tilt–chin lift
   c. open the airway manually using the jaw thrust maneuver
   d. leave the neck unstabilized if a cervical spine injury is suspected

10. The most common cause of respiratory distress in children is
    a. cardiac arrest
    b. airway obstruction
    c. asthma
    d. child abuse

SUGGESTED ACTIVITIES

- Create a teaching tool to educate peers or parents about one of the following:
  - falls
  - burns
  - choking
  - firearms
  - poisoning
  - vehicle/bicycle crashes
  - drowning
  - assault

- Describe and demonstrate how the procedure for performing CPR on an infant differs from the procedure for a child.

- Describe and demonstrate how the procedure for removing a foreign body obstruction from an infant differs from the procedure for a child.

- Discuss how the nurse can help parents express feelings of fear, anger, and guilt when a child is injured or poisoned, and list three ways of providing emotional support.

BIBLIOGRAPHY

American Heart Association. *Healthcare Provider's Manual for Basic Life Support.* Dallas: American Heart Association, 1988.

Budassi Sheehy, S. *Mosby's Manual of Emergency Care,* 3rd ed. St. Louis, MO: Mosby-Year Book, 1990.

Eichelberger, M. R., J. W. Ball, G. S. Pratsch, and E. Runion. *Pediatric Emergencies: A Manual for Prehospital Care Providers.* Englewood Cliffs, NJ: Brady/Prentice-Hall, 1992.

Emergency Cardiac Care Committee and Subcommittees, American Heart Association. Guidelines for cardiopulmonary resuscitation and emergency cardiac care. V. Pediatric basic life support. *Journal of the American Medical Association* 268, no. 16 (1992): 2251–2261.

Harris, P. *A Child's Story: Recovering through Creativity.* St. Louis, MO: Cracom Corporation, 1993.

Jones, N. E. Prevention of childhood injuries: Motor vehicle injuries. *Pediatric Nursing* 18, no. 4 (1992): 380–382.

Kottmeier, P. K. The battered child. *Pediatric Annals* 16, no. 4 (April, 1987): 343–351.

Rosenstein, B. J., and P. D. Fosarelli. *Pediatric Pearls: The Handbook of Practical Pediatrics.* St. Louis, MO: Mosby-Year Book, 1989.

Seidel, J., et al. Presentation and evaluation of sexual misuse in the emergency department. *Pediatric Emergency Care* 2 (1986): 157–164.

Willens, J. S. Strengthen your life-support skills. *Nursing 93* 23, no. 4 (1993): 54–58.

Wong, D. L. *Whaley & Wong's Essentials of Pediatric Nursing,* 4th ed. St. Louis, MO: Mosby-Year Book, 1993.

Hospitalization

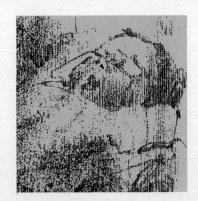

*P*reparing for Hospitalization

OBJECTIVES

AFTER STUDYING THIS CHAPTER, THE STUDENT SHOULD BE ABLE TO:

- DISCUSS THE ROLE OF THE NURSE IN PREPARING A CHILD AND FAMILY FOR HOSPITALIZATION.
- IDENTIFY THE TYPE OF INFORMATION NEEDED BY THE FAMILY OF THE HOSPITALIZED CHILD PRIOR TO ADMISSION.
- IDENTIFY INDICATORS OF STRESS AMONG SIBLINGS OF A HOSPITALIZED CHILD.
- IDENTIFY STRATEGIES THAT CAN BE USED TO PREPARE CHILDREN OF DIFFERENT AGES FOR HOSPITALIZATION.
- DISCUSS THE IMPORTANCE OF COMMUNICATION IN PREPARING CHILDREN OF DIFFERENT AGES FOR HOSPITALIZATION.

KEY TERMS

STRESSORS   RITUALS

DISBELIEF

ospitalization of a child can be planned or unplanned. For most children, regardless of the reason for admission, hospitalization is a fearful bewildering experience (Faller 1988). Even with preparation, it places stress on the child and the family. Unfamiliar sounds, smells, routines, and strangers; confinement; separation from parents and siblings; and loss of control are only a few of the **stressors** with which a child must cope during hospitalization.

PREPARING THE FAMILY FOR HOSPITALIZATION

Adequate preparation of the family can influence the child's adjustment to hospitalization, Figure 11–1. The focus of this preparation is to

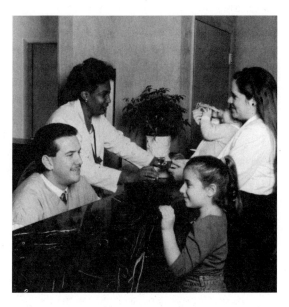

Figure 11–1   *Preadmission and day of admission activities can help prepare children and their families for the planned hospitalization.*

minimize stress and avoid crisis. A planned hospitalization can be an organized effort to comfort both the family and the child. Planning can involve a hospital teaching program that encompasses preadmission activities, day of admission activities, and discharge planning. The trend in many pediatric acute care settings is to include the family in a significant way (Brown and Ritchie 1990).

FAMILY ASSESSMENT

The first step in preparing the family is assessing their level of knowledge. What do they know? What do they need to know? Good communication skills and interviewing techniques are essential because the seriousness of the child's illness affects family reactions.

In the assessment process, the nurse should allow for a free exchange of information. This approach helps to build a positive relationship in which parents are able to talk openly about concerns and fears. It also gives the nurse an opportunity to learn the family structure, ages of siblings, and support systems that may already be present. Note the socioeconomic level and cultural and spiritual affiliation of the family, as well as the interaction between parents. Illness of a child can place additional stressors on the parents' relationship and reduce their ability to cope.

Throughout the assessment phase, reinforce to parents that they are an integral part of the child's recovery. Parenting the child should not change, and preparation for discharge should begin on admission. Observe and assess the parents' reaction to the child's illness. If the child has been diagnosed with an illness such as leukemia or cystic fibrosis that has long-term effects, parents may have difficulty believing that this is actually happening to their child. This **disbelief** is often coupled with anger and guilt. Anger, which may be directed at themselves or at others, is common. Parents may look for reasons for the onset of illness in their own actions or perceived shortcomings. Feelings of guilt can surface when parents anticipate their helplessness when confronted by their child's illness and pain.

The importance of the assessment phase should not be minimized. Hospitals in which preadmission teaching or conferences take place provide the nurse with an opportunity for conducting a planned interview.

PREADMISSION TEACHING AND INTERVIEW

Dialogue should be geared toward the parents' level of understanding. Language barriers and cultural patterns need to be considered to make teaching effective.

Ideally both parents should participate in the teaching process. Sometimes, however, one parent is more accepting and ready to participate than the other.

The information presented to parents should be honest and accurate. It should include anticipated reactions of the child to hospitalization. Telling the child about hospitalization can be traumatic for parents. How much do they say? What do they say? The answers to these questions will depend on the child's age and developmental level and the seriousness of the illness. Allow time between sessions for parents to formulate questions and develop strategies to help the child learn about hospitalization. Several resources are available to parents to help them formulate their approach, Figure 11–2. Particularly effective are books that can be read to the child in preparation for hospitalization, Figure 11–3.

Parents should be encouraged to participate in the care of the child during hospitalization. Mutual participation is ideal but not always practical. Parents may need to take turns visiting the child, particularly if there are other children at home. Working parents may find it difficult to care for their hospitalized child, so planning for extended family members to participate may be appropriate. Adjusting a work schedule may take some planning. But participation by parents will help ease feelings of helplessness, loss of control, and loss of the parenting role (Petrillo and Sanger 1980).

Be aware that in some cultures, adults other than the child's parents may provide important support to the child and family. Among Mexican Americans, for example, a godparent may be an important participant in

---

RESOURCE BOOKS

Curious George Goes to the Hospital, M. Rey and H. A. Rey, Houghton Mifflin Company.

Doctors and Nurses: What Do They Do? C. Green, Harper & Row Junior Books.

The Hospital Book, J. Howe, Crown Publishers.

Richard Scarry's Nicky Goes to the Doctor, R. Scarry, A Golden Book.

Why Am I Going to the Hospital? C. Ciliotta and C. Livingston, Lyle Stuart.

Your Child Goes to the Hospital: A Book for Parents, H. Love et al., Charles C. Thomas.

Note: Most major bookstores will special order books if they are not available on the shelf.

Figure 11–2   *Resource books to help prepare children for hospitalization*

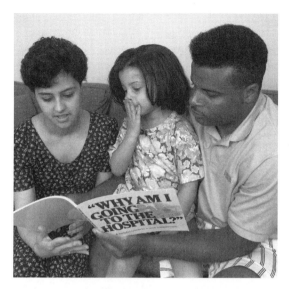

Figure 11–3 *Reading the child books that describe the hospital stay is one strategy that parents can use to prepare the child before admission.*

care of the hospitalized child. The presence of these support persons reduces the family's fear and anxiety and facilitates adjustment to the hospital setting (Giger and Davidhizar 1991). When extended family members or godparents will be present, it is important that they be identified to the staff.

Parents should be taught that the hospitalized child may exhibit uncharacteristic behaviors. That is, the child may be stubborn, overly quiet, sad, uncommunicative, or unruly. The child may cry without much provocation, and younger children, especially, may regress to behaviors such as bed wetting, thumb sucking, and use of the bottle or pacifier (Bolig and Weedle 1988). Hospitalization is particularly stressful for toddlers, who experience separation anxiety when parted from parents (see Chapter 13). Advising parents of these anticipated behavioral changes can help them cope when these behaviors occur.

During the preadmission interview, ask parents to describe the child's daily routine.

Ask about the child's toileting habits and the words ·used for toileting. It is important to know if the child takes an afternoon nap or if there is a favorite afterschool activity or television program. These **rituals** can be comforting and provide for emotional stability. Encourage parents to bring the child's favorite toys, blankets, books, or other objects from home. Figure 11–4 lists age-appropriate toys and activities that can be provided for the hospitalized child. Rooming-in also should be encouraged where it is permitted. The focus of this strategy is to minimize separation and maintain the appearance of the child's basic routine (Brown and Ritchie 1990).

Parents should be prepared for anticipated tests and procedures before admission and informed about pertinent preoperative and postoperative care. Blood workups and x-rays are common preadmission procedures. Information about anesthesia can be discussed at this time.

SIBLINGS

One area of teaching that is often neglected is the impact of hospitalization on the siblings of the hospitalized child. Age-appropriate information should be shared with the siblings. Clear, concise, truthful answers are best. Often, siblings feel neglected and less loved because the attention is on the hospitalized child. The parents' role should include listening to siblings and allowing them time to express their feelings and concerns. Time should be taken to praise them and reinforce their need to be loved (Craft and Craft 1989). Siblings often wonder if they will get sick too. Magical thinking is common among preschool children and may lead siblings at this developmental stage to believe that their thoughts and deeds caused the hospitalized child's illness. Rivalry, which may have existed before hospitalization, also can be a source of guilt and shame.

Separation does nothing to foster family ties, so siblings are encouraged to visit when

Anticipatory Guidance	
Age	**Toys/Activities**
Infant	Mobiles
	Cradle gyms
	Busy box
	Stuffed animals
Toddler	Stuffed animals
	Doctor's kit
	Dolls
	Picture books
	Simple puzzles
Preschool child	Balloons
	Puppets
	Crayons
	Toy hospital
	Books
	In-room television
School-age child	Playing cards
	Television
	Video games
	Transistor radio
	Books
	Simple games
	Cut outs
	Writing materials
	Art supplies
	Cuddly toys
Adolescent	Telephone
	Television
	Video games/movies
	Books
	Writing materials
	Art supplies
	Board games

Figure 11–4 *Anticipatory guidance: Age-appropriate toys and activities for hospitalized children*

possible. When visiting is not practical because of the age or emotional maturity of the siblings, they can send letters, pictures, photographs, cards, and even telephone the hospitalized child to maintain contact (Petrillo and Sanger 1980). Parents who are already having to cope with their own feelings and emotions have the added task of monitoring the support needed by the siblings.

Preparing the Child for Hospitalization

Preparation of the child for hospitalization is dependent on the child's age and stage of development. Telling the child about hospitalization, explaining procedures, and gaining cooperation are linked to the child's developmental readiness (Faller 1988). Timing of preparation is also age-dependent. Young children can be told about the planned hospitalization one to three days before admission, school-age children one week before admission, and adolescents as soon as the need for hospitalization is determined (Cowen 1993).

Theories of development proposed by Freud, Piaget, and Erikson provide a framework for anticipating responses of children at particular ages (refer to Chapter 7). Erikson's approach, based on psychosocial tasks or crises, is useful in developing age-appropriate approaches to children (Erikson 1963). Knowing what is normal can help nurses formulate the plan of care for children in stressful situations.

Using Erikson's theory as a framework, the following discussion provides both the family and nurse with information to meet the needs of the child before and during hospital admission.

Infant

According to Erikson, psychosocial tasks in the first year center on trust versus mistrust. At this stage, the infant can signal needs by crying or contentment. The infant's sense of self is closely tied to the caregiver. Talking to the infant, holding, and cuddling can lessen the traumatic experience of hospitalization. Encourage parents to room in, hold, feed, play, and provide some level of stimulation to the infant during hospitalization to encourage normal development.

TODDLER

From 1 to 3 years, psychosocial tasks focus on autonomy versus shame and doubt. The toddler is aware of hospitalization, separation, and loss of control. Parents and caregivers should explain in simple terms what is happening and how it will help to make the child better.

PRESCHOOL CHILD

The preschool years, from 3 to 6 years, are characterized by the psychosocial tasks of initiative versus guilt. The preschool child responds verbally and has many questions. Particular care must be given to explain hospitalization and procedures. Fear of bodily mutilation is common in this age group. At this age, the child responds well to prehospitalization programs. Introduce the child to the environment, particularly the unit or room, to help reduce the fear of the unknown. Emphasize healing and helping when discussing the need for hospitalization and procedures.

SCHOOL-AGE CHILD

The school-age years, from 6 to 12, are characterized by the psychosocial tasks of industry versus inferiority. The school-age child needs to have positive reinforcement. Be sure the child understands that hospitalization is not a punishment for something he or she did wrong. Self-confidence can be fragile, and trust at this stage is paramount. Preparation can involve simple books, diagrams, videotapes, and the opportunity to handle equipment (Cowen 1993).

ADOLESCENT

Adolescence, the period between 12 and 18 years, is characterized by the psychosocial tasks of identity versus role diffusion. Adolescents have an increasing sense of self and are influenced by peer groups and leadership. Hospitalization is particularly stressful because the adolescent is viewed as separate from the group. Visits from peers should be encouraged. Adolescents understand simple to complex medical terms and can be provided with verbal explanations, books, and diagrams to explain planned procedures (Cowen 1993). Adolescents have the ability to make decisions and should be involved in planning for hospitalization and given options, when appropriate.

NURSING CONSIDERATIONS IN PREPARING CHILDREN FOR HOSPITALIZATION

- Understanding growth and development milestones can assist the nurse in teaching and caring for the hospitalized child.
- In an ideal situation, in which hospitalization is planned, preadmission preparation should help meet parents' need to provide support and participate in care, as well as their needs for information and reinforcement. Siblings should have an opportunity to participate, ask questions, and continue to participate within the family circle.
- For the child, developmentally appropriate preparation can reduce stressors such as separation anxiety, fear of the unknown, and loss of control. A less-stressful experience, in turn, aids in the healing process.

Review Questions

A. Multiple choice. Select the best answer.

1. Interviewing the parent(s) is an integral part of the assessment process before the hospitalization of a child. Which of the following techniques is the best method to obtain information?
   a. Let parents direct the course of the interview.
   b. Give parents a checklist of questions.
   c. Talk to parents using open-ended questions.
   d. Quiz parents about how you can meet their needs.

2. The goal of the assessment process is to collect information and ultimately plan with the family a positive hospital experience. What would be the best first step?
   a. Use your interviewing skills to find out what the family knows about the child's hospitalization and illness.
   b. Be cordial and upbeat in your first meeting.
   c. Let parents take the inquiring role, since they know all about the child.
   d. Talk to only one parent at a time.

3. Preparing for the hospitalization of a child can create stress in the relationship of the parents. Even though it is best to talk to both parents, the nurse might interact primarily with one when the other parent
   a. keeps interrupting with questions
   b. refuses to participate in the discussion
   c. keeps projecting blame for the child's problem
   d. cries during the discussion

4. Participating in care is important for parents because
   a. it allows the parents to remain occupied
   b. parents know how to take care of the child better than the staff
   c. it is comforting for the child to have familiar caregivers
   d. it allows parents to monitor the staff

5. Many hospitals have preadmission programs and perform tests on an out-patient basis. The reason for this approach to child care is to
   a. save money
   b. introduce the family and child to the hospital in an organized manner
   c. help the staff form a relationship with the family
   d. get all the information needed before hospitalization

6. The role of the nurse in preparing the family for hospitalization is to
   a. provide support information as reinforcement for parents
   b. make sure the parents will not give false information to the child
   c. keep the child from being anxious about hospitalization
   d. allow the parents and child to pick out the room

7. Which of the following measures can be used to promote family harmony during a child's hospitalization?
   a. Siblings should not be told the truth about the hospitalization so that they do not worry too much.
   b. Parents should encourage and plan for visits by the siblings.
   c. Parents should have a significant other take care of the children at home because their time is limited.
   d. Parents should maintain a happy disposition.

8. Preparation for hospitalization for a child between the ages of 1 and 3 should include
   a. limiting parents' time with the child, since the child cries when they leave
   b. encouraging parents to keep the child neat and clean
   c. holding, cuddling, and talking to the child
   d. keeping the child in his or her own room to avoid exposure to any other illness

9. For children between the ages of 6 and 12, the preparation for hospitalization should include
   a. a truthful explanation in language that is nonthreatening
   b. an explanation that omits all the hurtful parts
   c. an explanation in terms they will not really understand to keep them from being afraid
   d. an explanation that is given only by the nurse, since she understands most about the illness

10. When an adolescent is hospitalized, the best preparation includes
   a. having a regular time for school friends to visit
   b. having the adolescent participate in decision making
   c. having the adolescent view all the procedures in which he or she will be involved
   d. limiting parents' visits, since the parents really do not understand this child

SUGGESTED ACTIVITIES

• Contact your local hospital's public relations department and inquire about the programs that are conducted to prepare for the hospitalization of a child. Make arrangements to view audiovisual materials that may be available.

• Practice communication techniques by role playing with classmates. Have a fellow student pick a developmental stage and diagnosis; then prepare the student for hospitalization.

• Contact a childcare center and arrange to observe normal child interactions. Compare and contrast the behaviors you observe with those of a hospitalized child.

• Read several of the books on the resource list in Figure 11–2 and develop a book review for each so that you can recommend particular books with some knowledge of their content.

BIBLIOGRAPHY

Bolig, R., and K. D. Weedle. Resiliency and hospitalization of children. *Child Health Care* 16, no. 4
(1988): 255–260.

Brown, J., and J. A. Ritchie. Nurses' perceptions of parent and nurse roles in caring for hospitalized children. *Child Health Care* 19, no. 1 (1990): 28–36.

Cowen, K. J. Hospital care for children. In D. Broadwell
Jackson and R. B. Saunders, eds. *Child Health
Nursing*. Philadelphia: J. B. Lippincott, 1993.

Craft, M. J., and J. L. Craft. Perceived changes in siblings of hospitalized children: A comparison of
sibling and parent reports. *Child Health Care* 18,
no. 1 (1989): 42–48.

Erikson, E. H. *Childhood and Society*, 2nd ed. New York:
W. W. Norton, 1963.

Faller, H. S. A child's perception of the hospital. *American
Journal of Maternal-Child Nursing* 13 (1988): 38.

Giger, J. N., and R. F. Davidhizar. *Transcultural Nursing:
Assessment and Intervention*. St. Louis, MO: Mosby-
Year Book, 1991.

Petrillo, M., and S. Sanger. *Emotional Care of Hospitalized
Children*, 2nd ed. Philadelphia: J. B. Lippincott,
1980.

Pontious, S. L. Practical Piaget: Helping children understand. *American Journal of Nursing* 82 (1982): 114–117.

CHAPTER

12

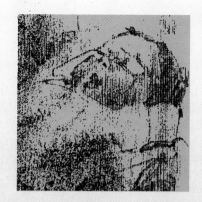

*A*ssessment

OBJECTIVES

AFTER STUDYING THIS CHAPTER, THE STUDENT SHOULD BE ABLE TO:

- IDENTIFY COMMON METHODS FOR MEASURING A CHILD'S PHYSICAL GROWTH.

- DESCRIBE THE VARIOUS METHODS AVAILABLE FOR MEASURING WEIGHT AND HEIGHT IN INFANTS, CHILDREN, AND ADOLESCENTS.

- DESCRIBE THE VARIOUS METHODS AVAILABLE FOR TAKING A CHILD'S TEMPERATURE.

- DESCRIBE THE RECOMMENDED METHODS FOR TAKING A CHILD'S PULSE.

- DEFINE SINUS ARRHYTHMIA AND EXPLAIN ITS SIGNIFICANCE TO PEDIATRIC ASSESSMENT.

- DESCRIBE METHODS FOR TAKING A CHILD'S BLOOD PRESSURE.

- DISCUSS NURSING CONSIDERATIONS IN PEDIATRIC ASSESSMENT.

KEY TERMS

HEAD CIRCUMFERENCE   SINUS ARRHYTHMIA

APICAL PULSE

175

outine pediatric assessment includes physical measurements (height, weight, head circumference, and chest circumference) and vital sign assessment (temperature, pulse, respirations, and blood pressure). Physical measurements help the nurse to determine whether a child's growth is within the normal parameters for his or her age. These measurements, along with vital sign assessment, provide valuable information that contributes to assessment of overall health status.

MEASUREMENTS

Measurement of physical growth in children is a key element in assessment of health status. Indicators of physical growth include height (length), weight, head circumference, and chest circumference. Values are plotted on growth charts, and the child's measurements in percentiles are compared with those of the general population (see the appendixes at the back of this textbook).

HEIGHT AND WEIGHT

Various devices are available for measuring height and weight in children. Infants and small children are weighed on an infant platform scale, which provides a measurement in ounces and grams, Figure 12–1. The scale has a platform with curved sides in which the child may sit or lie. Weigh the infant or child in as few clothes as possible, removing the diaper and shoes or slippers. A small sheet, cloth diaper, or paper towel should be placed on the scale before weighing the infant or child, to avoid the transfer of microorganisms from bare skin.

Infant length can be measured using an infant measuring board, which consists of a rigid headboard and movable footboard, Figure 12–2. Place the measuring board on a table and position the infant on his or her back on the board, with the head touching the headboard. Move the footboard up until it touches the bottom of the infant's feet.

An infant can also be measured on a pad

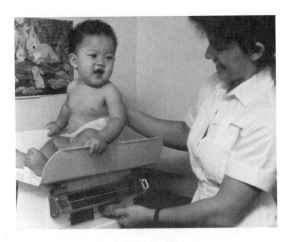

Figure 12–1   *Infant platform scale*

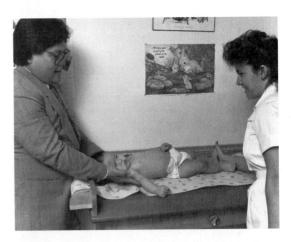

Figure 12–2   *Foot- and headboard for measuring the length of an infant*

by placing a pin into the pad or making a pencil mark at the top of the head and a second pin or mark at the heel of the extended leg. The length is the distance between the two pins. A tape measure can also be used.

A stature-measuring device may be used to measure height once the child is able to stand erect without support. The device consists of a movable headpiece attached to a rigid measuring bar and platform, Figure 12–3. A paper towel should be placed on the platform before use to avoid the potential transmission of microorganisms from bare feet.

HEAD CIRCUMFERENCE

Head circumference is usually measured in all children up to 3 years of age and in any child whose head size is questionable. Measure the head at its greatest circumference, slightly above the eyebrows and pinnae of the ears and around the occipital prominence at the back of the skull. Use a paper or metal tape, since a cloth tape may stretch and give a falsely small measurement, Figure 12–4. Generally head and chest circumference are equal at about 1 to 2 years of age.

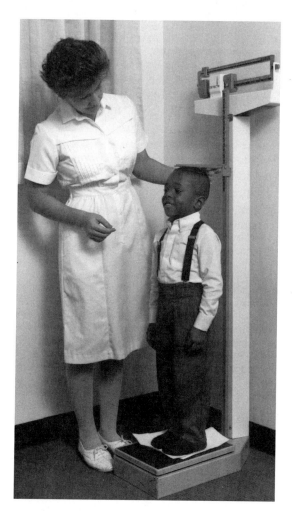

Figure 12–3 *Device to measure height in children*

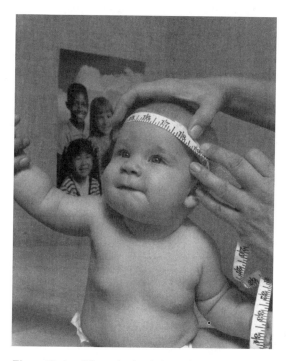

Figure 12–4 *Measuring head circumference*

CHEST CIRCUMFERENCE

Chest circumference is usually measured in children up to 12 months of age. Using a paper or flexible tape, measurefrom the midsternal area just under the child's nipples around the back, under the axillae, and around the chest. During childhood, chest circumference exceeds head size by about 5–7 cm (2–3 in.), Figure 12–5.

TEMPERATURE

Body temperature may be measured in Fahrenheit (F) or Celsius (C) through oral, rectal, axillary, or tympanic routes. Many types of thermometers are used. Mercury (glass) thermometers have been replaced in many institutions by digital thermometers, electronic thermometers, tympanic membrane sensors, and plastic strip thermometers, which provide accurate temperature readings in less time. Electronic thermometers can display temperature within 15 to 60 seconds, depending on the model used. A reading can be obtained by infrared tympanic membrane sensor in as little as 2 seconds. Recommendations for the length of time a mercury thermometer stays in place vary. The nurse should check the accepted procedure where he or she works.

ORAL TEMPERATURE

The oral route is used for children over 3 years of age, Figure 12–6. Caution the child against biting down on the thermometer. If a mercury thermometer is used, wait about 3 minutes before removing the thermometer. Do not take an oral temperature if the child has a history of seizures.

RECTAL TEMPERATURE

Rectal temperatures should be avoided, espe-

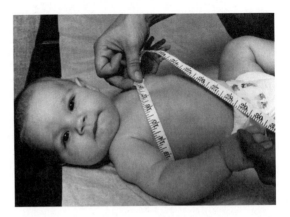

Figure 12–5   *Measuring chest circumference*

cially in newborns, because of the risk of rectal perforation but may be taken with caution in infants and toddlers when other methods or routes are not advised. Place the child prone or on the side, with the knees flexed. An infant can lie prone on a parent's lap, Figure 12–7. Do not force the thermometer. When using a mercury thermometer, allow approximately 3 to 5 minutes to obtain an accurate reading. Rectal temperatures are not indicated for children who have had rectal surgery or for those who have diarrhea.

AXILLARY TEMPERATURE

Axillary temperatures are often preferable to rectal or oral temperatures because they are safe and nonintrusive to take, as well as accurate. Place the mercury thermometer or probe in the axillary space and have the child hold the arm close to the trunk. If a mercury thermometer is used, keep in place for 5 minutes before reading, Figure 12–8.

PULSE

The **apical pulse**, which is heard at the apex of the heart, is generally preferred over other

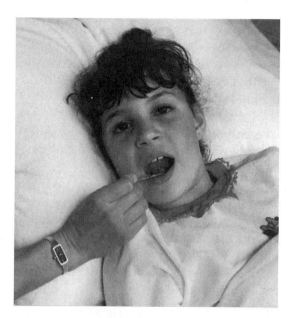

Figure 12–6   Measuring oral temperature

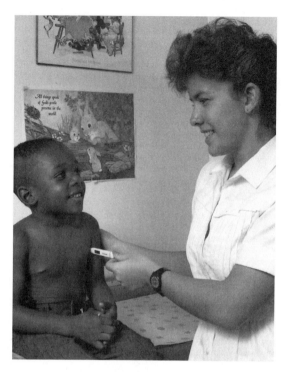

Figure 12–8   Measuring axillary temperature

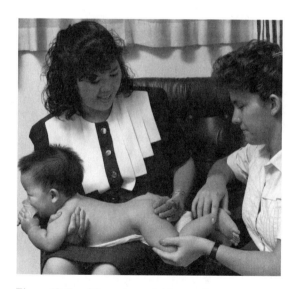

Figure 12–7   Measuring rectal temperature

pulse locations for infants and small children (under 5 years of age). A satisfactory pulse can

be taken radially (at the thumb side of the wrist, above the radial artery) in children over 2. Each "lub-dub" sound is counted as 1 beat. The pulse is counted for 1 full minute.

The normal pulse rate varies with age, decreasing as the child grows older, Figure 12–9. The heart rate may also vary considerably among children of the same age and size. The heart rate increases in response to exercise, excitement, anxiety, and fever and decreases to a resting rate when the child is still.

Listen to the heart rate, noting whether the heart rhythm is regular or irregular. Children often have a normal cycle of irregular rhythm associated with respiration called **sinus arrhythmia**. In sinus arrhythmia, the child's heart rate is faster on inspiration and slower on expiration. Record whether the pulse is normal, bounding, or thready.

Normal Heart Rate Ranges for Children

Age	Heart Rate Range	Average Heart Rate
Infants to 2 years	80–130	110
2 to 6 years	70–120	100
6 to 10 years	70–110	90
10 to 16 years	60–100	85

Figure 12–9

Respirations

In older children and adolescents, respiratory rate is counted in the same way as in an adult. In infants and young children (under 6 years of age), however, the diaphragm is the primary breathing muscle. Thus, respiratory rate is assessed by observing the rise and fall of the abdomen. Inspiration, when the chest or abdomen rises, and expiration, when the chest or abdomen falls, are counted as 1 respiration. Because these movements are often irregular, they should be counted for 1 full minute for accuracy. Normal respiratory rate varies with the child's age, Figure 12–10.

Normal Respiratory Rate Ranges for Children

Age	Respiratory Rate per Minute
1 year	20–40
3 years	20–30
6 years	16–22
10 years	16–20
17 years	12–20

Figure 12–10

Blood Pressure

Blood pressure measurement is part of routine vital sign assessment. In children 3 years of age and older, blood pressure should be measured annually.

Blood pressure may be measured using mercury gravity, electronic, or aneroid equipment. The size of the blood pressure cuff is determined by the size of the child's arm or leg. A general rule of thumb is that the width of the inflatable bladder should be forty percent of the circumference of the extremity used. If the cuff is too small, pressure will be falsely high; if too large, falsely low. Sometimes it is difficult to hear the blood pressure in an infant or small child. Use a pediatric stethoscope over pulse sites if possible.

If the pulse still cannot be auscultated, the blood pressure can be measured by touch. Palpate for the pulse. Keeping your fingers on the pulse, pump up the cuff until the pulse is no longer felt. Slowly open the air valve, watching the column of mercury, and note the number where the pulse is again palpated. This is called the palpated systolic blood pressure.

NURSING CONSIDERATIONS IN PEDIATRIC ASSESSMENT

- Assess parameters of normal growth: height, weight, chest circumference, and head circumference.
- Observe the child's overall appearance and posture.
- Evaluate the physical findings for degree of wellness.
- Observe the child's mobility during assessment procedures.

- Assess vital signs for degree of wellness.
- Observe how the family and child (patient) perceive and manage health.
- Use the opportunity presented by the pediatric assessment to observe the parent-child relationship.

REVIEW QUESTIONS

A. Multiple choice. Select the best answer.

1. Head circumference is
   a. not routinely measured in children over 3 years of age unless the head size is questionable
   b. usually measured with paper or metal tape
   c. usually measured with cloth tape
   d. normally exceeded by chest circumference in children under 2 years of age

2. The oral route is usually used to measure temperature in
   a. children over 3 years of age
   b. children with a history of seizures
   c. infants over 10 months of age
   d. children under 3 years of age

3. Axillary measurement of temperature is
   a. often preferred over rectal and oral methods
   b. more accurate than rectal or oral methods
   c. faster than oral or rectal methods
   d. indicated only for children over 6 years of age

4. The normal pulse rate for an infant is
   a. 70–120 b.p.m.
   b. 80–130 b.p.m.
   c. 90–140 b.p.m.
   d. 100–150 b.p.m.

5. When assessing respirations in infants and young children do all of the following except
   a. observe the rise and fall of the abdomen
   b. note whether breath sounds are clear on both sides of the chest
   c. check for flaring and/or retractions
   d. count rise and fall of chest or abdomen as separate respirations

B. True or false. Write *T* for a true statement and *F* for a false statement.

1. ___ The method chosen for taking a child's temperature will be influenced by the height and weight of the child.

2. ___ Chest circumference is usually measured in all children up to 3 years of age.

3. ___ The apical pulse is usually preferred over other pulse locations in infants.

4. ___ Sinus arrhythmia is an abnormal finding that should be reported immediately to the child's physician.

5. ___ Blood pressure should be measured annually in children 3 years of age and older.

SUGGESTED ACTIVITIES

• List and discuss the other types of observations that the nurse will want to make while taking measurements and assessing vital signs of a child.

• Review recommendations for taking temperatures of infants, toddlers, and children using different methods. Discuss the advantages, disadvantages, and precautions for each method.

• Interview three parents to find out what kinds of observations they make about the growth and development of their infants and children. Find out what their expectations are and how they arrived at those expectations. List any opportunities you identify for educating parents.

BIBLIOGRAPHY

Keir, L., B. A. Wise, and C. Krebs. *Medical Assisting: Administrative and Clinical Competencies*, 3rd ed. Albany, NY: Delmar Publishers, 1993.

Margolius, F. R., N. V. Sneed, and A. D. Hollerbach. Accuracy of apical pulse rate measurements in young children. *Nursing Research* 40, no. 6 (1991): 379–380.

Roche, A., et al. Head circumference reference data: Birth to 18 years. *Pediatrics* 7, no. 5 (1987): 706–712.

Seidel, H. M., J. W. Ball, J. E. Dains, and G. W. Benedict. *Mosby's Guide to Physical Examination*, 2nd ed. St. Louis, MO: Mosby-Year Book, 1991.

Wong, D. L. *Whaley & Wong's Essentials of Pediatric Nursing*, 4th ed. St. Louis, MO: Mosby-Year Book, 1993.

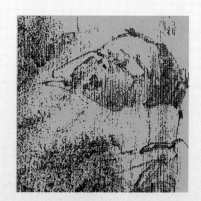

CHAPTER

13

The Hospitalized Child

OBJECTIVES

AFTER STUDYING THIS CHAPTER, THE STUDENT SHOULD BE ABLE TO:

- IDENTIFY THE STRESSORS OF HOSPITALIZATION FOR CHILDREN AT EACH DEVELOPMENTAL STAGE.
- DESCRIBE COMMON BEHAVIORAL REACTIONS TO THESE STRESSORS AT EACH DEVELOPMENTAL STAGE.
- DESCRIBE NURSING INTERVENTIONS TO MINIMIZE THE STRESS OF HOSPITALIZATION FOR CHILDREN.
- DISCUSS THE ROLE OF PLAY IN MINIMIZING THE STRESS OF HOSPITALIZATION.
- IDENTIFY NURSING INTERVENTIONS APPROPRIATE TO SUPPORT PARENTS, GRANDPARENTS, AND SIBLINGS DURING A CHILD'S HOSPITALIZATION.
- DISCUSS SCHOOLING NEEDS DURING HOSPITALIZATION.
- DISCUSS METHODS FOR PREPARING CHILDREN OF DIFFERENT DEVELOPMENTAL STAGES FOR PROCEDURES.
- IDENTIFY STRATEGIES TO HELP CHILDREN COPE WITH THE STRESSORS OF PROLONGED HOSPITALIZATION.
- DISCUSS THE IMPACT OF A CHRONICALLY ILL CHILD ON THE FAMILY.
- IDENTIFY RESOURCES THAT CAN HELP THE FAMILY OF A CHRONICALLY ILL CHILD COPE.

*h*ospitalization is a stressful experience for the child, parents, and siblings and has a profound effect on the family as a unit. In order to provide developmentally appropriate care, nurses must be familiar with age-specific responses to hospitalization and techniques to minimize hospital stressors.

STRESSORS OF HOSPITALIZATION

How a child reacts to the stressors of hospitalization is strongly influenced by his or her developmental stage. Erikson's stages of psychosocial development provide a framework for understanding these reactions (refer to Chapter 7). The major stressors of hospitalization for children of all ages include separation, loss of control, fear of bodily injury, and pain (Foster et al. 1989, Wong 1993).

SEPARATION FROM PARENTS AND FAMILIAR PEOPLE

Infant. Separation from familiar people and routines because of hospitalization is the most

184

disruptive stressor for infants. Young infants under 6 months of age display a response to a change in caretakers, but have not yet developed selective attachment to the primary caretaker. Infants under the age of 6 months who are separated from their mothers are likely to become quiet and subdued.

Providing for the care of the infant's basic needs is the priority of nursing care. Encourage parents to room-in with the infant and to participate in his or her care. These measures provide for continuity of the primary caregiver and help to maintain home routines as much as possible. Talking or singing to the infant, holding, rocking, and cuddling can also help to lessen the stressors of hospitalization.

After 8 months of age, infants have formed an intense attachment to the primary caretaker (usually the mother) and experience **separation anxiety** when separated from the caretaker. Older infants and toddlers who are separated from their mothers experience a pattern of responses that includes protest, despair, and detachment, Figure 13–1. These responses occur when the infant encounters strange people, strange events, and an absence of mothering (Bowlby 1969).

RESPONSE PATTERNS OF HOSPITALIZED CHILDREN	
1. **Protest**, a yearning and searching for the mother, characterized by sobbing, crying, and clinging as the mother tries to leave.	3. **Detachment**, an apparent loss of interest in the mother.
2. **Despair**, characterized by sadness, withdrawal, increasing protest at the mother's absence, and growing anger with her for staying away.	When reunited with the mother after a period of separation, the child exhibits intense anxiety, tends to be overpossessive, and is unwilling to be left alone, insisting on staying close to the mother any time he or she suspects the mother will be lost again.

Figure 13–1

During the initial phase of **protest**, the infant cannot be consoled and refuses any attention except from the parent. Crying may cease only with physical exhaustion.

When the act of protest fails to bring the parent back, the second phase, **despair**, becomes evident. The infant withdraws from events and people, rarely resisting anything that is done. This compliant behavior can be misunderstood to be an adaptation to the hospital experience. The infant is likely to cry intensely or have a temper tantrum when parents visit. This response is normal and does not indicate that the parents have no control over the infant or that the child is "better" when the parents are not around.

The third phase, **detachment**, usually occurs after prolonged separation and can result when an infant is cared for by a variety of nurses over an extended period in the hospital. The infant shows interest in the hospital surroundings and no longer appears upset when parents come and go. Although the infant appears to have adapted to the separation, in actuality he or she is repressing feelings for the parent.

It is important to explain to parents that separation anxiety is a normal response. Encourage the parents to room-in and participate in the

infant's care. If parents must leave, they should be honest about the need to do so. Bringing belongings from home such as familiar toys and blankets provides the infant with comfort objects.

Toddler and Preschool Child. The behaviors of protest, despair, and detachment continue to occur in response to separation during the toddler and preschool years. In the protest phase, the toddler cries out verbally, clings to parents, and tries to force the parents to stay. The toddler may attack strangers by kicking, biting, pinching, or hitting them. In the despair phase, the toddler is uncommunicative, passive, and uninterested in the environment. Regression to earlier behaviors, such as drinking from a bottle or needing to be diapered, is common. In the detachment phase, the toddler seems to have adjusted to hospitalization, appears happy and friendly, and is less demanding.

The preschool child may refuse to eat and have difficulty sleeping in response to separation. The child frequently asks when the parents will visit and cries quietly for parents when they are gone. Like the toddler, the preschool child may withdraw and regress to earlier behaviors. Breaking toys, hitting other children, and refusing to cooperate are common behaviors of the preschool child who is experiencing separation anxiety. Progression to the stage of detachment is uncommon.

Encourage parents of toddlers and preschool children to room-in and participate in the child's care, maintaining normal routines whenever possible. If parents must leave, encourage them to leave familiar objects such as a favorite toy or blanket with the child. Encourage the child to talk about the parents and home and to express feelings of protest. Avoid blaming or shaming the child for regressing to earlier behaviors. Give parents appropriate information so they can understand that the child's behavior is a normal response to separation. Provide comfort for the child by being physically present and spending time with the child.

School-Age Child. The school-age child is beginning to demonstrate an increased independence from parents. At this age, peers take on increased importance in how children see themselves. School-age children who are hospitalized and separated from their friends may react with feelings of loneliness, isolation, or depression. During hospitalization, school-age children need to have outlets for their energy and creativity. Playroom activities that enable them to be active and noisy may help in the adjustment to hospitalization. Parents remain important supports for the child. Although coping mechanisms are developing, under stress the child may revert to more dependent behaviors. Doing so may be distressing to the child, who is attempting to become more independent. Children and families need to understand that these responses to the stress of hospitalization are not unusual.

Adolescent. Adolescents have an increasing sense of self and are influenced by peer groups. Development of relationships and increased independence from parents are important at this stage. Hospitalization is particularly diffi-cult because the adolescent is separated from peer group support. Adolescents usually cope well with short-term separation from home and family. However, during hospitalization, visits and contacts from family and friends are important. Telephone calls can help maintain contact if visits are not possible. Adolescents may develop their own support group with other hospitalized adolescents. Nurses can help this process by encouraging adolescents to meet to discuss their health concerns.

LOSS OF CONTROL

A child who is hospitalized experiences loss of control over certain body functions and over the ability to perform activities of daily living. Behavioral and emotional responses to loss of control include whining, crying, hostility, frustration, and anger. The child may experience depression and apathy if he or she is not allowed to have some control over activities.

Infant. The infant who can sit, crawl, or walk experiences frustration with any physical limitation such as restraints, traction, or confinement to a crib. For this reason it is important to allow the infant as much mobility as possible. Loss of control also results from a change in usual routines, sights, sounds, and smells. Encourage usual family routines and rituals. Play activities and infant stimulation are necessary for continued development of social and motor skills.

Toddler. For the toddler, loss of control results from physical restriction, altered routines and rituals, and dependency (Wong 1993). Again, allow the toddler as much mobility as possible. Because toddlers rely on rituals to provide stability in their lives, maintaining home routines for eating, sleeping, bathing, toileting, and play is important, Figure 13–2. Disruption of these routines may result in regression to earlier behaviors. The toddler

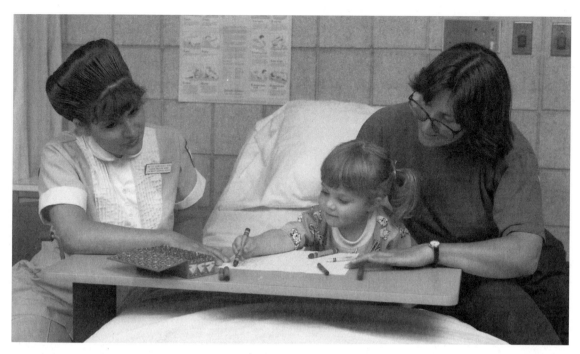

Figure 13–2   *Routine quiet play, such as coloring, can help the toddler cope with the stressors of hospitalization.*

may throw temper tantrums and be resistant to efforts of the caregiver. The parent's participation in the child's care should be strongly encouraged. Inform parents that some regression may occur and should be accepted without blaming the child.

Preschool Child.   The preschool child experiences loss of control in response to physical restriction, altered routines, dependency, and a loss of his or her sense of self-power (Wong 1993). Provide the preschooler opportunities to play, preferably activities that require the use of large muscle groups. If these activities are prohibited because of the child's physical condition, provide appropriate toys and games that allow the child to relieve some of the frustrations of limited mobility.

Preschool children have a tremendous sense of omnipotence and may think of illness and hospitalization as punishment for bad thoughts or deeds. This "magical thinking" results in an exaggerated and frightening view of what is happening to them. Preschoolers may experience feelings of shame, guilt, and fear. Talk to the child about the cause of the illness. Allow the child to be a part of the decision-making process whenever possible in order to provide some sense of control. Choices and decisions may be as simple as what color pajamas to wear or whether the child would prefer to take a medication from a spoon or a medicine cup.

School-Age Child.   Hospitalization threatens the school-age child's growing sense of independence. Having to wear pajamas all day or needing assistance with bathing or using a bed pan may be embarrassing and cause the child to feel that he or she has lost control. School-age children need to find ways in which to have some control in the hospital setting. They can be allowed to take part in making

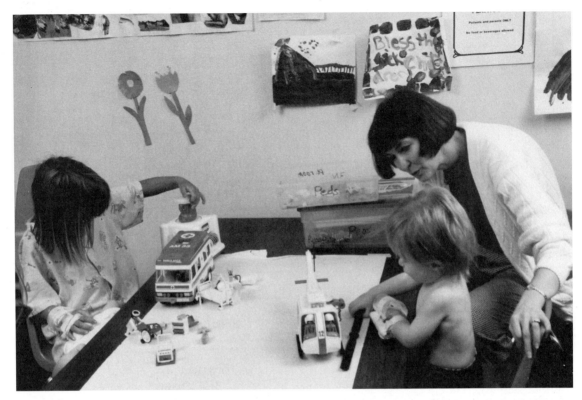

Figure 13–3   *This school-age child is able to express fears about her illness and hospitalization through play involving a toy hospital. A child life specialist looks on, assisting another child.*

decisions about activities of daily living or to choose a new hobby to investigate while they are in the hospital.

Children at this age may be reluctant to express concerns or ask questions out of fear of appearing to lack confidence. Help children talk about their concerns by leading them into conversations and letting them know that other children have the same concerns. Children can also be encouraged to express their concerns through games, puppet shows, or art, Figure 13–3. Explanations should be given in terms that are appropriate for the age of the child.

Adolescent.   The adolescent is often acutely aware of the loss of control that can occur in

the hospital. Adolescents want the nurse and others to relate to them as mature individuals and not to treat them as children. They can be helped to retain their identity by being allowed to wear their own clothes and to decorate their rooms with favorite objects and items. Setting aside an area in the hospital as a teen room with age-appropriate games, books, and other activities helps foster a sense of personal identity and independence, Figure 13–4. Allowing some flexibility in institutional rules can help the adolescent retain a sense of being in control. Letting an adolescent sleep in rather than being awakened for early morning assessments is an example of flexibility. Respecting the adolescent's privacy helps to support a sense of

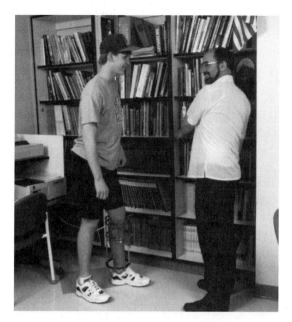

Figure 13–4 *A teen room provides age-appropriate activities for the hospitalized adolescent.*

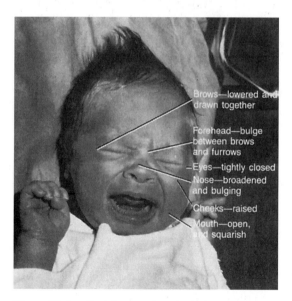

Brows—lowered and drawn together

Forehead—bulge between brows and furrows

Eyes—tightly closed

Nose—broadened and bulging

Cheeks—raised

Mouth—open, and squarish

Figure 13–5 *Facial expression of pain in an infant.* (From D. L. Wong. Whaley & Wong's Essentials of Pediatric Nursing, *4th ed. St. Louis, MO: Mosby-Year Book, 1993.*)

independence and control. Programs to maintain normal school and recreational activities also help to give the adolescent control.

BODILY INJURY AND PAIN

All children experience pain; the expression of pain, however, is directly related to a child's age and stage of development. Young children may not know what pain is and will need help describing it. They may refuse to admit pain because of fear of an injection or painful procedure. Parents are usually sensitive to their child's behaviors and should be encouraged to tell the nurse when the child is in pain. Appropriate pharmacological and nonpharmacological pain control methods should be used for children in all age groups and developmental stages (see Chapter 15).

Infant. The facial expression of distress is the most consistent indicator of pain in infants, Figure 13–5. Changes in vital signs may also alert the nurse. An older infant's responses to pain include loud crying, deliberate withdrawal of the body area, and the facial expression of discomfort. As the infant begins to have prior recall of painful experiences, apprehension and fear of painful events tend to increase. Encourage parents to stay with the infant and to hold and cuddle the infant to provide comfort.

Toddler. Toddlers frequently become overactive and restless with pain. They physically resist a painful stimulus, cry loudly, cling to the parent, and are immensely emotionally upset. Behavioral responses include grimacing, clenching the teeth, biting the lips, rubbing and opening the eyes wide, or acts of physical aggression such a biting, kicking, and hitting (Wong 1993). Encourage the toddler to express pain. Provide comfort measures as appropriate. Distraction and diversion are often useful.

Preschool Child. Preschool children are vulnerable to threats of bodily injury. Fear of bodily harm and mutilation is common and parents should be told that this response is normal at this developmental stage. Intrusive behaviors are very threatening. Preschool children may fear that all their blood will drain out after an injection. Painful procedures and pain may be viewed as punishment for wrongdoing. Allow the preschool child to act out fears with the use of dolls, dramatic play, and, for the older preschooler, with drawings and paintings. Encourage parents to stay with the child during procedures to provide comfort and security.

School-Age Child. School-age children may express concerns about bodily injury and pain by passive requests for help, talking about pain, or trying to delay events that may cause harm or pain to them. They may be afraid of not ever getting well again and of the effects the illness will have on their bodies. Allow the child to ask questions and discuss fears, and explain the child's illness and the reason for a procedure as well as the procedure itself in developmentally appropriate language.

Adolescent. The greatest stress of hospitalization for adolescents is the fear of bodily alterations. The nurse needs to be aware of concerns about bodily changes and be able to respond appropriately. Adolescents may fear losing control when they are in pain. Thus, they often react to pain by maintaining their self-control and giving little verbal response. They may be reluctant to discuss their pain, because discussing it would indicate an inability to maintain self-control. Adolescents may also think that nurses should know when they are in pain and that they should not have to ask for pain medication (Favaloro and Touzel 1990). Observe for signs of pain, such as changes in mobility, irritability, or being quiet and withdrawn.

NURSING CARE RELATED TO HOSPITALIZATION

SUPPORT SYSTEMS

An appropriate support system helps to reduce the fear and anxiety that accompany hospitalization of a child or sibling. Today's mobile families may not live near grandparents or other relatives and thus may lack this important support system. Parents may need to take turns spending time with the hospitalized child and juggle work and child care for other siblings. The single parent is especially stressed when a child is hospitalized. In some cultural groups it is common for other family members to assist the family who is experiencing hospitalization. Thus, grandparents, aunts and uncles, cousins, and other important people in the family's life may be present at home or in the hospital to provide support to the family.

SCHOOLING NEEDS

School is an important part of the life of the school-age child and adolescent. Children who are hospitalized, especially for frequent or extended admissions, should be helped to set aside time in which to study and complete schoolwork assignments. The nurse should also work with children and parents to determine whether the child's schooling needs are being met. Some children may need the services of a tutor to assist them with their assignments.

PREPARING FOR PROCEDURES

Preparing children for procedures helps to decrease their anxiety and fear and to increase their coping strategies in response to stressful situations (Broome 1990). Preparation for procedures is geared to the child's developmental level, which determines what information is given and when it is given (Bates and Broome 1986). Painful procedures should be performed in a separate treatment room, so that the child's room will be perceived as a safe place.

Infant and Toddler. Infants and toddlers do not understand lengthy explanations or anticipate actions that will happen to them. Immediately before a procedure is to be performed, give them short explanations and then continue with the procedure. Toddlers may benefit from handling equipment or small replicas of equipment before it is used on them. Dolls can be used to demonstrate what will happen during the procedure.

Preschool Child. Preschool children also benefit from handling equipment used in procedures. Puppets, cartoons, or stories can also be used to demonstrate procedures. Explain in simple terms close to the time at which the procedure will be performed how the procedure will affect the child.

School-Age Child. Plan to prepare the school-age child in advance of the scheduled time so the child has time to comprehend the information. Use diagrams, models, equipment, or videotapes and terminology the child can understand to explain and to prepare the child.

Adolescent. Adolescents require explanations and reasons for the procedure. If possible they should be involved in decision making and planning and given the opportunity to learn techniques to help them stay in control during the procedure. Encourage questions.

CHILDREN WITH CHRONIC DISEASES OR PROLONGED HOSPITALIZATIONS

Children with chronic diseases or prolonged hospitalizations are at risk for delays or regres-

sion in their development. Nurses along with other health team members can develop and implement plans of care that promote the child's development (Lipsi et al. 1991). The nurse should encourage communication and provide age-appropriate education to the child about the condition to help alleviate fears and concerns. Involve the child as much as possible with decisions and with activities related to self-care. Incorporating management of the condition into everyday activities helps normalize the child's lifestyle. Encourage parents to participate in the child's care, and promote interaction with siblings and peers. How the family and community respond to the child affects the child's perception of the illness. Encourage children to decorate their hospital rooms — with posters, pictures, cards, or displays of collections such as baseball cards — to make them feel more comfortable with their surroundings. Encourage children to develop new interests to help them occupy their time. Children can be helped to stay in control by developing and maintaining a routine schedule of activities throughout the day.

REHABILITATION

Rehabilitation care involves planning for the long-term needs of hospitalized children. Nurses should be involved in planning and implementing care for children who require rehabilitation in both acute-care hospitals and long-term care facilities.

FAMILY SUPPORT

Learning of a child's chronic illness often presents a crisis situation in families. Factors that determine how a family will respond include the nature, severity, and prognosis of the illness, the age and birth order of the child, the family's perception of the illness, religious beliefs, their ability to find some meaning in the illness, methods of coping, past experience, family structure, and available support systems. An illness that is progressive can be more difficult for the family to cope with than one that is not. Families adjust best with the support of relatives, friends, and community.

Parents' Responses. Parents who are told that their child has a chronic illness often react with shock and **denial**, or disbelief. They may not accept a diagnosis. Parents may be reluctant to obtain treatment for the child and may take the child to numerous physicians, hoping to confirm that the diagnosis was a mistake. Depending upon the severity of the illness, they may undergo stages of grieving (see Chapter 17). Parents may also experience guilt, especially if they feel responsible for the illness. Anxiety and confusion are common. The nurse needs to provide support, continued education, and guidance. Denial is an important stage in the adjustment process.

As parents begin to adjust, they may experience periods of increased sadness, anger, or guilt. They may exhibit anger directed toward the staff, spouse, or even the ill child. A parent may visit the child less frequently or reject the child emotionally. Overprotectiveness of the child, which can interfere with the child's need to develop initiative and self-esteem, is a more common parental response. Parents may engage in self-accusation. They may also feel shame, especially if the child's condition elicits pity, and may develop feelings of low self-esteem. One or both spouses may experience depression.

Spouses tend to cope differently; one may take longer to adjust than the other. Spouses may also have different views of how to care for the child. Parents can experience strength as they work together to reintegrate the child

into the family and to establish new goals for themselves, the child, and the family. They may focus on the positive aspects of the child and find meaning in the experience.

Stressors. A variety of stressors can affect the parents' ability to cope. A chronic illness often strains financial resources. One parent may have to leave work to care for the child. A parent may have to work two jobs to cover expenses. A single parent may not be able to leave work for extended periods of time to care for the child, causing feelings of guilt and anxiety. Time and energy spent caring for the child may result in restricted leisure activities and possible social isolation. Parents may worry about siblings. Each stage of the child's development is a reminder to the parent of the illness. Nurses need to anticipate these times and provide support.

Siblings' Responses. Factors such as age, developmental level, birth order, and number of children in the family as well as how parents react affect the way a sibling will respond. Younger children in particular may experience guilt, believing that they in some way caused the child's illness. Parents need to reassure siblings that the child's illness is not their fault. Young children may not understand the illness or the ill child's need for parental attention. Siblings may resent having to help care for the child or having to perform additional chores to enable the parents to do so.

Because the parents spend more time with the ill child, jealousy and anger are common reactions among siblings, who may engage in behaviors to demand attention from the parents. They may exhibit aggressiveness or develop physical symptoms, including symptoms similar to those of the ill child. A sibling may withdraw socially or reject the child. Siblings may experience difficulties in school. Parents need to devote time exclusively to siblings to consider the needs of all family members.

Siblings' responses can be positive as well. Siblings may help care for the child and make an effort to include the ill child in activities. They may exhibit cooperation, concern, and empathy. Parents should try to involve the siblings in the care of the ill child and in future plans as much as possible. Providing education about the child's condition will help siblings understand the time and attention needed to care for the child.

Role of the Nurse. The nurse plays an important role in the family's adjustment by providing guidance and support, Figure 13–6. The nurse serves as a role model for all family members. Being supportive and caring can help family members accept the child. The manner in which the nurse interacts with the child will help family members learn how to provide care.

The nurse can help parents focus on realistic expectations and goals. In addition, the nurse can help parents provide for the child's care and development as well as for the needs of the spouse and siblings. The nurse can encourage the family to be an advocate for the ill child, promoting education and opportunity within the community. The nurse should encourage the parents to find leisure time for themselves and for the family. The nurse

should be able to direct the family to available resources.

Resources. Resources are an important factor in the family's adjustment. Personal resources include age, intelligence, education, adaptability, optimism, past experience, and coping skills. Additional resources that can help the family cope include support from immediate family members, extended family, friends, community services, health care providers, organizations, and programs for the child such as alternative schooling and recreational programs. Families who live in urban areas may have better access to a greater number of community resources than those who live in rural areas. Parents who have children with similar conditions may be especially helpful in providing support. Support groups for parents and siblings provide a place for families to discuss similar concerns and strategies for coping. **Respite care**, in which trained health care providers assist the ill child, can enable parents and family to obtain needed leisure time.

Resources are also available to help prepare families for hospitalization of a child. The Association for the Care of Children's Health, 7910 Woodmont Avenue, Suite 300, Bethesda, Maryland 20814, is a national resource that provides such information.

PROVIDING SUPPORT FOR THE FAMILY OF A CHRONICALLY ILL CHILD

- Assess the family's ability to cope. Intervene when necessary.
- Develop a partnership with the parents, and provide support.
- Encourage communication among family members and with medical professionals.
- Provide age-appropriate educational information to family members.

- Consider the family's cultural, religious, and spiritual beliefs when providing guidance.
- Help the family to use resources or to develop their own.
- Examine personal attitudes about the child's condition.

Figure 13–6

REVIEW QUESTIONS

A. Multiple choice. Select the best answer.

1. Katie is 3 years old. She is hospitalized with idiopathic thrombocytopenic purpura. Katie's meals are served on a colorful plate with small utensils that fit easily in her hands. The dietary department has sent small portions of food on her tray. Katie's mother is rooming in and is present when you carry the tray into her room. You should

   a. hand the tray to her mother and ask her to feed Katie
   b. ask Katie who she would like to have help her with her tray
   c. feed Katie, using the small utensils
   d. allow Katie to feed herself

2. Micah is 30 months of age and has been potty trained for 6 months. He is hospitalized for surgical treatment of chronic otitis media. Micah has wet the bed three times since the surgical procedure 12 hours ago. His mother is angry because she had successfully potty trained him before he "came in here." You should

   a. explain to his mother that regression to earlier behaviors is common with hospitalization
   b. cut back on the fluids you are giving him, especially the sodas
   c. get a box of disposable diapers and put one on him
   d. tell the mother it's not your fault he is wetting the bed

3. Connor, 5 years old, is hospitalized with diabetes mellitus. Connor begins to cry when the nurse tries to give him his medication. The most appropriate nursing action is to

   a. tell Connor if he is a "big boy" he can have a lollipop after the procedure
   b. explain to his parents that boys this age always refuse to take medication
   c. encourage Connor to communicate his feelings, and provide comfort
   d. inform Connor and his parents that he will have to cooperate

4. When planning care for adolescents in the hospital, the nurse should include all of the following except
   a. privacy
   b. area for them to gather for group activities
   c. allowing them to wear their own clothes
   d. maintaining strict rules restricting visitors

5. Which of the following is the most significant stressor of hospitalization for adolescents?
   a. fear of pain
   b. separation from family
   c. fear of altered body image
   d. fear of bodily injury

6. Which of the following is a positive response among children to having a chronically ill sibling?
   a. empathy
   b. mimicking symptoms of the illness
   c. aggressive behavior
   d. overprotectiveness of the ill child

7. Parents of a chronically ill child need to remain focused on
   a. the child's illness
   b. their own personal needs
   c. the needs of all family members, including the ill child
   d. the procedures of health care professionals

8. The first reaction of parents to learning that a child is chronically ill is usually
   a. depression
   b. denial
   c. social isolation
   d. resolution

B. True or false. Write *T* for a true statement and *F* for a false statement.

1. ___ It is best for everyone if the parents stay outside the treatment room rather than with the toddler during a procedure.

2. ___ A nursing intervention to get a preschooler to take his medication is to tell him to "be a good boy" like his roommate, Jonathan.

3. ___ Infants do not need pharmacological agents for pain control because they experience only minimal pain.

4. ___ Procedures should be explained to children in terms appropriate for their developmental level.

5. ___ Preparing children for painful procedures decreases their fear.

SUGGESTED ACTIVITIES

- Care for hospitalized children of different developmental stages. Compare and contrast children's reactions to illness and hospitalization. Record your findings in a journal.

- Invite the parents of a chronically ill child to speak to the class about the needs of families and siblings during hospitalization and after returning home.

- Invite the parents and siblings of a child who was admitted to the hospital because of an emergency situation to talk about their fears and needs during this time of crisis.

- Invite a pediatric staff nurse to discuss common reactions of children to hospitalization and nursing care to minimize the stressors of hospitalization.

- Make a list of community resources for families with chronically ill children. Identify support groups, resources provided by hospitals, and health organizations.

- Interview a nurse who works with families of chronically ill children about strategies that have proven successful in promoting their adjustment.

BIBLIOGRAPHY

Bates, T., and M. Broome. Preparation of children for hospitalization and surgery: A review of the literature. *Journal of Pediatric Nursing* 1, no. 4 (1986): 230–239.

Betz, C. L., M. Hunsberger, and S. Wright. *Family-Centered Nursing Care of Children*, 2nd ed. Philadelphia: W. B. Saunders, 1994.

Bowlby, J. *Attachment and Loss*, vol. 1. New York: Basic Books, 1969.

Bowlby, J. *Attachment and Loss*, vol. 2. New York: Basic Books, 1973.

Broome, M. Preparation of children for painful procedures. *Pediatric Nursing* 16, no. 6 (1990): 537–541.

Carson, D., J. Fravely, and J. Council. Children's prehospitalization conceptions of illness, cognitive development, and personal adjustment. *Child Health Care* 21, no. 2 (1992): 103–110.

Favaloro, R., and B. Touzel. A comparison of adolescents' and nurses' postoperative pain rating and perceptions. *Pediatric Nursing* 16, no. 4 (1990): 414–417, 424.

Foster, R. L., M. M. Hunsberger, and J. J. Anderson. *Family-Centered Nursing Care of Children*. Philadelphia: W. B. Saunders, 1989.

Lipsi, K., K. Clement-Shafer, and C. Rushton. Developmental rounds: An intervention strategy for hospitalized infants. *Pediatric Nursing* 17, no. 5 (1991): 433–437, 468.

Marks, M. G. *Broadribb's Introductory Pediatric Nursing*, 4th ed. Philadelphia: J. B. Lippincott, 1994.

Marlow, D. R., and B. A. Redding. *Textbook of Pediatric Nursing*, 6th ed. Philadelphia: W. B. Saunders, 1988.

Mott, S., S. James, and A. Sperhac. *Nursing Care of Children and Families*. Redwood City, CA: Addison-Wesley, 1990.

Murray, R. B., and J. Zentner. *Nursing Assessment and Health Promotion: Strategies through the Life Span*. Norwalk, CT: Appleton and Lange, 1993.

Pillitteri, A. *Maternal and Child Health Nursing*. Philadelphia: J. B. Lippincott, 1992.

Scipien, G. M., M. A. Chard, J. Howe, M. U. Barnard. *Pediatric Nursing Care*. St. Louis, MO: Mosby–Year Book, 1990.

Servonsky, J., and S. R. Opas. *Nursing Management of Children*. Boston: Jones and Bartlett Publishers, 1987.

Smeltzer, S. C., and B. G. Bare. *Brunner & Suddarth's Textbook of Medical–Surgical Nursing*, 7th ed. Philadelphia: J. B. Lippincott, 1992.

Vessey, J., and M. Mahon. Therapeutic play and the hospitalized child. *Journal of Pediatric Nursing* 5, no. 5 (1990): 328–333.

Whaley, L., and D. Wong, eds. *Nursing Care of Infants and Children*, 4th ed. St. Louis, MO: Mosby-Year Book, 1991.

Wong, D. L. *Whaley & Wong's Essentials of Pediatric Nursing*, 4th ed. St. Louis, MO: Mosby-Year Book, 1993.

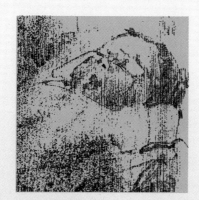

CHAPTER

14

Routine Pediatric Procedures

OBJECTIVES

AFTER STUDYING THIS CHAPTER, THE STUDENT SHOULD BE ABLE TO:

- PREPARE CHILDREN AT DIFFERENT DEVELOPMENTAL STAGES FOR PROCEDURES.

- IDENTIFY THE REQUIREMENTS FOR OBTAINING INFORMED CONSENT IN CHILDREN.

- SAFELY RESTRAIN, HOLD, TRANSPORT, AND POSITION A CHILD FOR PROCEDURES.

- ADMINISTER MEDICATIONS TO CHILDREN CORRECTLY AND SAFELY BY DIFFERENT ROUTES.

- APPLY A URINE COLLECTION BAG AND OBTAIN A URINE SPECIMEN.

- ADMINISTER OXYGEN TO A CHILD, USING VARIOUS DELIVERY SYSTEMS.

- SUCTION A TRACHEOSTOMY TUBE IN A CHILD.

- SUCTION AN INFANT'S NOSE USING A BULB SYRINGE.

- ASSIST WITH THE INSERTION OF A NASOGASTRIC OR GASTROSTOMY TUBE.

- ADMINISTER A GAVAGE FEEDING TO A CHILD.

197

KEY TERMS

CRADLE HOLD   UPRIGHT HOLD

FOOTBALL HOLD

*N*urses who care for hospitalized children need to be familiar with a variety of pediatric procedures performed routinely in the hospital setting. This chapter highlights variations and precautions for the following procedures: informed consent, restraints and positioning, medication administration, specimen collection, oxygen administration, suctioning, nasogastric and gastrostomy tubes, and gavage feeding.

INFORMED CONSENT
FOR CHILDREN

If a child is a minor, a parent or legal guardian must give written consent for any procedure or treatment. If the parent is unavailable, the person who is assuming the responsibility for the child can give consent for emergency treatment providing he or she has written permission from a parent or legal guardian to authorize care. Verbal consent can be given by a parent or guardian over the telephone provided that two witnesses are listening to the consent. There must be written and signed documentation of the phone call. An emancipated minor may give consent as a mature minor.

PREPARING CHILDREN
FOR PROCEDURES

Children should be prepared for procedures on the basis of their age, developmental stage, and ability to understand what is being explained to them. The nurse should be honest about the activities and discomfort associated with the specific procedure in order to develop a trusting relationship with the child. Involving parents when appropriate can provide support and comfort to the child (see Chapter 13).

INFANT

The infant feels pain and shows signs of anxiety during procedures. Give a pacifier or bottle and hold the infant close to provide comfort.

TODDLER

Explain the procedure to the toddler just before it is to be performed. Use simple words and objects, if appropriate. Provide distraction during the procedure and reward the toddler after the procedure is over. Encourage the toddler to express feelings. Provide comfort and support.

PRESCHOOL CHILD

Provide the preschool child with simple verbal explanations about procedures. Let the child handle equipment if possible. Answer all questions as honestly as possible. Preschool children fear bodily harm and mutilation and find invasive procedures threatening. The child may think that a painful procedure is punishment for something he or she did wrong. Encourage the child to talk about fears and anxieties.

SCHOOL-AGE CHILD

The school-age child understands treatments and procedures. Use terminology the child can easily comprehend. The school-age child also fears bodily injury and needs to be encouraged to talk about fears and anxieties.

ADOLESCENT

The adolescent understands explanations about procedures. Answer any questions he or she may have. The adolescent will react to pain by trying to act stoic while maintaining self-control. Encourage the adolescent to discuss fears and anxieties if he or she is willing. Coping methods such as imagery, breathing, or relaxation techniques can be helpful. Involving the adolescent in the decision-making process, when possible, can help the teenager retain a sense of being in control.

RESTRAINTS AND POSITIONING

HIGH-TOP CRIB

Infants and toddlers are usually placed in high-top cribs to protect them from injury in the hospital environment, Figure 14–1.

ELBOW RESTRAINTS

Elbow restraints are used to keep a child from

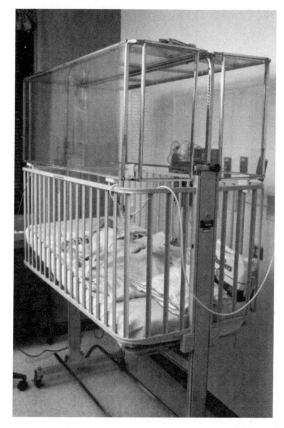

Figure 14–1   High-top crib

bending an elbow or touching the face, neck, or head. A commercially manufactured restraint or a modified armboard can be used. To apply an elbow restraint:

1. Place the armboard on the ventral side of the arm, extending from midhumerus to midforearm.
2. Wrap Kling around the armboard.
3. Tape in place, Figure 14–2.

PAPOOSE BOARD

The papoose board is a commercially manufactured body restraint consisting of a metal board with cloth wrappings lined with Velcro

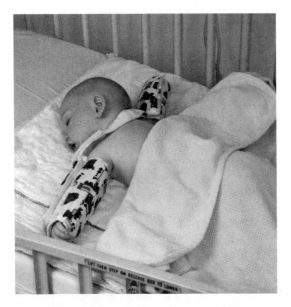

Figure 14–2   *Elbow restraints*

fasteners. The board immobilizes the child's arms and legs. To use a papoose board:

1. Place a towel, small sheet, or small bath blanket over the board.
2. Place the child supine with head at the top of the board.
3. Place the cloth wrappings around the child, securing the Velcro.

MUMMY RESTRAINT

The mummy restraint is used to immobilize an infant's arms and legs. To apply a mummy restraint:

1. Fold down the top corner of a small blanket. Place the infant diagonally on the blanket with neck at the fold, Figure 14–3a.
2. Bring one side of the blanket over the infant's arm, shoulder, and chest, and secure beneath the body, Figure 14–3b. Bring the bottom corner up over infant.
3. Bring the other side over the infant and wrap securely, Figure 14–3c.

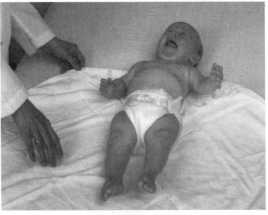

a.

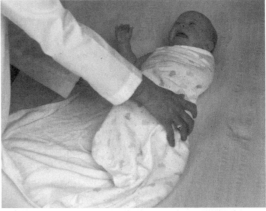

b.

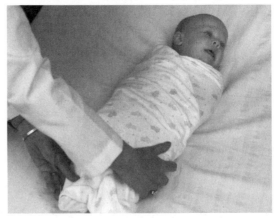

c.

Figure 14–3   *Mummy restraint*

HOLDING AND TRANSPORTING INFANTS

Hospitalized infants need to be held as well as transported to other areas within the hospital. Three positions for safely holding and transporting infants are the **cradle**, **football**, and **upright holds**.

Cradle Hold. The infant is held with head resting in the bend of the nurse's elbow with back supported. The infant's thigh is held by the carrying arm, Figure 14–4a.

Football Hold. The infant's body is supported on the nurse's forearm. The infant's head and neck rest in the nurse's palm. The rest of the infant's body is securely held between the nurse's body and elbow, Figure 14–4b.

Upright Hold. The infant is held upright against the nurse's chest and shoulder. The infant's buttocks are supported by one of the nurse's hands. The other hand and arm support the infant's head and shoulders, Figure 14–4c.

POSITIONING FOR A LUMBAR PUNCTURE

A lumbar puncture is used to measure cerebrospinal fluid (CSF) pressure, obtain a sample of CSF, or administer medications, anesthetics, air, or radiopaque contrast material. To position a child for lumbar puncture:

1. Place the child on the side (lateral recumbent) with knees pulled to abdomen and neck flexed to the chin. The back should be arched. An infant can be held in this position by leaning over and holding the neck, buttocks, and thighs in your hands, Figure 14–5. An infant can also be placed in a sitting position with head flexed on the chest. An older child can sit up with neck flexed to the chin and spine arched forward. Lean

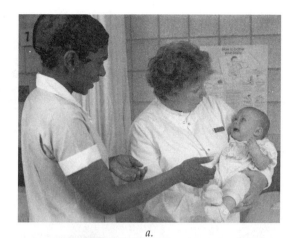

a.

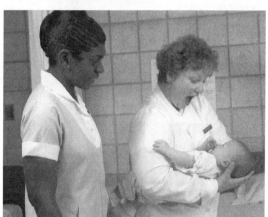

b.

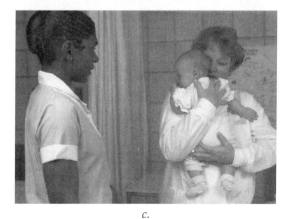

c.

Figure 14–4 *(a) Cradle hold. (b) Football hold. (c) Upright hold.*

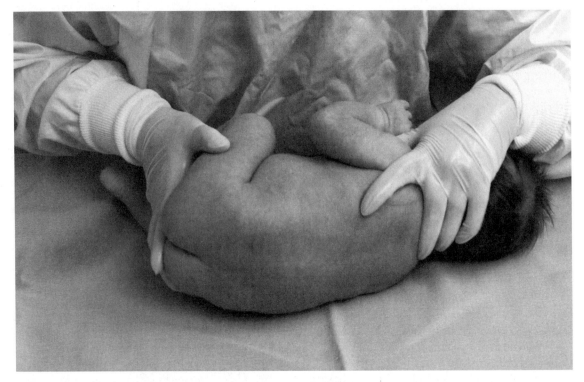

Figure 14–5   *Positioning infant for a lumbar puncture*

over the child with your entire body, using your forearms against the child's legs and buttocks and around the shoulders and head, being careful not to interfere with respiratory effort.

Medication Administration

The nurse should follow the "Five Rights" of proper drug administration before any medication is given:

1. Right drug
2. Right patient
3. Right time
4. Right route
5. Right dose

Routes of Administration

Oral Route. The method of administration depends on the child's age. Liquid medications can be administered by placing small amounts of liquid along the side of an infant's mouth using a plastic syringe, calibrated dropper, medicine cup, or spoon. Wait for the infant to swallow before administering more liquid. Give medications slowly. Alternatively, medication can be put in a nipple from which the infant then sucks. Tablets can be crushed and mixed in juice, syrup, or strained fruit. Toddlers and preschool-age children may need to be held firmly on the nurse or parent's lap.

PRECAUTION: Never put medications into the infant's formula. The infant may not consume the entire feeding, or may ingest so slowly that the medication loses potency. Never give oral medications to a crying child. Aspiration may result. Do not hold the child's nose closed.

Intramuscular Route

1. The recommended injection site for children under 3 years of age is the vastus lateralis. The gluteal sites can be used after the child is walking, if hospital policy permits.
2. Have another nurse, assistant, or parent restrain the child during the injection.
3. Put on clean gloves. Locate injection site.
4. Clean the site with alcohol or Betadine using a firm outward circular motion.
5. Firmly grasp the muscle between the thumb and fingers to stabilize and isolate the muscle.
6. Using a dartlike motion, insert the needle quickly at a 90-degree angle. Pull back on the plunger. If no blood is present, inject the medication, withdraw the needle, and massage the area with a dry gauze pad.

   PRECAUTION: Do not cap needle. Discard in a puncture-resistant container using universal precaution recommendations.

Intravenous Route

Preparation

1. Check the intravenous site for patency, redness, blanching, and edema. IV site should be well stabilized.
2. Check specific dilution recommendations.
3. Check medication compatibility with intravenous fluids that the child is receiving.
4. Check administration rate.
5. Check length of time drug can be administered.

Administration

1. Intravenous medications for children should be put in a volutrol, burette, or soluset and administered through a continuous infusion pump for accurate administration.
2. Set time of infusion.
3. Monitor site during infusion for signs of infiltration.
4. Flush line with a compatible solution after medication has infused.

Eye Drops

1. Place the child in a supine or sitting position with head extended.
2. Put on clean gloves.
3. Pull the child's lower lid down while your other hand rests on the child's head.
4. Place drops or ointment into the lower conjunctival sac starting from the inner canthus.
5. Close the eyelids to prevent leakage of medication after administration.
6. Blot the inner canthus of the eye and position the child's head in the midline to prevent excessive medication from getting into the other eye.

Ear Drops

1. Place the child in a supine position with head turned exposing the ear upward.
2. For a child under 3 years of age, pull the pinna gently down and back to straighten the ear canal.
3. For the child older than 3 years, pull the pinna up and back.
4. Instill drops into the ear canal.
5. Have the child remain in the same position for a few minutes to help the medication drain into the ear canal.
6. A cotton plug may be put loosely in the ear to stop medication from draining out.

SPECIMEN COLLECTION

BLOOD

Blood samples of children are obtained by venipuncture or capillary stick. The child is restrained in a supine position on a bed, preferably not the patient's bed, or stretcher.

Venipuncture. The sites most frequently used are the antecubital fossa and forearm. The dorsum of the hand or foot may also be used. The external jugular and femoral vein are used when it is difficult to obtain blood from traditional sites.

Capillary Stick. The sites include the plantar surface of the heel for newborns and children under the age of 1 year, the great toe, the ear lobe or the palmar surface of the tip of the third or fourth finger for children over 1 year. The site may be warmed first.

> **PRECAUTION:** Use universal precautions when drawing blood from any patient.

URINE

Infant. Urine collection bags are used to obtain a urine specimen from infants and toddlers who are not yet toilet trained. The bags are clear plastic with adhesive tabs. To apply a collection bag correctly:

1. Put on clean gloves.
2. Wash and thoroughly dry the perineum, genitalia, and surrounding skin.
3. Remove paper covering adhesive, Figure 14–6a.
4. Attach the bag, using the adhesive tabs — for girls stretch the perineum and apply the bag around the labia; for boys place the penis and scrotum inside the bag, Figure 14–6c. Sometimes, the penis only is placed inside the bag.
5. Seal tightly to protect against leaks. Put the child's diaper back on carefully.
6. Check the bag frequently and as soon as the child urinates, gently pull the bag away from the skin.

OXYGEN ADMINISTRATION

FACE MASK

A face mask delivers increased concentrations of oxygen effectively. Several types of masks are available. The mask should extend from the bridge of the child's nose to the cleft of the chin. The mask should fit snugly on the face, but no pressure should be put on the eyes.

NASAL CANNULA

The nasal cannula delivers a low flow and low concentration of oxygen. The prongs of the cannula are placed in the child's nares, allowing the child to be mobile.

BLOW-BY

Blow-by oxygen is used when the child needs low concentrations of oxygen with humidification. The oxygen cannula is held under the child's nose.

TRACHEOSTOMY COLLAR

A tracheostomy collar is a plastic collar that goes over a tracheostomy tube. It provides humidified air or oxygen and keeps the airway warm and moist.

> **PRECAUTION:** Watch for fluid collection in the tubing and take precautions so that fluid does not drain into the tracheostomy.

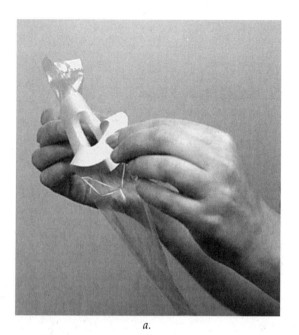

a.

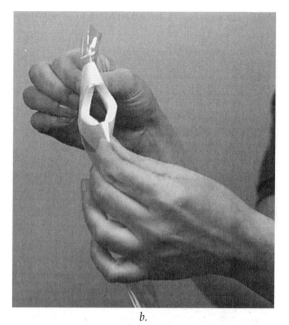

b.

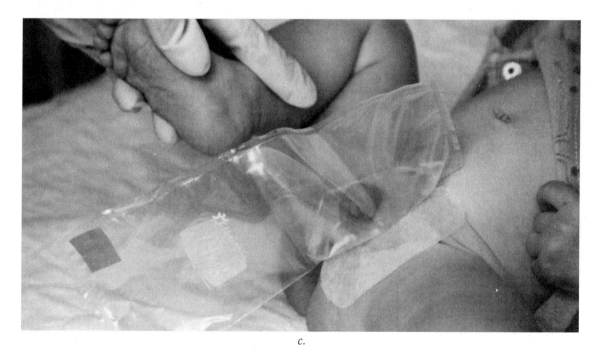

c.

Figure 14–6   *Applying a urine collection bag. (a) Removing paper covering adhesive. (b) Bending and opening the collection bag. (NOTE: Although gloves are recommended when placing a urine collection bag on an infant, it is difficult to remove the paper covering using gloves. Gloves must be worn, however, when touching the infant's perineal area.) (c) Collection bag applied.*

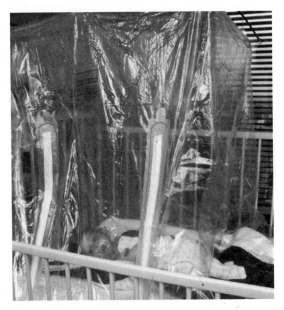

Figure 14–7   *Child in mist tent*

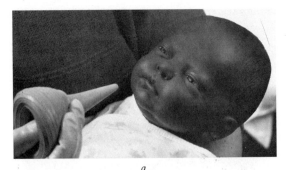

a.

b.

Figure 14–8   *(a) Squeezing the bulb syringe.*
(b) Releasing the bulb syringe.

MIST TENT (OXYGEN TENT)

The mist tent delivers oxygen concentrations of 35% to 40% and is an effective way to deliver humidified oxygen, Figure 14–7. Tuck the tent under the mattress to reduce oxygen loss. Check the child's clothes and blankets frequently and change when damp.

SUCTIONING

Suctioning may be necessary to maintain a patent airway in a pediatric patient. Children with tracheostomies will require tracheostomy tube suctioning. Infants, who are obligatory nose breathers, may require suctioning to remove excessive nasal secretions.

USING A BULB SYRINGE

A bulb syringe is used to suction excess secretions from an infant's nose. To use a bulb syringe:

1. Squeeze the bulb before placing the tip into the infant's nose, Figure 14–8a.
2. Place the tip of the bulb syringe into the infant's nares or mouth.
3. Be sure there is a seal and release the bulb, Figure 14–8b.
4. Remove the syringe and expel the contents.
5. Repeat as needed to clear airway.

NASOGASTRIC AND GASTROSTOMY TUBES

Nasogastric tubes are inserted to provide liquid feedings for the child who cannot swallow, to decompress the stomach, or to wash out (or lavage) the stomach. Gastrostomy tubes are inserted to provide liquid feedings to the child requiring long-term tube feeding.

PROCEDURE

Suctioning a Tracheostomy Tube

Purpose: Tracheostomy tube suctioning is required to keep the airway open and free of mucous plugs and increased secretions.

Equipment:

- Catheter kit containing sterile suction catheter, sterile cup, and sterile gloves. The size of the catheter used for suctioning depends on the size of the tracheostomy tube in place. The diameter of the catheter should be one-half the diameter of the tracheostomy tube.
- Sterile normal saline
- Clean gloves
- Bedside equipment should include replacement tracheostomy tubes, Ambu bag, oxygen, and suction equipment.

Preparation:

1. Turn on the wall suction. Set as ordered.
2. Turn on oxygen source and attach to the Ambu bag.

Procedure:

1. Put the sterile glove on your dominant hand. Put a clean glove on the other hand.
2. Using sterile technique, remove the catheter from the paper sheath and attach to suction.
3. To test suction equipment, place end of catheter in a cup of sterile saline.
4. Hyperventilate the child before and after suctioning with 100% oxygen if ordered by the physician.
5. Insert the catheter with the suction port open no more than 0.5 cm below the edge of the tracheostomy tube, Figure 14–9a.
6. Withdraw the catheter slowly, rotating the catheter while covering the suction port, Figure 14–9b.
7. Remove catheter and irrigate with sterile water.
8. If secretions are thick, a few drops of sterile saline (0.5 to 2 mL) injected into the tube can help to loosen them.
9. Suction after saline instillation.
10. Suction as needed until airway is clear.

PRECAUTION: Do not suction for longer than 5 to 10 seconds at a time. Allow the child to rest between aspirations to prevent hypoxia. Monitor respiratory status.

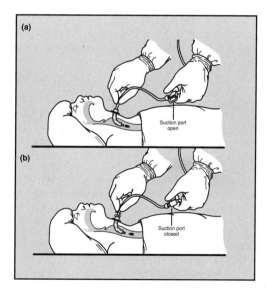

Figure 14–9   *Tracheostomy suctioning. (a) Insertion, port open. (b) Withdrawal, port closed. (From D. L. Wong. Whaley & Wong's Essentials of Pediatric Nursing,* 4th ed. St. Louis, MO: Mosby-Year Book, 1993.)

GASTROSTOMY TUBES

Gastrostomy tubes are surgically placed in the stomach in children needing long-term feedings. To provide proper gastrostomy tube care:

1. Monitor the insertion site for any irritation or infection.
2. Clean area daily and apply an antibiotic ointment.
3. Apply a dressing when needed.
4. Tape the tube carefully to prevent the tube from dislodging and causing erosion or enlargement of the insertion site.
5. Clamp the tube when not in use.

GASTROSTOMY FEEDING BUTTON

The gastrostomy button is a small flexible device that may be used instead of a gastrostomy tube in a child requiring long-term tube feedings.

PROCEDURE

Nasogastric Tubes

Purpose: Nasogastric tubes are inserted through the nose into the stomach and are used for alimentation or decompression and emptying of the stomach.

Equipment:

- Appropriate-size tube
- Suction
- Tape
- Stethoscope
- 20-mL syringe, gauze, and clean gloves

Preparation:

1. Place the child in a supine position. Elevate the head of the bed, if possible.
2. Measure the distance from the tragus of the ear to the mouth and then to the xiphoid process to determine the distance to the stomach. Mark the tube with a piece of tape.

Procedure:

1. Put on clean gloves.
2. Lubricate the tube with water-soluble lubricant or sterile water.
3. Insert the tube into the child's nares or mouth.
4. If using the nose, advance the tube along the floor of the nasal passages.
5. If using the mouth, direct the tube toward the back of the throat.
6. Have the child swallow, if possible, while the tube is being inserted to make placement easier.
7. Advance the tube until you have reached the mark.
8. Check the tube for placement by aspirating stomach contents and checking pH or by injecting a small amount of air through the syringe while auscultating over the stomach. Growling sounds indicate the tube is properly placed.
9. Tape securely in place and attach to the child's nose or cheek with tape. Document tube placement as well as the amount and nature of aspirated contents.
10. To remove the tube, place the child in Fowler's position. Unfasten the tape, and gently pull from the oropharynx.

A well-established gastrostomy site is required. A mushroom-like tip holds the button in place, and two flat wings help to keep it against the abdominal wall. A one-way valve inside the button at the gastric opening prevents reflux of stomach contents.

GAVAGE FEEDING

A gavage feeding is given through a tube that has been placed into the stomach through either the nose or mouth. The size of the tube used for the feeding depends on the thickness of the feeding and the size of the child.

PROCEDURE

Gavage Feeding

Purpose: Infants and children are fed by gavage because of congenital anomalies, to supplement oral feedings, and after surgery. Feedings can be intermittent or continuous, and administration can be performed by gravity or pump. (Refer to Chapter 3 and Figure 3–5.)

Equipment:

- Sterile water for irrigation of the tube
- A stethoscope to check tube placement
- An asepto syringe or 10-, 20-, or 30-mL syringes
- The formula or solution
- If the feeding is to be administered by gravity, an IV pole may be used.

Procedure:

1. Place the infant or child in an upright position if possible. If not, place the child on the back or right side with head and chest elevated.
2. Check the placement of the tube before each feeding by aspirating stomach contents and by injecting a small amount of air through the syringe while auscultating over the stomach. Growling sounds indicate the tube is properly placed. Feeding may need to be held if residual is significant. Replace residual.
3. Formula should be administered at room temperature.
4. Start the flow slowly to ensure patency. The feeding should take approximately 30 minutes to complete. If administering feeding by gravity, raise or lower syringe to regulate flow rate.
5. Flush the tube with sterile water (1–5 mL, depending on the tube's size).
6. Clamp the tube. If the tube is to be removed, clamp or pinch and withdraw quickly.
7. Position the child on the right side after feeding for about 1 hour to prevent aspiration or vomiting and to facilitate gastric emptying.
8. Document the amount and type of feeding, including residual, duration of the feeding, placement of the tube, and patient response to the procedure.

Review Questions

A. Multiple choice. Select the best answer.

1. In which of the following positions is the infant supported along the forearm?
    a. cradle hold
    b. football hold
    c. mummy hold
    d. upright hold

2. Todd, 5 years old, is scheduled to receive an intramuscular injection. The preferred administration site for a child of Todd's age is the
    a. vastus lateralis
    b. gluteus maximus
    c. vastus medialis
    d. biceps brachii

3. The diameter of the catheter used for suctioning a tracheostomy tube should be
    a. one-quarter the diameter of the tube
    b. one-third the diameter of the tube
    c. one-half the diameter of the tube
    d. two-thirds the diameter of the tube

4. Which of the following delivery modes would provide the highest concentration of oxygen?
    a. face mask
    b. nasal cannula
    c. mist tent
    d. blow-by

5. Which of the following is a nontraditional venipuncture site that is used when drawing blood is difficult?
    a. antecubital fossa
    b. dorsum of the hand
    c. dorsum of the foot
    d. femoral vein

B. True or false. Write *T* for a true statement and *F* for a false statement.

1. ___ Toddlers benefit from simple explanations of procedures.

2. ___ When administering ear drops to a 4-year-old child, pull the pinna down and back.

3. ___ Oral medications should never be put in an infant's formula.

4. ___ When suctioning a tracheostomy tube, the nurse may safely apply suction for up to 15 seconds at a time.

5. ___ The formula used for gavage feeding should be administered at room temperature.

SUGGESTED ACTIVITIES

- Select a procedure. Practice explaining the procedure to children of different developmental stages. What differences are necessary?

- Spend time in an out-patient department or emergency room observing how children are restrained for procedures.

- Practice carrying and transporting a life-size infant doll or mannequin.

- Make a list of the different routes for administering medications to children and identify safety precautions that should be taken.

- List the differences in technique when applying a urine collection bag to a boy or girl.

- Practice using a bulb syringe on an infant mannequin.

BIBLIOGRAPHY

Bindler, R. M., and L. B. Howry. *Pediatric Drugs and Nursing Procedures.* Norwalk, CT: Appleton and Lange, 1991.

Broadwell Jackson, D., and R. B. Saunders. *Child Health Nursing.* Philadelphia: J. B. Lippincott, 1993.

Heiney, S. P. Helping children through painful procedures. *American Journal of Nursing,* November (1991): 20–24

Rice, J., and E. G. Skelley. *Medications and Mathematics for the Nurse,* 7th ed. Albany, NY: Delmar Publishers, 1993.

Skale, N. *Manual of Pediatric Nursing Procedures.* Philadelphia: J. B. Lippincott, 1992.

Speer, K. M., and C. L. Swann. *The Addison-Wesley Manual of Pediatric Nursing Procedures.* Redwood City, CA: Addison-Wesley, 1993.

Wong, D. L. *Whaley & Wong's Essentials of Pediatric Nursing,* 4th ed. St. Louis, MO: Mosby-Year Book, 1993.

CHAPTER

15

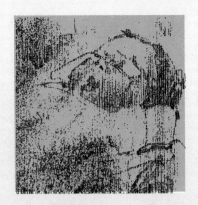

The Pediatric Surgical Patient

OBJECTIVES

AFTER STUDYING THIS CHAPTER, THE STUDENT SHOULD BE ABLE TO:

- DEFINE THE ROLE OF THE NURSE IN THE PREOPERATIVE AND POSTOPERATIVE CARE OF THE PEDIATRIC SURGICAL PATIENT.
- IDENTIFY SIGNIFICANT STRESSORS ASSOCIATED WITH SURGERY THAT PRODUCE ANXIETY FOR CHILDREN.
- DESCRIBE NURSING CARE THAT MAY REDUCE THE PSYCHOLOGICAL AND PHYSICAL STRESS OF SURGERY FOR THE CHILD AND FAMILY.
- DESCRIBE PREOPERATIVE NURSING PROCEDURES.
- DISCUSS THE IMPLICATIONS OF PREOPERATIVE TEACHING FOR THE POSTOPERATIVE RECOVERY PERIOD.
- DESCRIBE POSTOPERATIVE NURSING CARE OF THE CHILD.
- DISCUSS PEDIATRIC POSTOPERATIVE PAIN MANAGEMENT.
- IDENTIFY NURSING CONSIDERATIONS IN DISCHARGE PLANNING FOR THE POSTSURGICAL PEDIATRIC PATIENT.

*C*onditions requiring surgery are as stressful for children and families as hospitalization (refer to Chapters 11 and 13). With today's focus on cost containment and advances in surgical technology, nurses do not have a great deal of time to prepare children and their families for the surgical experience. Pediatric surgery can take place in a traditional hospital setting, in an out-patient surgical suite associated with the hospital, or in a free-standing surgical center. Many children now go home soon after recovery from anesthesia. The nurse needs to assist the child through the surgical experience and help the child return to optimal functioning.

PREOPERATIVE CARE

Preoperative care is the care given to the child and family in preparation for the forthcoming surgery. Children require emotional and physical preparation as part of preoperative care. The specific care will depend on the reason for the surgery and the individual needs of the child. Figure 15–1 summarizes preoperative nursing care of the child.

PSYCHOLOGICAL ASPECTS

Providing emotional support is as important as the preparation given for hospital procedures. When planning care, the nurse should be aware of the six stressors that produce anxiety for the child before and after surgery: (1) admission, (2) blood testing, (3) the day before surgery, (4) preoperative injections, (5) transport to the operating room, and (6) return from the postanesthesia area (Visintainer and Wolfer 1975).

Preoperative teaching is designed to reduce preoperative anxiety and promote a positive postoperative outcome. Rehearsing surgical events with the inclusion of known stressors has been shown to decrease the trauma of the surgical experience. Preoperative teaching helps children use their coping skills and feel in control of a difficult situation (Kennedy and Riddle 1989). In addition, children who receive emotional support and understand procedures generally experience fewer complications of surgery than children who do not receive support or information (Yale 1993). Materials used and timing of delivery must take into account the child's developmental stage:

NURSING CARE PLAN: Preoperative Care

NURSING DIAGNOSIS	GOAL(S)
Anxiety or fear (child) related to surgery (separation anxiety, fear of the unknown, or lack of knowledge)	Before surgery, the child will demonstrate minimal insecurity and anxiety. The child will be relaxed before entering the operating room.
Anxiety or fear (parents) related to potentially life-threatening condition of child	The parents will be able to explain the child's forthcoming surgery and the hoped-for response.
Risk for injury related to surgery	Before the child goes to surgery, legal authorization will be signed and included on the chart. Before surgery, all necessary physical preparation will be completed.

Figure 15–1 *Nursing care plan for preoperative care of the child undergoing surgery*

NURSING INTERVENTION	RATIONALE
Before the surgery, explain what will be happening and what the child's role will be. Use age-appropriate terminology and teaching materials.	Knowledge decreases anxiety, which in turn decreases the amount of medication needed for anesthesia and promotes postoperative recovery.
Orient the child to unfamiliar surroundings. Explain where the parents will be.	
Administer preoperative medication (preferably oral) if ordered. Place the child in a quiet room. Allow parents to stay with the child. Allow parents and a favorite toy or object to accompany the child.	Intramuscular injections are stressful. Allowing parents and significant objects to accompany the child utilizes the child's own coping strategies and decreases separation anxiety.
Include important family members in preoperative teaching.	Increased knowledge decreases anxiety. When the parents feel secure and trusting the child is more likely to feel secure as well.
Discuss informed consent with parent or legal guardian.	Parent or legal guardian must give verbal or written consent for surgery for children under 18 years of age (with exceptions).
Check document for correct surgical procedure and correct date. Witness signature of parent or legal guardian. Place on chart.	
Administer any preparations designed to cleanse the bowel, antibiotics, and preoperative medications, as ordered.	Enemas or irrigating solutions cleanse the bowel of normal bacteria. Antibiotics help prevent infection. Preoperative medications may be used to calm the patient, control pain, or help the patient cope with anesthesia.
Dress the child in hospital gown (if possible allow to wear underwear or pajama bottoms).	Clothing must be unrestrictive to allow full visualization during surgery. Underclothing or pajama bottoms are very important to children and can be removed after anesthesia.

Figure 15–1 *continued*

NURSING DIAGNOSIS	GOAL(S)
Risk for injury related to surgery *(continued)*	During surgery, the child will experience no complications due to aspiration, allergies, anemia, bleeding, or infection.

The child will arrive safely in the operating room. |

Figure 15–1 *continued*

- *Infants* and toddlers can be told about the procedure as it begins.
- *Preschoolers* benefit from rehearsals and trips to the areas involved before surgery.
- *School-age children* benefit from films in which peers model behavior. They can be taught about the surgical procedure and routine up to a week before the surgery.

- *Adolescents* can be taught about the surgical procedure as soon as it is scheduled. Provide clear explanations and teach stress-reduction techniques. Discuss particular fears related to surgery (anesthesia, venipuncture).

If pain is an expected result of the surgical procedure, children need to be honestly told of

NURSING INTERVENTION	RATIONALE
Remove any makeup, prostheses, or ortho-dontic devices.	All items that could harm the child during surgery must be removed.
Bathe child, groom hair, and brush teeth. Check for loose teeth. Record any skin lesions or breaks in the skin.	Bathing decreases the number of microorganisms on the skin. Bathing is also comforting.
Prepare operative site according to physician's orders.	Antimicrobial soaps and removal of hair further decrease the chance of infection.
Give the child nothing to eat or drink after the time designated by the physician's orders. Have the child void before taking preoperative medication.	Undigested food if vomited could be inhaled into the lungs causing aspiration pneumonia.
Take and record vital signs.	Changes in vital signs may indicate pain or fever. They also provide a baseline for comparison in recovery period.
Check laboratory reports for hemoglobin, white blood count, reduced platelets, or prolonged bleeding time.	Surgery would be postponed if there was a potential for hemorrhage related to inability of the blood to clot.
Check identification band. Put side-rails up or use safety straps when conveying. Do not leave child unattended.	Children are susceptible to injury during transport, especially when premedicated for surgery.

Figure 15–1   *continued*

the possibilities beforehand. They need to know that the pain will not last long. Older children are capable of using imaging or relaxation techniques to cope with painful situations (Berde 1989).

Parents will be anxious and need support and guidance before and after the surgical procedure. Including parents in the child's preoperative teaching helps them understand and cope with their child's responses to the experience. Although not always permitted, the presence of parents before surgery has a calming effect on the child. Many hospitals allow parents to stay with the child until the induction of the anesthesia and then to be present when the child awakens from anesthesia, Figure 15–2. Parents should be offered the option of staying with their child when policy permits.

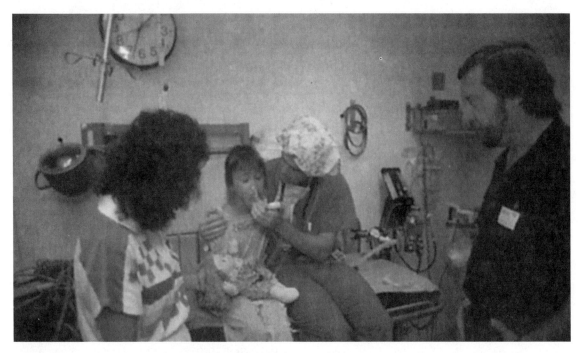

Figure 15–2 *Parents with child undergoing anesthesia (From D. L. Wong.* Whaley & Wong's Essentials of Pediatric Nursing, *4th ed. St. Louis, MO: Mosby-Year Book, 1993.)*

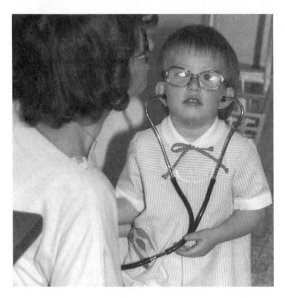

Figure 15–3 *Allowing the child to play with hospital equipment helps to lessen anxiety.*

Most children when asked state that they want their parents present (Murphy 1992).

Allowing children the opportunity to see and play with equipment, such as stethoscopes, blood pressure cuffs, and oxygen masks, helps to lessen their anxiety, Figure 15–3. Sometimes it is helpful to rehearse the child's surgery using a favorite doll. Drawings are an enjoyable activity for children of all ages and can offer invaluable information about a child's perceptions and fears, Figure 15–4. This information can help nurses to correct misconceptions and lessen the child's anxieties before surgery (O'Malley and McNamera 1993).

PHYSICAL ASPECTS

In addition to psychological care, children usu-

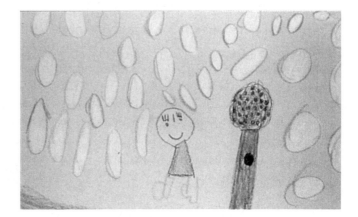

a.

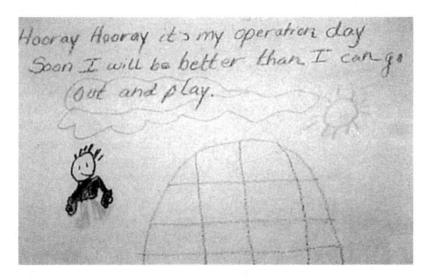

Hooray Hooray it's my operation day
Soon I will be better than I can go
out and play.

b.

Figure 15–4 *These two drawings illustrate children's conceptions of the surgical experience. (a) Trees drawn with knotholes represent a child's fear of invasive procedures. (b) This child's mother has added her feelings about surgery to his drawing. (From M. E. O'Malley and S. T. McNamera. Children's drawings. AORN Journal 57, 1993.)*

ally require various types of physical care before surgery. The steps of the preoperative process are usually arranged in what is known as a **preoperative checklist**, Figure 15–5. When preparing the child for surgery, the nurse notes when each step of the checklist has been accomplished.

The physician determines the fluid and nutritional needs of the child before surgery. Generally, no milk or solid foods are given after midnight of the night before surgery. But clear liquids (if ordered) can be given up to about two hours before surgery. Infants in particular should not go for longer than four hours

SAMPLE PREOPERATIVE CHECKLIST

- Consent forms witnessed, signed, and in chart

- Identification band in place

- Laboratory tests completed and results in chart

- Allergies clearly noted in chart

- Vital signs obtained and recorded

- NPO before surgery

- Voided before surgery

- Prescribed medications given

- Eyeglasses and any prostheses, including orthodontic devices, removed

- Mouth checked for loose teeth

- Operative site bathed and cleansed, if ordered

Figure 15–5

without fluids. In order for the child to be well hydrated, an intravenous line is started. Careful attention must be given to IV drip rates to avoid overhydration.

POSTOPERATIVE CARE

Postoperative care includes the physical as well as emotional care given in the postanesthesia room (PAR; also referred to as the postanesthesia care unit or the recovery room) and on the nursing unit during recovery from the surgical procedure. After the surgical procedure, the child is closely monitored in the postanesthesia area. Once sufficiently recovered from anesthesia, the child is either transferred back to the room or discharged home. The child should be awake, alert, and have stable vital signs, and any nausea, vomiting, or pain should be under control before release from the postanesthesia area. Figure 15–6 summarizes postoperative nursing care of the child.

TRANSFERRING THE CHILD

When a child is transferred from the postanesthesia area back to the room, the transferring nurse is responsible for giving a report on the child's status, including: (1) what was done during the surgery, (2) what anesthesia was administered, (3) whether any medications have been given, and (4) what orders the physician has written. The child's level of consciousness, vital signs, dressings and wounds, tubes, IV lines, and comfort level are assessed.

ARRIVAL ON NURSING UNIT

Close supervision is important. Changes in vital signs or behavior may signal life-threatening complications such as shock, hemorrhage, or malignant hyperthermia. Priority assessments during this period are airway, breathing, and circulation. Careful documentation and communication are essential (Whaley and Wong 1991).

PAIN MANAGEMENT

A common misconception is that children have a higher pain threshold than adults. They do not. Children are, however, often undermedicated for postoperative pain because of their inability to provide a description of pain.

The child's level of comfort should be assessed, and analgesics given accordingly. Change in behavior is the best indicator that a child may need pain medication. Assessment tools such as the Faces rating scale (Figure 15–7) can help the nurse and the child determine the quality of the child's postsurgical pain (Wong and Baker 1988). The nurse asks the child to pick the face that most closely describes the pain he or she is feeling. Keep in mind that fear of injections may prevent a child from acknowledging pain. Reassure the child that pain medication does not have to involve a "shot."

Effective **pain management** occurs when medications are given at regular intervals rather than on an as-needed basis. Children as young as 7 years of age benefit from patient-controlled analgesia (a drug-delivery system that allows patients to administer pain medication as they need it).

Nonpharmacological pain control methods may be used with analgesics, to increase their effectiveness, or alone when the child has minimal pain. These methods include distraction, cutaneous stimulation (rubbing, massage), transcutaneous electrical nerve stimulation (TENS), relaxation, hypnosis, imagery, and application of heat and cold. The presence of parents is also an important source of comfort for children in pain.

Pain needs to be controlled in order for the child to be able to perform effectively **postoperative exercises**, such as coughing and deep breathing, early ambulation, or leg exercises. These exercises stimulate circulation and respiration, thereby preventing atelectasis and blood stasis. Children who receive adequate pain management have less anxiety and recover more quickly than those who do not (Bender et al. 1990).

Mastery over painful and stressful events is important to children. During the recovery period, they need time to work through the experience. Play, drawing, and storytelling provide excellent means for expression and allow the child to discuss fears and perceptions.

WOUND CARE

Children usually return from surgery with surgical dressings in place. Compression is accomplished with elasticized bandages. If bleeding is controlled, the wound may be covered with a clear dressing. This dressing protects the wound, allows healing, and is easily viewed and cleaned (Failla and Vega-Cruz 1991).

The initial surgical dressing is usually not changed by the nurse, but it can be reinforced if bleeding occurs. Careful measurements and documentation regarding the dressing and drainage are essential. Any drains connected to the wound should be assessed for patency and amount of drainage. Careful aseptic technique must be exercised when handling or changing dressings.

DISCHARGE PLANNING

Discharge planning should include parents, other caregivers, and the extended family, as appropriate. The child's developmental stage, parents' educational level, and the extent of the surgery must be considered when giving discharge instructions. Reinforce verbal instructions about wound care, diet, activity, and pain management with written instructions. Additional considerations include proximity of the home to health care services, available support services, and the financial needs of the family (Hamilton and Vessey 1992).

NURSING CARE PLAN: Postoperative Care

NURSING DIAGNOSIS	GOAL(S)
Risk for injury related to surgery or anesthesia	The child will return safely from surgery with least amount of stress possible.
	The child's wound will heal and be free of infection.
	The child will not develop complications of surgery.
Pain	The child will rest quietly and exhibit minimum evidence of pain.

Figure 15–6   *Nursing care plan for postoperative care of the child undergoing surgery.*

Nursing Intervention	Rationale
Place the child in bed in position of safety and comfort. Follow physician's orders.	Measures to provide safety and comfort minimize trauma of transfer to hospital room.
Perform careful handwashing. Keep wound clean and dry.	Handwashing is the first line of defense against microorganisms.
Follow hospital procedure regarding changing dressings. Apply antibacterial medications as ordered. Record any unusual appearance or drainage.	Clean dry dressings inhibit growth of microorganisms. Antimicrobial medications and soaps fight infection. Redness, drainage, or swelling may be signs of infection.
Change diapers carefully to prevent contamination.	Careful disposal of diapers decreases the child's chance of developing an infection.
Check carefully for excessive bleeding. Monitor carefully for stable vital signs. Assist with early ambulation. Help the child to void.	Early detection of complications allows for prompt intervention. Common complications of surgery may be shock, respiratory depression, hemorrhage, and infection. Changes in vital signs may be the first clue. Early ambulation increases circulation and stimulates respiration.
Keep the child NPO until awake.	Until bowel sounds return nothing should be given by mouth to decrease the chance of aspiration and gastric distention.
Assess pain frequently using assessment tools as well as physiological responses (e.g., heart rate and blood pressure).	Children may have difficulty communicating that they have pain. Unrelieved pain has negative physical and psychological effects.
Administer analgesics as prescribed and evaluate their effectiveness. Administer antiemetics as ordered. Include nonpharmacological pain relief (e.g., ice, imaging, and breathing techniques).	Prevention of pain is best. Severe pain is difficult to manage. Continuous administration of opioid analgesics gives optimum pain relief.

Figure 15–6   *continued*

NURSING DIAGNOSIS	GOAL(S)
Risk for fluid volume deficit	The child will take in and retain sufficient fluids to maintain adequate hydration.
Altered nutrition: potential for less than body requirements	The child will receive adequate nourishment.

Figure 15–6 continued

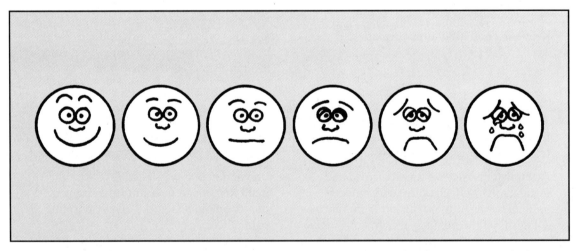

Figure 15–7 *Faces rating scale (From D. L. Wong. Whaley & Wong's Essentials of Pediatric Nursing, 4th ed. St. Louis, MO: Mosby-Year Book, 1993.)*

NURSING INTERVENTION	RATIONALE
Check for signs of dehydration (e.g., shiny, tight dry skin, less output than expected for age).	Skin should be warm, dry and supple.
Obtain weight measurement daily. Record intake and output. Weigh all diapers.	Helps ensure an accurate record of fluid status. An infant should have 6 to 8 wet diapers a day.
Offer fluids as soon as ordered or as child can tolerate them.	
Encourage the child with favorite drinks, ice chips, frozen pops (no red drinks or frozen pops if bleeding needs to be evaluated).	Providing favorite drinks improves fluid intake.
Ensure a nutritious diet appropriate to individual recovery pace and age.	A well-balanced diet promotes healing.

Figure 15–6   *continued*

NURSING CARE RELATED TO THE PRE- AND POSTOPERATIVE PERIOD

- Provide knowledgeable nursing care during the pre- and postoperative period.
- Anticipate stressful pre- and postoperative events and give appropriate nursing care to lessen the trauma of known stressors.
- Provide honest, developmentally appropriate explanations of pre- and postoperative procedures and routines.
- Prepare the child for pre- and postoperative procedures and allow him or her to rehearse, handle equipment, and visit the surgical area.
- Assess the child's understanding of preoperative teaching. (For example, have the child point to the part of the body that will be operated on.)
- Monitor the child postoperatively for changes in vital signs and assist in postoperative exercises.
- Observe the child for pain and use both pharmacological and nonpharmacological interventions for pain control.

REVIEW QUESTIONS

A. Multiple choice. Select the best answer.

1. The nurse caring for a pediatric surgical patient is responsible for
    a. ordering preoperative medications
    b. determining the child's fluid and nutritional intake
    c. assisting the child through the surgical experience
    d. informing the child and family about the advantages and risks of the surgery

2. To help decrease the trauma of the surgical experience for the pediatric patient, the nurse should
    a. avoid telling the child about the effects of surgery
    b. allow the child to rehearse surgical events
    c. relate information about the surgical procedures as if the child were an adult
    d. discuss informed consent with the parent or legal guardian

3. Of the following preoperative information, which would be most important for psychological support of an infant?
    a. favorite foods
    b. normal comforting pattern
    c. birth date
    d. number of siblings

4. The pediatric surgical patient can be expected to perceive which of the following as the most stressful?
    a. preoperative teaching, visiting the operating room, examining a stethoscope
    b. meals, parental visitation wearing a hospital gown
    c. roommates, primary care nurse, transport to the laboratory
    d. admission, blood testing, transport to surgery on a cart

5. The nurse demonstrates nursing interventions to lessen the psychological trauma of the child and family when he or she
    a. asks the parents to leave during preoperative procedures
    b. includes the parents during preparation of the child for the preoperative procedure
    c. keeps hospital equipment out of sight until the procedure has begun
    d. gives significant toys to family member for safe keeping

6. Of the following, which would be important for the anesthesiologist to know?
    a. the child's normal bedtime
    b. the child's last bowel movement
    c. the child's loose third molar
    d. the child's favorite sport

7. Timmy, 4 years old, clings to his teddy bear and refuses to get onto the surgical cart. What is the best solution?
    a. Firmly tell Timmy he must get on the cart — it is hospital policy.
    b. Postpone the surgery until Timmy is ready to go.
    c. Ask the physician to come talk to Timmy.
    d. Allow Timmy's parents to pull him to surgery in the unit wagon.

8. All of the following are normal preoperative procedures except
    a. antibacterial bath
    b. preoperative medication
    c. completion of preoperative checklist
    d. blood transfusion

9. The nurse prepares to receive a pediatric patient from the postanesthesia area. The priority assessment will be
   a. pain level
   b. respiratory status
   c. intravenous infusion site
   d. patency of drainage tubes

10. When will the nurse give the child something to drink?
    a. as soon as the child is awake
    b two hours after admission to room
    c. as soon as the child is awake enough to swallow and the physician's orders permit
    d. eight hours after surgery

11. Early ambulation after surgery accomplishes which of the following?
    a. diverts the child from the surgical pain
    b. stimulates respiratory and circulatory function
    c. assures early hospital dismissal
    d. increases the chance of postsurgical complications

SUGGESTED ACTIVITIES

- Speak with a nurse who has cared for pediatric surgical patients about how these children have described the surgical experience (choose a specific age group: toddler, preschool child, etc.). Identify stressors and actions that might help to alleviate a child's fear and anxiety.

- Collect and compare several pre- and post-operative checklists. What items do all checklists have in common? How do they differ? Make suggestions for additions or deletions.

- Write for the following free materials:
  - Faces scale (send a stamped self-addressed business envelope to Ms. C. Baker, 4412 St. Thomas Drive, Oklahoma City, OK 73120)
  - Pain management materials (AHCPR Publications Clearinghouse, P.O. Box 8547, Silver Spring, MD 20907; or call 1-800-358-9295)

BIBLIOGRAPHY

Acute Pain Management Guideline Panel. *Acute Pain Management in Infants, Children, and Adolescents: Operative and Medical Procedures. Quick Reference Guide for Clinicians.* AHCPR Pub. No. 92-0020. Rockville, MD: Agency for Health Care Policy and Research, Public Health Service, U.S. Department of Health and Human Services, 1992.

Bender, L. H., K. Weaver, and K. Edwards. Postoperative patient-controlled analgesia in children. *Pediatric Nursing* 16 (1990): 549–557.

Berde, C. B. Pediatric postoperative pain management. *Pediatric Clinics of North America* 36 (1989): 921–937.

Failla, S., and P. Vega-Cruz. Ask the O.R. *American Journal of Nursing* 91 (1991): 26–27.

Hamilton, B., and J. Vessey. Pediatric discharge planning. *Pediatric Nursing* 18 (1992): 475–478.

Jacox, A., B. Ferrell, G. Heidrich, N. Hester, and C. Measkowski. Managing acute pain. *American Journal of Nursing* 92 (1992): 49–55.

Kennedy, D., and I. Riddle. The influence of the timing of preparation on the anxiety of preschool children experiencing surgery. *Maternal-Child Nursing Journal* 18 (1989): 117–131.

Konings, K. Preop use of Golytely in pediatrics. *Pediatric Nursing* 15 (1989): 473–474.

Murphy, E. K. OR nursing law: Issues regarding parents in the operating room during their children's care. *AORN Journal* 56 (1992): 120–124.

O'Malley, M. E., and S. T. McNamera. Children's drawings. *AORN Journal* 57 (1993): 1074–1089.

Visintainer, M. A., and J. A. Wolfer. Psychological preparation for surgical pediatric patients: The effects of children's and parents' stress responses and adjustment. *Pediatrics* 56, no. 2 (1975): 187–202.

Whaley, L. F., and D. L. Wong. *Nursing Care of Infants and Children*, 4th ed., pp. 1184–2101. St. Louis, MO: Mosby-Year Book, 1991.

Wong, D., and C. Baker. Pain in children: Comparison of assessment scales. *Pediatric Nursing* 14, no. 1 (1988): 9–17.

Yale, E. Preoperative teaching strategy. *AORN Journal* 57 (1993): 901-908.

CHAPTER
16

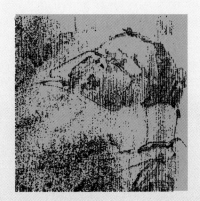

*F*luid and Electrolyte Therapy

Objectives

After studying this chapter, the student should be able to:

- Explain how normal fluid and electrolyte balance is maintained.
- Describe the different fluid compartments of the body.
- Explain why the young have a higher risk of fluid and electrolyte imbalances than adults.
- List nursing considerations in providing oral and parenteral fluid and electrolyte replacement therapy.

Key Terms

HOMEOSTASIS

INSENSIBLE PERSPIRATION

SENSIBLE PERSPIRATION

INTRACELLULAR FLUID

EXTRACELLULAR FLUID

INTRAVASCULAR FLUID

INTERSTITIAL FLUID

ELECTROLYTES

ater is the largest single component of body fluid. Without water life ceases. Fluid in the body also contains electrolytes, which are necessary for cell function. The amount, distribution, and movement of fluids and electrolytes have a profound effect on the functioning of every system within the body, including the transmission of nerve impulses, the contraction and relaxation of muscles, and the rate of metabolic processes.

MAINTENANCE OF FLUID BALANCE

In health, the body maintains a condition of **homeostasis**, or equilibrium of the internal environment. Fluid intake and loss are balanced. Newborns generally meet all of their fluid needs by drinking breast milk or formula. Older children consume a variety of fluids and solid foods to provide water to the body. A small amount of water is released during the metabolism of nutrients.

Total body water as a percentage of weight varies with age. In newborns, about 77% of body weight is water. The percentage decreases to about 60% by the first or second year of life. While this percentage is the same as it is for young and middle-aged adults, the distribution of body fluids in children differs from that of adults until puberty.

NORMAL FLUID LOSSES

The major regulator of fluid balance is the kidney. The kidney responds to changes in the volume and composition of body fluid by altering the amount and composition of the urine it excretes. For the first two years of life, the immature kidney responds poorly to changes in fluid status and is unable to concentrate urine effectively. This results in high urine output and a great need for water.

Water is also lost through the skin, either by **insensible** (unnoticed) **perspiration**, or evaporation, or by **sensible** (noticeable) **perspiration**, or sweating. Infants and young children have a much larger body surface area in relationship to their weight than adults do. The amount of water lost through the skin is significant in the very young.

Water is also lost through respiration and excretion. Insensible fluid loss occurs when water vapor is exhaled. Small amounts of water are lost in feces. Metabolic rate and heat production are higher in infants and young children, resulting in a greater amount of water needed to remove wastes.

FLUID COMPARTMENTS

Fluid is distributed in the body among three different compartments. These compartments are not discrete sacs but areas in the body where fluid is found. The composition of the fluid varies among compartments.

Intracellular fluid is found within the cells and, except in very young infants, comprises the largest quantity of fluid in the body. **Extracellular fluid** is found outside the cells. Infants and young children have a significantly higher percentage of extracellular fluid than adults do, which predisposes them to more rapid fluid loss. Figure 16–1 illustrates age-related fluid distribution changes in the body.

There are two types of extracellular fluid. **Intravascular fluid** is found within the blood vessels. Clinical laboratory tests normally report the composition of intravascular fluid. **Interstitial fluid** is found in the spaces between cells in tissue.

ELECTROLYTES

Electrolytes are substances that dissociate into ions when dissolved. Each ion carries either a positive or negative charge. The major body electrolytes are shown in Figure 16–2. Electrolytes are distributed unevenly among the different fluid compartments, but the total number (in milliequivalents) of anions must equal the total number of cations in each compartment.

Besides playing specific roles in metabolism and body function, electrolytes influence the movement of water from one compartment to another by **osmosis**. Osmosis is the movement of a solvent (liquid in which another substance, or solute, can dissolve) from an area of lesser solute (e.g., electrolyte) concentration to an area of greater solute concentration to achieve a balance of concentrations. When fluid imbalances occur, electrolyte imbalances are also likely to be present.

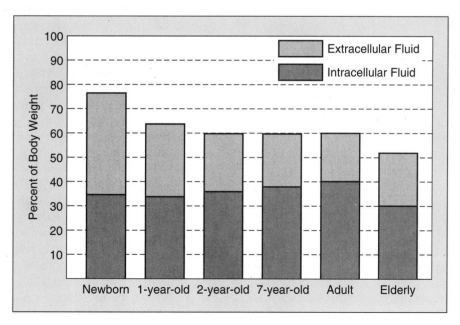

Figure 16–1   *Age-related fluid distribution changes*

DISTRIBUTION OF THE MAJOR IONS IN BODY FLUIDS		
Ion	**Intravascular Fluid (mEq/L)**	**Intracellular Fluid (mEq/L)**
Na^+	135–145	10
K^+	3.5–5.0	141–150
Ca^{++}	4.5–5.5	—
Mg^{++}	1.3–2.1	40
Cl^-	95–108	5
HCO_3^-	22–26	10
HPO_4^-	1.7–2.6	100
SO_4^-	1	14
Organic acids	5	—
Protein	16	75

Figure 16–2

DISTURBANCES IN FLUID AND ELECTROLYTE BALANCE

Fluid and electrolyte imbalances result from either altered intake or abnormal loss of fluids. Because children have smaller fluid reserves than adults, fluid volume deficits such as dehydration are more common than fluid volume excesses such as edema.

DEHYDRATION

Dehydration occurs when fluid output exceeds fluid intake. Dehydration can develop very rapidly in the young. The most common causes of dehydration in children are diarrhea and vomiting. Dehydration can also be caused by fever, excessive sweating, and restricted fluid intake. When gastrointestinal fluid is lost, electrolytes are also lost. Electrolyte imbalances, therefore, can occur in conjunction with dehydration. In the treatment of dehydration, it is essential that the nurse maintain accurate fluid intake and output records, Figure 16–3. Every effort should be made to collect and record information about all urine, vomitus, and liquid stools. A soiled diaper should be weighed and the weight compared with that of an unsoiled diaper. Refer to Chapter 24 for a discussion of symptoms, treatment, and nursing care for dehydration.

FLUID AND ELECTROLYTE REPLACEMENT

Oral replacement of fluids and electrolytes is always preferable to parenteral (intravenous) replacement therapy when the child's condition permits. Commercial oral replacement fluids such as Pedialyte or Infalyte provide a balance of water, major electrolytes, and glucose. Other fluids such as water, fruit juices, and decarbonated soft drinks provide partial replacement. Fruit juices and soft drinks, however, are not indicated to replace fluids lost from diarrhea because their high sugar content can exacerbate this condition. Milk (other than breast milk) or formula, which may not be tolerated, should be avoided as initial replacement fluids for infants.

A child should never be forced to consume needed oral fluids. Children who require oral fluids may be encouraged or gently persuaded to drink beverages. The nurse may offer small amounts of liquids at frequent intervals. It takes patience and ingenuity to administer fluids to small children. Incorporating play can help. Toddlers may need assistance in drinking from a cup. Ice chips or Popsicle bits are sometimes accepted more willingly than liquids.

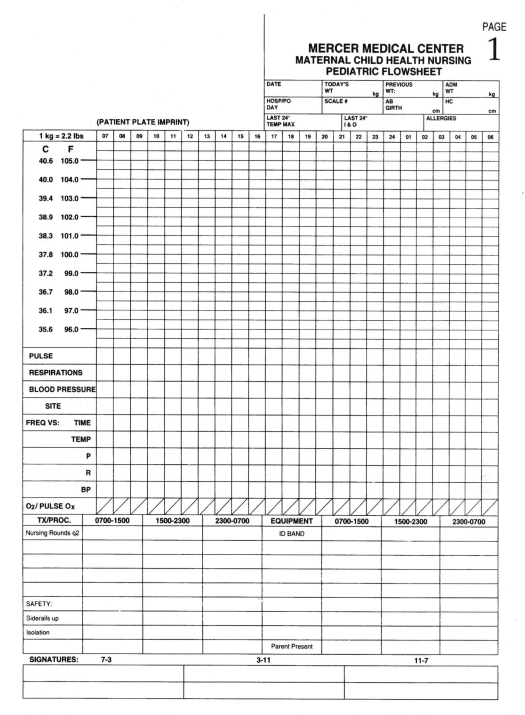

Figure 16–3   *Twenty-four hour fluid intake and output record. (Courtesy of Mercer Medical Center, Trenton, NJ)*

MERCER MEDICAL CENTER
MATERNAL CHILD HEALTH NURSING
PEDIATRIC FLOWSHEET

PAGE

2

(PATIENT PLATE IMPRINT)

STANDARD FINDING
IV SITE: intact surrounding skin, no signs of infiltration or phlebitis, line patent

DATE	A				B				C				SITE ASSESS	IV FLUSH (CONC)	MEDS
	BUR VOL / FILL	PUMP VOLUME REMAIN	HR / CUM	RATE	BUR VOL / FILL	PUMP VOL REMAIN	HR / CUM	RATE	BUR VOL / FILL	PUMP VOL REMAIN	HR / CUM	RATE			
06															
07															
08															
09															
10															
11															
12															
13															
RESET 14															
8° TOTAL															
15															
16															
17															
18															
19															
20															
21															
RESET 22															
8°/16° TOT															
23															
24															
01															
02															
03															
04															
05															
RESET 06															
8°/24° TOT															

Figure 16–3   *continued*

PAGE

3

MERCER MEDICAL CENTER
MATERNAL CHILD HEALTH NURSING
PEDIATRIC FLOWSHEET

DATE

(PATIENT PLATE IMPRINT)

STOOL STANDARD ABBREVIATIONS

a) L = loose	d) G = green	g) B = brown	j) Ⓜ = moderate
b) M = meconium	e) S = seedy	h) R = mucousy	k) Ⓢ = small
c) Y = yellow	f) W = watery	i) Ⓛ = large	

	INTAKE						OUTPUT								
	DIET	PO	NG/GT HRLY / CUM	PLACEMENT CHECK / FEED BAG CHANGE		INTAKE TOTAL	URINE	URINE TESTS	FOLEY CARE	STOOL	STOOL TESTS	COMBO	EMESIS		OUTPUT TOTAL
06															
07															
08															
09															
10															
11															
12															
13															
14															
8° TOTAL															
15															
16															
17															
18															
19															
20															
21															
22															
8°/16° TOT															
23															
24															
01															
02															
03															
04															
05															
06															
8°/24° TOT															

Figure 16–3   continued

PAGE

MERCER MEDICAL CENTER
MATERNAL CHILD HEALTH NURSING
PEDIATRIC FLOWSHEET

4

DATE

(PATIENT PLATE IMPRINT)

ASSESSMENTS / FREQUENCY   **OBSERVATION**

	TIME												
NEUROLOGICAL	TIME												
RESPIRATORY	TIME												
CARDIOVASCULAR	TIME												
ABDOMEN/GI	TIME												
GU	TIME												
MUSCULOSKELETAL	TIME												
SKIN	TIME												
PAIN	TIME												
OTHER	TIME												

TIME   **SIGNIFICANT FINDINGS \ NURSING OBSERVATIONS \ PATIENT OUTCOMES**

Standard Findings

Neurological: spontaneous eye opening, brisk pupil response, free spontaneous movement of extremities, verbalization and orientation appropriate for age, anterior fontanelle soft and flat for age no syncope, no eye drainage

Respiratory: regular unlabored respirations, no cough, clear & equal air movement in all lung fields, chest movement symmetrical, no nasal discharge or flaring, no ear discharge, throat free of soreness and exudate, no retractions

Cardiovascular: heart rate regular and no murmur, color pink. capillary refill < 2 sec, peripheral pulses strong and equal, blood pressure appropriate for age, afebrile, no peripheral edema present

Abdomen/GI: soft & nondistended, active bowel sounds (5-34/min), no emesis, no loose or diarrhea stools

GU: no frequency, burning, itching, no hematuria, no vaginal discharge, testes descended

Musculoskeletal: intact sensation, able to move all joints, no deformities

Skin: tears present, mucous membranes moist, skin warm and dry, no signs of breakdown/infection/rash, no bruises, scars, no pallor, cyanosis, jaundice, skin turgor quick, no tenting

Pain: able to participate in ADL's, arousable, no narcotic side effects, pain scale zero

Other: endocrine: lab work WNL for age

Key:
  S = Patient meets standard findings
  A = Patient does not meet standard findings - document assessment
  NC = (No change) Assessment unchanged from previous findings

Figure 16–3   *continued*

INTRAVENOUS REPLACEMENT THERAPY

Intravenous (IV), or parenteral, replacement therapy is used to replace lost fluids and electrolytes and to provide nutrition and maintenance fluids as well as a vehicle for administering medications or blood products. A secondary effect of intravenous therapy is that the gastrointestinal system is rested, reducing the opportunity for fluid loss through vomiting and diarrhea. Intravenous replacement therapy is used when oral therapy is impossible or not indicated; it may also be used in conjunction with oral replacement therapy to ensure fluid and electrolyte balance. Intravenous sites vary depending upon the situation and include the veins of the hand, foot, wrist, or arm, and for infants the veins of the scalp, Figure 16–4.

Many commercial solutions are available to meet specific replacement needs. The physician prescribes the amount and type of solution over time and the route by which it is administered. The nurse is responsible for safely and effectively administering the prescribed solution in the correct amount, at the specified rate, by the prescribed route.

Devices to control the rate of infusion, such as those that deliver microdrops, may also be used. Even with these devices, however, the nurse must monitor for changes in the infusion rate, signs of infection, and signs of fluid volume overload, including swelling at the infusion site, moist rales in the lungs, confusion, and behavioral changes.

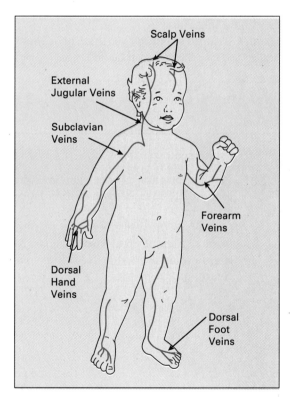

Figure 16-4 *Superficial vein sites commonly used for intravenous infusion*

TOTAL PARENTERAL NUTRITION

Total parenteral nutrition (TPN), or hyperalimentation, supplies all the nutrients that a child needs. A mixture of glucose, electrolytes, protein, lipids, vitamins, minerals, trace elements, and water is administered most often through a central venous line that has been surgically inserted directly into the superior vena cava through the subclavian or jugular vein. Lipids may be given separately. Medications are administered through a peripheral site.

The nurse is responsible for maintaining sterility and for frequent monitoring and assessment. Complications from TPN replacement therapy include infection, hyperglycemia (excessive blood glucose), and thrombosis resulting from dislodging of the catheter and fluid loss. Emotional support and appropriate explanations should be provided to children receiving TPN, or IV replacement fluids, and to their families.

REVIEW QUESTIONS

A. Multiple choice. Select the best answer.

1. Infants have more difficulty regulating fluid loss than adults because their
   a. metabolic reactions are immature
   b. kidneys are less able to concentrate urine
   c. fluid intake habits are more irregular than those of adults
   d. sense of thirst is underdeveloped

2. Fluid is lost in appreciable quantities through
   a. the skin
   b. nerve impulses
   c. osmosis
   d. the eyes

3. Dehydration in children is most commonly caused by
   a. inadequate fluid intake
   b. fever
   c. vomiting and diarrhea
   d. edema

4. Which of the following supplies all of the nutrients a child needs?
   a. intravenous rehydration
   b. fruit juice
   c. food high in protein
   d. total parenteral nutrition

5. Carlo, age 18 months, is receiving intravenous fluids. The nurse should
   a. return every hour to check for swelling at the infusion site
   b. ask Carlo's parents to help monitor the infusion rate
   c. stay with Carlo and periodically listen to his chest, take his pulse, and monitor his behavior
   d. tie Carlo's hands so that he cannot remove the infusion needle

---

B. True or false. Write *T* for a true statement and *F* for a false statement.

1. ___ Homeostasis refers to the optimal functioning of the body.
2. ___ The kidneys of children under two years of age do not concentrate urine well.
3. ___ Metabolic rate and heat production are lower in young children than in adults.
4. ___ The composition of intracellular fluid is normally measured in clinical laboratory tests.
5. ___ Osmosis is the movement of a solvent from an area of greater solute concentration to an area of lesser solute concentration.

SUGGESTED ACTIVITIES

- Role play a child about to receive intravenous fluids. The child is accompanied by a parent. The nurse will explain the procedure to both the parent and the child to prepare them for this experience.

- Visit a pediatric unit of a hospital. Talk with nurses about what strategies work to get a reluctant toddler to drink. Write a paragraph, analyzing which strategies you feel are best and why.

BIBLIOGRAPHY

Kee, J. L. and B. J. Paulanka. *Fluids and Electrolytes with Clinical Applications: A Programmed Approach*, 5th ed. Albany, NY: Delmar Publishers, 1994,

Metheny, N. M. *Fluid and Electrolyte Balance: Nursing Considerations*, 2nd ed. Philadelphia: J. B. Lippincott, 1992.

Weldy, N. J. *Body Fluids and Electrolytes: A Programmed Presentation*, 6th ed. St. Louis, MO: Mosby–Year Book, 1992.

Wong, D. L. *Whaley & Wong's Essentials of Pediatric Nursing*, 5th ed. St. Louis, MO: Mosby–Year Book, 1995.

The Dying Child

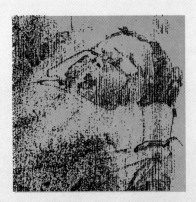

*C*aring for the Dying Child

OBJECTIVES

AFTER STUDYING THIS CHAPTER, THE STUDENT SHOULD BE ABLE TO:

- IDENTIFY THE CHILD'S CONCEPT OF DEATH AT VARIOUS DEVELOPMENTAL STAGES.
- DEFINE THE STAGES OF GRIEVING, ACCORDING TO KUBLER-ROSS.
- DESCRIBE COMMON RESPONSES OF PARENTS OF A DYING CHILD.
- DESCRIBE COMMON RESPONSES OF SIBLINGS OF A DYING CHILD.
- DISCUSS SOURCES OF SUPPORT FOR THE DYING CHILD AND FAMILY.
- DESCRIBE HOSPICE CARE.
- OUTLINE NURSING CONSIDERATIONS IN THE CARE OF THE DYING CHILD.

KEY TERMS

MAGICAL THINKING   HOSPICE CARE

ANTICIPATORY GRIEVING

the death of a child is difficult for both families and health care providers to face. The life of a child who dies is often viewed as having been unjustly cut short. Helping dying children and their families to cope with and accept the child's death is one of the greatest challenges facing nurses. To provide effective and supportive care, the nurse must understand children's perceptions of death at varying ages, stages of grieving, and parental and sibling responses. The nurse should also be knowledgeable about resources that can provide support to the family of a dying child.

CHILDREN'S PERCEPTION OF DEATH AND DYING

As we grow older, we learn about death from our environment and those around us. Death is a part of life. We begin to develop a concept of death that changes with each developmental stage. Some children are exposed to death when a family member dies. Other children learn about death by observing the life cycles of the insects, birds, and animals around them. All children experience life uniquely and develop at individual rates. Furthermore, all children express and handle feelings and cope with illness and death in their own way.

INFANCY AND TODDLERHOOD

Concept of Death. Infants and toddlers appear to have no real concept of death. Because young children live in the present, it is impossible for them to comprehend the absence of life. Death is perceived as a separation from loved ones.

Reactions to Death and Dying. Infants respond to the behaviors of those around them. Thus, they may respond with distress to the emotional and physical distress of others, especially their parents' reactions of sadness, anxiety, depression, or anger.

Toddlers, who lack a true concept or understanding of death, will persist in seeking to speak with or visit a person who has died. It is important to emphasize that the dead person will return only in the child's thoughts and memories.

Terminally ill toddlers fear separation from their parents. Because ritualism is extremely important in the toddler's life, any change in the ill child's routines can produce anxiety. Parents should be with the child as much as possible.

PRESCHOOL YEARS

Concept of Death. During the preschool period, between 3 and 5 years of age, children gradually develop the concept of nonexistence, of "life" and "not life." However, death is seen as reversible and temporary. Death may be seen as a kind of sleep, a temporary separation. To the preschooler, death is unpleasant because it separates people.

Reactions to Death and Dying. Preschool children have a tremendous sense of omnipotence, which leads them to believe that their thoughts and deeds can cause an event to occur. This belief is termed **magical thinking**. They may think that their thoughts caused the death of another. Similarly, preschoolers who become seriously ill may believe that the illness is punishment for their thoughts and actions.

The terminally ill preschooler's greatest fear concerning death is separation from parents. Preschoolers may fear going to sleep and never waking up. They may also associate "going to sleep" under anesthesia for surgical procedures with death (for example, a pet may have been "put to sleep"). For this reason, the presence of parents during painful or traumatic procedures is often helpful.

School-Age Years

Concept of Death. Children between the ages of 5 and 9 tend to personify death. Death is seen as a person such as an angel, ghost, God, skeleton, or a monster, who is either living or dead, with either good or bad intentions, who causes people to die. Children may have nightmares about these figures. They tend to believe that their own death can be avoided by personal ingenuity and efforts (for example, by running faster than death or locking the door to keep death out). From age 9 or 10 through adolescence, children begin to comprehend that death is inevitable, universal, and irreversible, and that they too will die someday, Figure 17–1.

Reactions to Death and Dying. School-age children continue to attribute the cause of death to misdeeds or bad thoughts and feel intense guilt and responsibility for the event. They tend to fear the possibility of death more than its occurrence. Bodily mutilation is especially feared.

It is important for school-age children to assimilate all the facts about death into a concrete logical framework. They want to know what happens to the dead body, who dresses it, and how the body feels. This information helps them to understand what will happen to them if they should die.

To achieve independence, self-worth, and self-esteem, seriously ill school-age children need to understand what is happening to them, to participate in their own care, and to be able to make decisions. Dying represents a loss of control over every aspect of living. Anticipatory preparation is effective and very necessary. Fear, exhibited as verbal uncooperativeness, may be erroneously interpreted as rude, impolite, or stubborn behavior. In reality, this verbal behavior is a plea for control and power.

Adolescence

Concept of Death. Adolescents have a mature understanding of death and yet still are influenced by remnants of magical thinking. Possible feelings of guilt and shame can be alleviated by making it clear that thoughts and activities do not cause diseases such as cancer.

Reactions to Death and Dying. Adolescents have more difficulty than other age groups in dealing with death. Some teenagers cope with death by expressing appropriate emotions, talking about the loss, and resolving the grief.

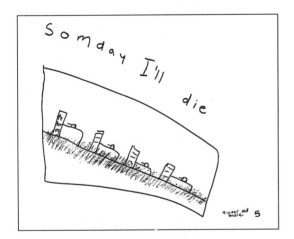 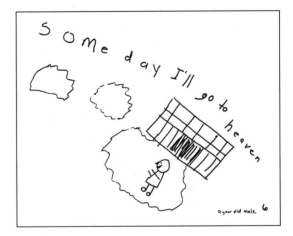

Figure 17–1   *These pictures illustrate the school-age child's concept of death. (Courtesy of Darlene McCown, Ph.D., R.N., P.N.P.)*

Others may appear undisturbed by the event, extremely angry, or unusually silent and withdrawn. Expect and accept these personal expressions of anger, fear, and sadness. Nurses can also be role models for parents in communicating with the adolescent.

The developmental task of adolescence is to establish an identity by finding out who one is, what one's purpose is, and where one belongs. Adolescents strive for group acceptance as well as independence from parental constraints. The crisis of a life-threatening illness may make an adolescent feel isolated from peers and unable to communicate with parents for emotional support. Any suggestion of being different or of ceasing to be is a threat.

Often the adolescent becomes emotionally attached to a nurse or physician. Parents may not understand this attachment and may even resent it. Reassure them that this is a normal occurrence for many adolescents who face a life-threatening illness.

The physical changes that occur with a life-threatening illness are especially troublesome for adolescents, who are oriented to the present. Physical changes are of more concern than the prognosis for future recovery.

It is important to allow the adolescent maximum self-control and independence during hospitalization. Answer questions honestly. Respect the need for privacy and solitude.

Stages of Grieving

The stages of grieving identified by Elisabeth Kubler-Ross (1969) can be applied to older school-aged children and adolescents with a life-threatening illness, as well as their parents and siblings. These stages represent behaviors that surface as the individual attempts to cope with the anticipated loss, and are not necessarily sequential.

- *Denial* and *isolation* are the initial reactions, during which the individual reacts with shock and disbelief. Denial serves as a protective buffer against overwhelming anxiety.

- *Anger* usually follows denial and is a reaction that occurs with the recognition of the reality of the diagnosis. Anger may be expressed as envy and resentment of the living. It may also be displaced onto others: "The doctor is no good"; "The nurse's didn't care." This stage may occur and recur anytime during the course of an illness.

- *Bargaining* occurs when the individual tries to postpone the inevitable. The individual usually bargains for an extension of life, preferably without pain.

- *Depression* may center on past losses, such as loss of hair from chemotherapy, or on anticipated losses, such as impending death.

- *Acceptance*, the final phase, is a time of inner peace and resolution in which the individual is no longer angry or depressed, recognizing that death is a certainty. This stage occurs only if the individual works through the earlier stages of grieving.

Parents' Responses

Death of a loved one is always painful. The death of a child, however, is especially difficult to accept. Because we expect to live to old age and associate dying with having lived a full life, children's deaths are viewed as unnatural and even unfair.

When a child dies unexpectedly, the parents are at first overwhelmed, experiencing shock and disbelief. The grieving process may last for weeks, months, or even years. Parents need reassurance that their feelings are normal and expected. If the death was preventable, parents will need to deal with feelings of guilt before they can begin to resolve and accept the loss.

When a child is diagnosed with a terminal illness, most parents react with shock at the time the diagnosis is given. This reaction is commonly followed by denial, and then guilt.

"If only we'd come to the doctor sooner" is a common reaction. Anger is typical. Parents may displace anger onto others, particularly health care professionals. Nurses who care for the child may be seen as competitors for the child's attention. It is important that nurses respect the parents' feelings and allow for these expressions of anger.

Anticipatory grieving occurs individually as each parent begins to accept the loss of the child and increases in intensity until the child's death. Typically, the mother is most intensely involved with the ill or dying child. The father may feel left out or escape by concentrating on work. During the anticipatory grieving phase, it is important for the nurse to help parents maintain a bond with and provide comfort for their child.

Siblings' Responses

Siblings of terminally ill children experience changes in family routines as parents spend time with the ill child, often away from the home and possibly in another community. Even very young children who do not fully understand the implications of death are aware that something serious is going on. They experience not only separation from their brother or sister, but also separation from their parents.

The healthy siblings may feel unloved and respond by increasing their demands on parents. They may express feelings of resentment, anger, anxiety, depression, fear of the ill child's death, fear of their own death, jealousy, guilt, psychological and physical isolation from their parents, and a wide variety of behaviors aimed at obtaining attention from the parents (Walker 1990). These behaviors occur at a time when the parents are already under stress from the emotions and responsibilities of caring for the dying child. It is important to reassure siblings that they will continue to be loved and cared for.

Young children are unable to understand cause-and-effect relationships. They may think that they caused the death, viewing death as a punishment or the result of their angry thoughts. Siblings may express angry feelings toward the child who has died. Anger also may be turned inward, resulting in depression. It is important that parents recognize that anger is a normal part of the grief process and anticipate and accept these feelings.

As appropriate, siblings should be encouraged to visit the ill child. If they wish to participate, they should also be included in care of the dying child.

Common Stressors of Terminal Illness

Children who experience a life-threatening illness usually have some awareness that they are seriously ill, whether or not their parents or health care providers have actually discussed their condition with them. Potential stressors for terminally ill children include inadequate information about their disease and its treatment, not understanding what they hear, and not being informed as the disease progresses (Hymovich and Hagopian 1992). Dying children need to be able to share in honest communication. It is inadvisable to lie to children in an effort to "protect" them from the knowledge that they are dying. How, when, and what children are told are extremely important (Walker 1993).

Resources for Care of the Ill or Dying Child

Support Groups

Support groups can provide emotional support to the parents and siblings of ill or dying children. These groups, composed of families who are coping with or have experienced a similar illness or loss, provide a forum for expressing and understanding feelings of grief and loss (Wheeler and Limbo 1990). Family support systems and friends are also very important during the crisis of the illness and after the death of a child.

SPIRITUAL SUPPORT

Spiritual beliefs about life and death become more important as the child and family begin to face the reality of the child's death. These beliefs can provide great comfort and support (Mott et al. 1990). Parents and other family members may request the presence of clergy or hold prayer sessions for the dying child. Nurses must take care to support the beliefs of the family and not impose their own personal beliefs on others.

HOSPICE AND HOME CARE

Hospice care provides holistic care and support for the terminally ill patient. This care may take place in the family's home, in a hospice center, or in a facility that applies the hospice concept. The goal of hospice care is to enable the individual to live life as fully as possible; free of pain; with respect, choices, and dignity; supported and cared for by his or her family. In this caring atmosphere, the patient and family can be assisted in the grieving process and in the preparation for death.

Hospice care of children is provided by an interdisciplinary team that provides a continuum of care and facilitates the role of the parents as the primary caregivers. Whether the care takes place in the home or in a hospice center, the hospice team is available to the family around the clock. Hospice care includes pain control measures and emotional support for the child and family members.

NURSING CONSIDERATIONS

EMOTIONAL NEEDS OF THE DYING CHILD

The dying child has the same emotional and developmental needs as other children of the same age and requires an environment that meets those needs. A key component of nursing care is promoting the child's and family's feelings of trust and security in the hospital staff. This is especially important when caring for the dying child. Perhaps the most important nursing intervention is that of explaining what death is, if the child asks. Nurses should answer only those questions asked by the child and should ensure that their answers are appropriate to the child's developmental stage (Petix 1987). An understanding of the child's experiences with death or dying can help the nurse communicate. Figure 17–2 is a nursing care plan for the child who is terminally ill or dying.

AWARENESS OF PERSONAL FEELINGS

The nurse develops a close relationship with the child and family who are facing death. The death of a child can be especially difficult for nurses who, like others in our society, do not expect children to die. There is a sense of helplessness and failure when a child dies. It is important that the nurse understand his or her perceptions of death and dying and realize that these perceptions have been defined by circumstances and specific situations in his or her life.

Nurses often react in much the same way as the family when a child is diagnosed with a fatal illness. Denial serves to protect the nurse from being overwhelmed by the reality of impending death. Anger may be expressed when the nurse finds that he or she has been assigned to care for the terminally ill child. Nurses may also feel anger toward family members who are demanding and seemingly

NURSING CARE PLAN: Terminally Ill or Dying Child

Nursing Diagnosis	Goal(s)	Nursing Intervention	Rationale
Anticipatory grieving (family)	The family will receive comfort and supportive care from the nursing staff.	Identify the family's stage of grieving. Convey an attitude of caring to the family.	The stage of grieving affects how the nurse relates to the family's actions and concerns.
		Give parents and siblings an opportunity to express and clarify feelings.	Provides the family with a safe outlet for feelings and clarifies concerns that may be unnecessary.
		Provide information about the child's status.	Being informed about the child's status increases the family's sense of security and control.
		Help the family deal with their feelings.	Providing an opportunity to express and clarify feelings may help to minimize stress.
		Involve family members in planning the child's care and in decision making when possible.	Participation enables family members to come to terms with the reality of the child's illness.
		Provide privacy for the family and provide for the physical comfort of the child and family.	Communicates genuine concern for the child and family.

Figure 17–2   *Nursing care plan for the child who is terminally ill or dying*

NURSING DIAGNOSIS	GOAL(S)	NURSING INTERVENTION	RATIONALE
		Encourage family members to talk to the child.	Having parents explain and talk with the child about the illness and hospitalization experience opens family communication.
Fear and anxiety	The child will experience a reduction in fear and anxiety through the empathetic care of the nursing staff.	Be open and honest in communication with the child: • Answer only the questions asked. • Explain death to the child, if asked. • Tell the truth in simple terms. • Use the language of the child.	The child who is informed about the illness and treatment feels less isolated and is better able to cope.
		Be a good listener and observer.	Provides a safe, acceptable outlet for feelings.
		Give the child the opportunity to discuss fears and prognosis. Reassure the child that he or she will not be left alone to die.	Acknowledgment of the child's fears and concerns decreases fear and anxiety and prevents the child from experiencing feelings of isolation and alienation.

Figure 17–2   *continued*

Nursing Diagnosis	Goal(s)	Nursing Intervention	Rationale
Ineffective family coping	The family will identify stressors of the child's illness and possible coping strategies.	Encourage the family's involvement in the child's care, as desired, and assist them to care for their child.	Involvement gives family members a sense of control and comfort in knowing they did something to help the child.
		Provide opportunities for expression and clarification of feelings.	Allowing the family to communicate feelings helps them to accept and deal with their emotions.
		Include siblings in discussions of the child's prognosis and course of the disease. Include what is known about the disease; emphasize that none of the siblings' thoughts or actions could have caused it and that other family members won't "catch" the disease.	Siblings have increased feelings of self-worth when they assume responsibilities for the ill child. Including siblings makes them feel less isolated and reassures them that someone cares about them and about what is happening to them.
		Explore with the family the stressors they have experienced and discuss how they have coped.	Helps the family to identify coping skills that have worked for them and gives them courage to face what is ahead.

Figure 17–2   *continued*

unappreciative of their care. Recognition of these feelings may lead to a sense of guilt. Nurses may experience alternating feelings of hope and despair. Another common reaction is ambivalence. Nurses need to accept that they cannot be all things to all people and they need support too. The nurse's role is unique, and the privilege of providing care, comfort, and compassionate support to a child and family can be very fulfilling.

REVIEW QUESTIONS

A. Multiple choice. Select the best answer.

1. Samantha, 11 years of age, is terminally ill with leukemia. One quiet night Samantha asks the nurse, "What will it be like when I die?" The best response by the nurse would be,
   a. You need to have your parents explain that to you.
   b. Samantha, everything is going to be okay. You don't need to worry.
   c. I'm too busy to talk about such hard times right now. I'll be back later.
   d. Samantha, tell me what you think it will be like.

2. A preschool child who becomes very ill is likely to perceive this illness as
   a. punishment for bad thoughts or deeds
   b. a bogeyman who has come to get him
   c. insignificant
   d. frightening because it may lead to body mutilation

3. Nine-year-old Mario is dying of osteosarcoma. He tells the nurse that he doesn't want his friends to think he looks "different" from anyone else. The nurse working with Mario realizes that his fear associated with dying is fear of
   a. being separated from his parents
   b. rejection
   c. mutilation
   d. losing his hair

4. Krista's grandmother has died. When her parents go to check on Krista at bedtime, her door is locked. She tells her parents that she is afraid of the "ghost that took Grandma away." In what age group is this concept of death common?
   a. toddlerhood
   b. preschool age
   c. early school age
   d. adolescence

5. Jamie is crying and states that it is her fault that her baby brother died. During what developmental period are children likely to feel guilt that their bad thoughts or deeds are sufficient to have caused an illness or death?
   a. toddlerhood
   b. preschool years
   c. early school age
   d. adolescence

B. True or false. Write *T* for a true statement and *F* for a false statement.

1. ____ Of all age groups, the school-age child by far has the most difficult time dealing with death, including his or her own death.

2. ____ The adolescent is less concerned with present physical changes than with the prognosis for future recovery.

3. ____ Siblings may respond with a wide range of emotions during the dying child's illness.

4. ____ Young children are unable to understand cause-and-effect relationships.

5. ____ Young children know they are seriously ill even if no one has discussed this fact with them.

Suggested Activities

- Schedule clinical hours with a nurse who specializes in pediatric oncology. Observe strategies that he or she uses with children of different developmental stages.

- Review case situations of nurses working with dying children and discuss what the nurse may be feeling, as well as appropriate interventions in these situations.

- Interview a nurse or social worker who works with children who have life-threatening illnesses about the emotional aspects of working with these children and their families.

- Speak with a grief counselor about family responses to the death of a child.

- Read a book written by parents of a child who has died to understand their perspective.

Bibliography

Armstrong-Dailey, A. Children's hospice care. *Pediatric Nursing* 16, no. 4 (1990): 337–339, 409.

Bowden, V. Children's literature: The death experience. *Pediatric Nursing* 19, no. 1 (1993): 17–21.

Bowlby, J. *Attachment and Loss*, vol. 1. New York: Basic Books, 1969.

Bowlby, J. *Attachment and Loss*, vol. 2. New York: Basic Books, 1973.

Castiglia, P. Death of a sibling. *Journal of Pediatric Health Care* 2, no. 4 (1988): 211–213.

Foster, R. L., M. M. Hunsberger, and J. J. Tackett Anderson. *Family-Centered Nursing Care of Children*. Philadelphia: W. B. Saunders, 1989.

Gibbons, M. B. A child dies, a child survives: The impact of sibling loss. *Journal of Pediatric Care* 6, no. 2 (1992): 65–72.

Hymovich, D., and G. Hagopian. *Chronic Illness in Children and Adults: A Psychosocial Approach.* Philadelphia: W. B. Saunders, 1992.

Kubler-Ross, E. *On Death and Dying.* New York: Macmillan, 1969.

Lawson, L. V. Culturally sensitive support for grieving parents. *Maternal Child Nursing* 15 (March/April, 1990): 76–79.

McCown, D. When children face death in a family. *Journal of Pediatric Health Care* 2, no. 1 (1988): 14–19.

Mott, S., S. James, and A. Sperhac. *Nursing Care of Children and Families.* Redwood City, CA: Addison-Wesley, 1990.

National Institute of Mental Health. *Caring about Kids: Talking to Children about Death.* Publication no. (ADM) 79-838. Washington, D.C.: U.S. Department of Health, Education and Welfare, 1979.

Petix, M. Explaining death to school-age children. *Pediatric Nursing* 13, no. 6 (1987): 394–396.

Phillips, M. Support groups for parents of chronically ill children. *Pediatric Nursing* 16, no. 4 (1990): 404–406.

Walker, C. Siblings of children with cancer. *Oncology Nursing Forum* 17, no. 3 (1990): 355–360.

Walker, C. L. The child who is dying. In D. Broadwell Jackson and R. B. Saunders, eds. *Child Health Nursing.* Philadelphia: J. B. Lippincott, 1993.

Whaley, L., and D. Wong. *Nursing Care of Infants and Children*, 4th ed. St. Louis, MO: Mosby-Year Book, 1991.

Wheeler, S. R., and R. Limbo. Blueprint for a perinatal bereavement support group. *Pediatric Nursing* 16, no. 4 (1990): 341–347.

Wong, D. L. *Whaley & Wong's Essentials of Pediatric Nursing*, 4th ed. St. Louis, MO: Mosby-Year Book, 1993.

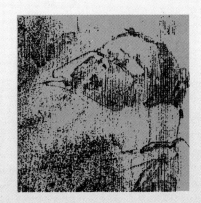

CHAPTER

18

Sudden Infant Death Syndrome

OBJECTIVES

AFTER STUDYING THIS CHAPTER, THE STUDENT SHOULD BE ABLE TO:

- STATE THE INCIDENCE OF SIDS IN THE UNITED STATES.
- IDENTIFY MATERNAL AND INFANT FACTORS THAT APPEAR TO PLACE INFANTS AT RISK FOR SIDS.
- DESCRIBE COMMON RESPONSES OF FAMILIES OF INFANTS WHO DIE FROM SIDS.
- IDENTIFY SPECIFIC INTERVENTIONS FOR THESE FAMILIES.
- IDENTIFY SUPPORT GROUPS AVAILABLE FOR FAMILIES OF AN INFANT WHO DIES OF SIDS.
- IDENTIFY NURSING CARE RELATED TO THE FAMILY OF AN INFANT WITH SIDS.

KEY TERMS

SUDDEN INFANT DEATH
  SYNDROME (SIDS)
CRIB DEATH

COT DEATH
SLEEP APNEA

$\mathcal{S}$udden infant death syndrome (SIDS), also called **crib death** or **cot death**, is the sudden death of an infant under 1 year of age that remains unexplained following a complete autopsy investigation and review of the history. SIDS is the leading cause of death in children between the ages of 1 and 12 months in the United States. Between 7,000 and 8,000 infants die of SIDS each year.

CAUSE

The cause of SIDS is unknown, although the following pattern of risk factors appears to predispose an infant to SIDS: low socioeconomic status, mother younger than 20 years, multiple pregnancies with short intervals between births, twin or triplet birth, male infant, and low birth weight. Other factors that have been linked with SIDS are:

- *Season and time of day*: SIDS occurs most often in winter and between midnight and 9 A.M.
- *Sleep*: Most deaths are unobserved and are thought to occur during sleep.
- *Illness*: SIDS is often preceded by a mild upper respiratory illness.
- *Race*: It is most common among Native American infants, followed by black, hispanic, and white infants; the lowest incidence is among Asian infants.
- *Family recurrence*: It is four to five times more common among siblings of an infant who died of SIDS, although no genetic link has been found (Rudolph 1991).

Research has focused on the possibility that SIDS infants have as-yet-unidentified neurological or respiratory alterations that result in abnormal breathing. For the past 20 years, researchers have also investigated whether there is a connection between SIDS and **sleep apnea**. Sleep apnea is the cessation of breathing for brief periods during sleep. The link between the prone (abdominal) sleeping position and an increased risk of SIDS prompted the American Academy of Pediatrics to recommend that healthy infants sleep supine or on the side. The exceptions are infants with respiratory problems or infants with gastric reflux who require special positioning. Infants with a history of sleep apnea who have required resuscitation, and siblings of SIDS victims often are monitored at home in an effort to prevent SIDS. The majority of SIDS victims, however, have no symptoms before death.

FAMILY RESPONSES

Typically the infant is found in the morning, dead in the crib. Parents may find the infant huddled in a corner, underneath the sheet or blanket, with blood-tinged, frothy fluid coming from the nose and mouth. The infant's position and wet, stool-filled diaper indicate a sudden, convulsive death. Parents commonly report having heard no cries or other sounds of distress during the night.

The first response of parents is to call for help. Efforts may be made to resuscitate the infant. When these fail, the focus of emergency personnel is shifted to the family. Parents commonly feel guilt, confusion, grief, and anger, and question whether they could have done something to prevent the infant's death. For this reason, police and emergency personnel should be able to provide appropriate information about SIDS; in particular, that the cause of SIDS is unknown, it occurs unexpectedly, and it cannot be predicted or prevented.

Figure 18–1 provides a summary of nursing interventions that can be used in assisting the family of an infant who has died of SIDS.

Providing Support for the Family of a SIDS Infant

- Provide private area for parents and support persons to say "goodbye." Obtain a rocking chair and enough chairs for family and friends present. Place a "Do Not Disturb" sign on the door.

- Wrap the infant in a clean blanket, comb the hair, wash the face, swab the mouth, and apply petroleum jelly to the lips before bringing the infant to parents.

- Make sure parents are seated and an ammonia ampule is available (in case they faint) before placing infant on the lap. Gently remind them that the

infant's skin will feel cool and bluish "blood" bruises may be visible.

- Provide a lock of hair, handprints, and footprints of the infant to the parents for a memory book. Obtain these while preparing the infant for viewing; offer them before the family leaves the hospital.

- Collect all personal items belonging to the infant and any written information (names of resource persons, SIDS support groups) for the parents to take with them before they leave the hospital.

Figure 18–1

Support Groups

SIDS affects all family members, including the siblings and grandparents of the infant. Many hospitals have follow-up programs in which nurses call or visit the family to provide support and answer questions about the infant's death. Other individuals who were close to the infant, such as babysitters, may also benefit from psychological support and counseling.

Group therapy is recommended for all families of SIDS victims. Most communities have a local support group that includes other parents of SIDS victims. Nurses can also refer parents to the National Foundation for Sudden Infant Death Syndrome, 8240 Professional Place, Landover, MD 20785; telephone (301) 459-3388, 24-hour hotline (800) 221-7437.

Nurses are often deeply affected by the death of a seemingly healthy infant and should be encouraged to express their feelings about the infant's death and the resuscitation effort.

Nursing Care Related to Family of Infant with SIDS

- Remember that an autopsy is required by law in most states when a child's death is unexplained.
- Reassure parents of a confirmed SIDS infant that they are not responsible for the infant's death and would not have been able to prevent it.
- Help the family begin the grief process.
- Provide emotional support for parents, siblings, and other family members.
- Refer parents to appropriate local support groups.
- Recommend resources for obtaining information about SIDS.
- Consider child abuse as a cause of death when an infant dies unexpectedly (even if the thought makes you uncomfortable).

REVIEW QUESTIONS

A. Multiple choice. Select the best answer.

1. Sudden infant death syndrome is characterized by which of the following?
   a. involves the death of an infant under 1 year
   b. occurs most often between 9 P.M. and midnight
   c. is explained only after a complete autopsy
   d. is preceded by high-pitched cry of infant

2. Which of the following is a risk factor that appears to predispose an infant to sudden infant death syndrome?
   a. low socioeconomic status of parent(s)
   b. high birth weight
   c. older mother
   d. female infant

3. Which of the following does not refer to sudden infant death syndrome?
   a. SIDS
   b. sleep apnea
   c. cot death
   d. crib death

4. In the United States, sudden infant death syndrome is the leading cause of death in children between 1 and 12 months of age. How many deaths does it cause each year?
   a. 7,000–8,000
   b. 3,000–6,000
   c. 70,000–80,000
   d. 30,000–60,000

5. Research on sudden infant death syndrome finds which of the following factors to be linked to its occurrence?
   a. It occurs most often in summer.
   b. It is most common among Asian infants.
   c. It is often preceded by diarrhea and vomiting.
   d. It is more common among siblings of an infant who died of SIDS.

6. Which of the following is typical of sudden infant death syndrome?
   a. Infant appears to have been neglected by parents.
   b. Blood-tinged, frothy fluid is found coming from nose and mouth.
   c. Infant's death is preceded by a severe viral illness.
   d. Infant is found stretched out, face up, with back arched upward.

7. What information should a nurse tell parents concerned about sudden infant death syndrome?
   a. Continuous monitoring can prevent these deaths.
   b. Research will soon identify the cause.
   c. It cannot be predicted.
   d. It can be prevented through altered nutritional and lifestyle practices.

8. The nurse can play a key role in helping the grief-stricken parents by doing which of the following?
   a. counseling the family to avoid viewing the infant
   b. avoiding mention of the need for an autopsy
   c. allowing the family to hold or touch the infant, if desired
   d. suggesting that family members put the death behind them and move on with their lives

9. The nurse might recommend any of the following support resources for parents and others close to the deceased infant except
   a. National Foundation for Sudden Infant Death Syndrome
   b. group therapy
   c. hospital follow-up programs
   d. Alcoholics Anonymous

10. Research into the cause of sudden infant death syndrome has centered on the following
    a. a connection with sleep apnea
    b. gastrointestinal alterations
    c. infant alcoholism
    d. congenital anomalies

SUGGESTED ACTIVITIES

- Discuss your feelings about death with your classmates. Identify ways in which those feelings will help or hinder you in dealing with people who have different beliefs. List methods you can use to help make your reactions more effective and supportive.

- Discuss with your classmates your feelings about the sudden and unexplained death of an infant. Identify ways in which this type of death differs from others. List ways in which you can demonstrate your sensitivity.

- Interview someone who has been involved in a professional capacity with the death of an infant from SIDS. Find out what problems health care workers have in dealing with the sudden, unexplained death of an infant. Discuss ways in which you can prepare yourself or support other health care workers for this situation.

- The nurse must consider child abuse as a possible cause of death when an infant dies unexpectedly. Discuss how you would handle this possibility in an actual situation with the family of a child who had just died.

BIBLIOGRAPHY

Broadwell Jackson, D., and R. B. Saunders, eds. *Child Health Nursing*. Philadelphia: J. B. Lippincott, 1993.

Rudolph, A. M. *Rudolph's Pediatrics*, 19th ed. Norwalk, CT: Appleton & Lange, 1991.

Wong, D. L. *Whaley & Wong's Essentials of Pediatric Nursing*, 4th ed. St. Louis, MO: Mosby-Year Book, 1993.

Zylke, J. W. Sudden infant death syndrome: Resurgent research offers hope. *Journal of the American Medical Association* 262 (1989): 1565.

Common Pediatric Conditions

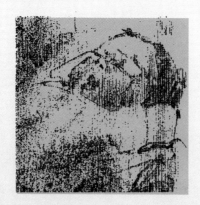

CHAPTER

19

Communicable and Infectious Diseases

Objectives

AFTER STUDYING THIS CHAPTER, THE STUDENT SHOULD BE ABLE TO:

*   Differentiate between communicable and infectious diseases.
*   Describe the links in the chain of infection.
*   List the four stages of infection.
*   Identify measures that health care providers can take to prevent the spread of infection.
*   Describe several types of isolation and explain their use.
*   Identify several communicable and infectious diseases of childhood, including their causative agents, transmission, incubation period, contagious period, prevention, signs and symptoms, treatment, and nursing care.
*   Discuss the cause, incidence, and symptoms of acquired immunodeficiency syndrome, and describe the treatment and nursing care of children with this disorder.

KEY TERMS

COMMUNICABLE DISEASES

INFECTIOUS DISEASES

HOST

CHAIN OF INFECTION

CAUSATIVE AGENT

PATHOGEN

RESERVOIR

PORTAL OF EXIT

TRANSMISSION

DIRECT CONTACT

INDIRECT CONTACT

PORTAL OF ENTRY

SUSCEPTIBLE HOST

PRODROMAL PHASE

BARRIER

ISOLATION

Communicable diseases are diseases that are spread from one person to another either directly or indirectly. **Infectious diseases** are diseases that are caused by microorganisms that invade the body and then reproduce and multiply. Disease is caused by damage to the cells, secretion of a toxin, or an antigen-antibody reaction (combining of antibody and antigen resulting in antibody production) in the **host** (a person who harbors the infectious organism). Infectious diseases are the fifth most common cause of death in the United States and account for half of all health care visits (Foster et al. 1989, Grimes 1991). By law, many communicable diseases must be reported to the local health department.

THE INFECTIOUS PROCESS

THE CHAIN OF INFECTION

The process of the development of infectious disease in humans is called the **chain of infection**. This chain must be intact for an organism to produce an infectious disease. Conversely, to prevent infection, one of the links of the chain must be broken. The links are the causative agent, reservoir, portal of exit, transmission, portal of entry, and susceptible host, Figure 19–1.

The **causative agent** (also called a **pathogen**) is the organism that causes the disease. The most common causes of disease in children are viruses, bacteria, parasites, and fungi. The **reservoir** is where the organism grows and reproduces. The reservoir can be someone with the disease, someone carrying the disease, an animal, or the environment.

The **portal of exit** refers to the method by which the infectious organism leaves the reservoir. It can leave through bodily secretions from the respiratory, genitourinary, or intestinal tract; feces; blood; saliva; tears; draining wounds; and vaginal secretions.

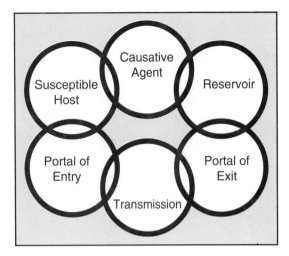

Figure 19–1   The chain of infection

Transmission is the spread of pathogens, by either direct contact or indirect contact, by airborne spread, by inanimate objects (such as soil, food, bedding, towels, and combs), or by vectors (such as insects). **Direct contact** refers to actual physical contact (body-to-body), as in the spread of sexually transmitted diseases. **Indirect contact** occurs as a result of organisms that live on animate or inanimate objects, which become common vehicles with the potential to infect many people.

The **portal of entry** is the means by which the organism enters the host. It may enter through breaks in the skin or mucous membranes, ingestion, inhalation, or across the placenta in utero. A **susceptible host** is a person at risk for contracting an infectious disease. Several risk factors contribute to the individual's susceptibility to infection and to the severity of the resulting disease. These include:

- age
- sex
- pre-existing diseases and conditions
- immunizations and vaccinations
- heredity
- efficiency of immune system

- nutritional status
- living conditions

STAGES OF INFECTION

Infection occurs in four identifiable stages: the latent period, incubation period, communicability period, and disease period. The length of each stage varies, depending on the pathogen and the susceptibility of the host. The latent period begins when the body is invaded by the pathogen and ends when the person begins to shed the pathogen (communicability period). The incubation period begins when the pathogen invades the body and ends when the disease process starts. During this period, the pathogen multiplies within the individual. The communicability period begins when the latent period ends and continues for as long as the pathogen is present. The disease period follows the incubation period. During incubation, the individual may or may not have symptoms (Grimes 1991). The earliest phase of the developing disease or condition is referred to as the **prodromal phase**.

INFECTION CONTROL
AND PRECAUTIONS

STANDARD PRECAUTIONS

An essential component of disease prevention is infection control. The Centers for Disease Control and Prevention (CDC) recommends that blood and body fluid precautions be used for all patients. Nurses need to protect themselves from exposure to infectious agents in the blood or other body fluids of patients. This protection involves the use of a **barrier**, such as gloves, gown, mask, and protective eyewear. The goal of standard precautions is to minimize the risk of exposure to the blood and body fluids of all patients regardless of their isolation precaution status or diagnosis. Standard precautions to take in all clinical settings are presented in Figure 19–2.

STANDARD PRECAUTIONS
FOR INFECTION CONTROL

Wash Hands (Plain soap)
Wash after touching **blood, body fluids, secretions, excretions,** and **contaminated items.** Wash immediately **after gloves are removed** and **between patient contacts.** Avoid transfer of microorganisms to other patients or environments.

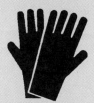

Wear Gloves
Wear when touching **blood, body fluids, secretions, excretions,** and **contaminated items.** Put on **clean** gloves just **before touching mucous membranes** and **nonintact skin.** Change gloves between tasks and procedures on the same patient after contact with material that may contain high concentrations of microorganisms. Remove gloves promptly after use, before touching noncontaminated items and environmental surfaces, and before going to another patient, and wash hands immediately to avoid transfer of microorganisms to other patients or environments.

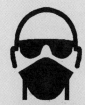

Wear Mask and Eye Protection or Face Shield
Protect mucous membranes of the eyes, nose and mouth during procedures and patient-care activities that are likely to generate **splashes** or **sprays** of **blood, body fluids, secretions,** or **excretions.**

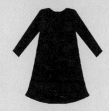

Wear Gown
Protect skin and prevent soiling of clothing during procedures that are likely to generate **splashes** or **sprays** of **blood, body fluids, secretions,** or **excretions.** Remove a soiled gown as promptly as possible and wash hands to avoid transfer of microorganisms to other patients or environments.

Patient-Care Equipment
Handle used patient-care equipment soiled with **blood, body fluids, secretions,** or **excretions** in a manner that prevents skin and mucous membrane exposures, contamination of clothing, and transfer of microorganisms to other patients and environments. Ensure that reusable equipment is not used for the care of another patient until it has been appropriately cleaned and reprocessed and single use items are properly discarded.

Figure 19–2 *(Courtesy of BREVIS Corporation)*

Environmental Control
Follow hospital procedures for routine care, cleaning, and disinfection of environmental surfaces, beds, bedrails, bedside equipment and other frequently touched surfaces.

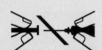

Linen
Handle, transport, and process used linen soiled with **blood, body fluids, secretions,** or **excretions** in a manner that prevents exposures and contamination of clothing, and avoids transfer of microorganisms to other patients and environments.

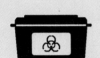

Occupational Health and Bloodborne Pathogens
Prevent injuries when using needles, scalpels, and other sharp instruments or devices; when handling sharp instruments after procedures; when cleaning used instruments; and when disposing of used needles.

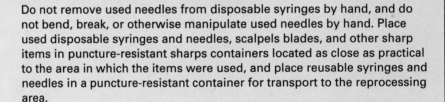

Never recap used needles using both hands or any other technique that involves directing the point of a needle towards any part of the body; rather, use either a one-handed "scoop" technique or a mechanical device designed for holding the needle sheath.

Do not remove used needles from disposable syringes by hand, and do not bend, break, or otherwise manipulate used needles by hand. Place used disposable syringes and needles, scalpels blades, and other sharp items in puncture-resistant sharps containers located as close as practical to the area in which the items were used, and place reusable syringes and needles in a puncture-resistant container for transport to the reprocessing area.

Use **resuscitation devices** as an alternative to mouth-to-mouth resuscitation.

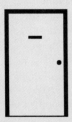

Patient Placement
Use a **private room** for a patient who contaminates the environment or who does not (or cannot be expected to) assist in maintaining appropriate hygiene or environmental control. Consult Infection Control if a private room is not available.

Figure 19–2   *continued*

ISOLATION

Children are placed in short-term **isolation** for infectious diseases, for chemotherapy, and because of immunodeficiency diseases. The CDC has established isolation guidelines, based on the mode of transmission, designed to protect patients and staff from acquiring communicable diseases. The purpose of placing a child in isolation is to interrupt the chain of infection by preventing the transmission of microbes. The type of isolation or precaution used depends on the disease and its mode of transmission. The CDC has identified the following three levels of precaution:

- Contact Precautions
- Droplet Precautions
- Airborne Precautions

The recommendations associated with each type of transmission are shown in Figures 19–3, 19–4, and 19–5.

The nurse must follow hospital policy where he or she works for isolation guidelines, procedures, and precautions. All hospital health care providers and personnel need to be responsible for and practice proper isolation techniques to protect patients, the environment, and themselves. The most important of these techniques are:

- *Handwashing*: the most important means of preventing the spread of infection for all isolation precautions
- *Gowns*: worn to prevent self-contamination
- *Gloves*: worn whenever there is exposure to body fluids
- *Face mask*: worn whenever there is exposure to droplet secretions
- *Equipment*: disposable equipment should be used whenever possible
- *Needle safety*: needles should be placed in an appropriate rigid, puncture-resistant container or receptacle
- *Containment of articles:* contaminated articles (linens, equipment, trash) should be bagged, labeled, and disposed of according to hospital guidelines for specific isolation precautions
- *Patient transport:* limited to essential purposes

Children in isolation are at risk for loneliness and depression from lack of social interaction. The following nursing interventions can help to prevent or reduce this social isolation.

- Encourage parents and siblings to visit and to bring in the child's favorite washable toys from home.
- Encourage patients, especially teenagers, to call friends.
- Reassure small children that they can talk to the nurse using the intercom in their room.
- Spend extra time with the child, reading a story or playing a game.
- Provide diversionary activities.

Be sure the child and parents understand that they must abide by the isolation precautions for the safety of the patient and others.

COMMUNICABLE AND INFECTIOUS DISEASES OF CHILDHOOD

Figure 19–4 describes communicable and infectious diseases of childhood, along with their treatment and nursing care. The incidence of some of these diseases has dropped because of the development of vaccines that are routinely administered to children (see Chapter 25). Improved preventive measures have reduced the incidence of other diseases. Nurses who work in pediatrics should become familiar with the signs and symptoms, as well as possible complications, of these diseases.

ACQUIRED IMMUNODEFICIENCY SYNDROME

Description. Acquired immunodeficiency syndrome (AIDS) is a multisystem disorder that occurs in adults and children infected with human immunodeficiency virus (HIV-1), one of a family of viruses called retroviruses.

CONTACT PRECAUTIONS
(in addition to Standard Precautions)
VISITORS: Report to nurse before entering.

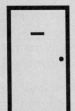

Patient Placement
Private room, if possible. Cohort if private room is not available.

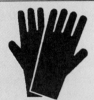

Gloves
Wear gloves when entering patient room.
Change gloves after having contact with infective material that may contain high concentrations of microorganisms (**fecal** material and **wound drainage**). **Remove** gloves before leaving patient room.

Wash
Wash hands with an **antimicrobial** agent immediately after glove removal. After glove removal and handwashing, ensure that hands do not touch potentially contaminated environmental surfaces or items in the patient's room to avoid transfer of microorganisms to other patients or environments.

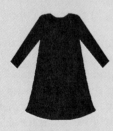

Gown
Wear gown when entering patient room if you anticipate that your clothing will have a substantial contact with the patient, environmental surfaces, or items in the patient's room, or if the patient is **incontinent,** or has **diarrhea,** an **ilestomy,** a **colostomy,** or **wound drainage** not contained by a dressing. **Remove** gown before leaving the patient's environment and ensure that clothing does not contact potentially contaminated environmental surfaces to avoid transfer of microorganisms to other patients or environments.

Patient Transport
Limit transport of patient to essential purposes only. During transport, ensure that precautions are maintained to minimize the risk of transmission of microorganisms to other patients and contamination of environmental surfaces and equipment.

Patient-Care Equipment
Dedicate the use of noncritical patient-care equipment to a single patient. If common equipment is used, clean and disinfect between patients.

Figure 19–3 *Strict isolation is used for children with diseases such as smallpox, diphtheria, and chickenpox. (Courtesy of BREVIS Corporation)*

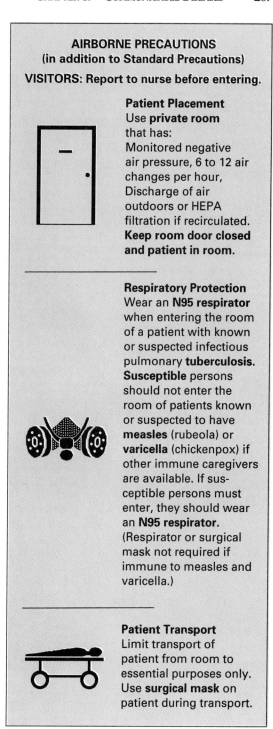

DROPLET PRECAUTIONS
(in addition to Standard Precautions)

VISITORS: Report to nurse before entering.

Patient Placement
Private room, if possible. Cohort or maintain spatial separation of **3 feet** from other patients or visitors if private room is not available.

Mask
Wear mask when working within **3 feet** of patient (or upon entering room).

Patient Transport
Limit transport of patient from room to essential purposes only. Use **surgical mask** on patient during transport.

Figure 19–4

AIRBORNE PRECAUTIONS
(in addition to Standard Precautions)

VISITORS: Report to nurse before entering.

Patient Placement
Use **private room** that has: Monitored negative air pressure, 6 to 12 air changes per hour, Discharge of air outdoors or HEPA filtration if recirculated. **Keep room door closed and patient in room.**

Respiratory Protection
Wear an **N95 respirator** when entering the room of a patient with known or suspected infectious pulmonary **tuberculosis.** **Susceptible** persons should not enter the room of patients known or suspected to have **measles** (rubeola) or **varicella** (chickenpox) if other immune caregivers are available. If susceptible persons must enter, they should wear an **N95 respirator.** (Respirator or surgical mask not required if immune to measles and varicella.)

Patient Transport
Limit transport of patient from room to essential purposes only. Use **surgical mask** on patient during transport.

The virus causes gradual destruction of the body's immune system. As a result, the patient becomes immunocompromised and is at risk for serious infection and invasion by any pathogen.

HIV is transmitted through sexual contact, sharing contaminated needles, and through injection or transfusion. HIV has been found in blood, semen, vaginal secretions, and in breast milk (in low concentrations). Approximately 80% of HIV-infected children are under the age of 13 years (Rudolph 1991).

Text Continues on Page 279

Figure 19–5

COMMUNICABLE AND INFECTIOUS DISEASES OF CHILDHOOD

Disease

Chickenpox

Agent: Varicella, herpes zoster virus

Transmission: Airborne; direct contact with an infected person

Incubation period: 10–21 days (average of 14–15 days)

Communicability period: From 1 to 2 days before the onset of the rash to 5–6 days after

Prevention: Isolation of infected patients; live attenuated varicella vaccine (see Chapter 9)

Signs and Symptoms

1–2 days before the rash, patient develops a low-grade fever and malaise. Rash starts as macules on an erythematous base, progresses to papules, and then to clear fluid-filled vesicles approximately 2–4 mm in diameter. Unruptured vesicles become purulent and dry and crust over. Crust may remain for 1–3 weeks. Lesions are not confined to the skin and can develop on any mucosal surface. Fever is present during rash peak and disappears by the time vesicles have dried or crusted over.

Treatment and Nursing Care

Maintain strict isolation in hospital.

Provide relief of itching (oatmeal baths, Caladryl lotion, Benadryl, cool environment).

Fever management.

Encourage fluids (fruit-flavored popsicles, soft drinks, ice cubes).

Keep children busy so they don't have time to itch (coloring, painting, finger-painting, playing games).

Keep patient's fingernails short and clean.

Diphtheria

Agent: Corynebacterium diphtheriae

Transmission: Droplet (from active cases or carriers)

Incubation period: 1–7 days

Communicability period: Variable (usually 2 weeks), until bacilli are no longer present in discharge and lesions

Prevention: Active immunization with diphtheria toxoid (see Chapter 9)

Respiratory tract and skin infections. Disease can be either mild or severe. Sore throat, difficulty swallowing, low-grade fever. THROAT: Erythema, localized exudate or a membrane, which may occur as a patch, cover entire tonsil, or spread to cover the soft and hard palates and the posterior portion of the pharynx. Membrane may be whitish and wipe off easily or be thick, blue-white to gray-black, and adhere. Attempts to remove the membrane result in bleeding. Enlarged cervical lymph nodes.

Maintain strict isolation in hospital.

Corticosteroids.

Antibiotics.

Fever management.

Airway maintenance.

Monitor breathing pattern and effort.

Provide oxygen as prescribed.

Figure 19–6

COMMUNICABLE AND INFECTIOUS DISEASES OF CHILDHOOD

Disease	Signs and Symptoms	Treatment and Nursing Care
Erythema infectiosum (fifth disease) *Agent*: Parvovirus B19 *Transmission*: Droplet *Incubation period*: 6–14 days *Communicability period*: Unknown *Prevention*: None	First symptom is a rash, which appears in three stages. FIRST STAGE: Red, maculopapular, coalesces on the cheeks, looking like a "slapped face" with circumoral pallor; disappears in 1–4 days. SECOND STAGE: A day after face rash appears, a red maculopapular rash appears on arms, legs, and trunk; rash proceeds from proximal to distal surface; can last 1 week or more. THIRD STAGE: Rash fades but can reappear if skin is irritated or exposed to heat or cold.	No specific treatment. Provide comfort measures. Temperature control (acetaminophen). Relieve itching with antipruritics. Explain the three phases of the rash to parents.
Hepatitis B (HBV) *Agent*: Hepadnaviridae *Transmission*: Direct or indirect contact with blood, semen, sexual contact; by direct access to the circulation through breaks in the skin or passages through mucous membranes, blood products, infected needles, infected mothers to newborns, person-to-person spread, interpersonal contact over long periods of time, between siblings and adults *Incubation period*: 45–180 days (average of 60–90 days) *Communicability period*: During incubation period and throughout clinical course of disease *Prevention*: Hepatitis B vaccine (see Chapter 9)	Onset is insidious, including malaise, weakness, anorexia. Diagnosis can be made only by serological testing.	Maintain strict isolation in hospital. Maintain bed rest. Maintain fluid balance. Provide high-caloric liquids, encourage small frequent feedings. Watch for bruising and bleeding. Educate parents about the disease and its transmission and make clear that untreated infection can result in chronic active hepatitis and cirrhosis.

Figure 19–6   continued

Communicable and Infectious Diseases of Childhood

Disease

Lyme disease (tickborne bacterial infection)

Agent: Borrelia burgdorferi spirochete

Transmission: Tick bite; ticks live in wooded areas and grasslands; infected ticks are carried by wild animals (birds, mice, raccoons, deer) and by domestic animals (cats, dogs, horses, cows); tick bite is not painful; tick transmits infected spirochetes when it draws blood for nourishment.

Incubation period: 3–32 days

Communicability period: Not communicable

Prevention: Avoid tick-infested areas; wear appropriate dress outdoors (long pants; socks that overlap pant cuffs, closed-toe shoes); use bug repellents; frequently inspect clothing, skin, and hiking equipment after return from tick-infested areas

Signs and Symptoms

INITIAL SIGNS: Slowly expanding red rash called erythema migrans. Starts as a flat or raised red area. May progress to partial central clearing ("bull's eye"), or develop blisters or scabs in the center, or have a bluish discoloration. OTHER EARLY SIGNS WITH OR WITHOUT RASH: Fatigue, headache, stiff neck, jaw discomfort, pain or stiffness in muscles or joints, slight fever, swollen glands or conjunctivitis. If untreated, can result in arthritis, joint pain and swelling, and heart and nervous system complications.

Treatment and Nursing Care

Antibiotics (tetracycline or doxycycline for children over 8; penicillin or erythromycin for younger children).

Remove tick carefully: Using tweezers, grasp tick as close to its mouth as possible. Be careful not to crush the tick's body. Pull gently until the tick releases itself. Apply an antiseptic to the bite area.

Reassure parents that not all ticks carry the spirochete that causes Lyme disease.

Figure 19–6   *continued*

COMMUNICABLE AND INFECTIOUS DISEASES OF CHILDHOOD

Disease	Signs and Symptoms	Treatment and Nursing Care
Measles (rubeola) *Agent*: Paramyxovirus group (a single-stranded RNA virus) *Transmission*: Airborne; large respiratory droplets; close contact between patients and susceptible persons *Incubation period*: Average 10–12 days (range of 8–16 days) *Communicability period*: One of the most contagious diseases; infectious during prodromal phase and for the first few days of the rash (from 4 days before to 4 days after the onset of the rash) *Prevention*: Live attenuated virus vaccine (see Chapter 9)	Fever, malaise, followed by cough, coryza, and conjunctivitis. Maculopapular rash usually appears approximately 14 days after infection and typically 2–4 days after onset of prodromal symptoms. Rash starts on the face and hairline and then spreads to the trunk and extremities. Temperature elevation occurs 1–3 days after rash onset. Rash lasts 5–7 days. BUCCAL MUCOSA: small bluish-white spots on a red background (Koplik's spots) seen on buccal mucosa 2 days before and after the onset of the rash.	Maintain strict isolation in hospital until day 5 of rash. Maintain bed rest. Relieve itching with antipruritics. Fever management. Encourage fluids. Advise parents that child's eyes can be sensitive to light.
Mononucleosis (acute viral infection) *Agent*: Epstein-Barr virus (EBV) of the herpesvirus family *Transmission*: Direct contact with infected oropharyngeal secretions (saliva, kissing) *Incubation period*: 4–6 weeks (30–50 days) *Communicability period*: Saliva remains infective for up to 18 months *Prevention*: None	Febrile illness, sore throat, malaise, fatigue, myalgia, generalized lymphadenopathy, splenomegaly. Symptoms resolve within 2–3 weeks.	Corticosteroids (prednisone). Maintain bed rest. Treat sore throat and fever. Advise parents that it may take up to 3–4 weeks for child to feel normal.

Figure 19–6   continued

COMMUNICABLE AND INFECTIOUS DISEASES OF CHILDHOOD

Disease	Signs and Symptoms	Treatment and Nursing Care
Mumps (infectious parotitis) *Agent*: Myxovirus group (RNA virus) *Transmission*: Droplet; direct contact *Incubation period*: 14–21 days (average of 18 days) *Communicability period*: Virus may be excreted 7 days before to 9 days after clinical onset of disease *Prevention*: Live attenuated virus vaccine (see Chapter 9)	PRODROMAL PHASE: Anorexia, headache, vomiting, myalgia lasting 12–48 hours. Mild to moderate fever, painful unilateral or bilateral parotid gland swelling, orchitis. Inflammation of other salivary organs.	Maintain strict isolation in hospital. Corticosteroids, if indicated. Antipyretics (acetaminophen) for pain and fever. Encourage fluids. Maintain bed rest.
Pertussis (whooping cough) *Agent*: Bordella pertussis *Transmission*: Droplet; one of the most contagious diseases *Incubation period*: 7–10 days (range of 4–21 days) *Communicability period*: Begins approximately 1 week after exposure and ends within 4 to 6 weeks; child is most infectious during the early stages *Prevention*: Active immunization with killed-cell vaccine (see Chapter 9)	Spasmodic, paroxysmal coughing (the sudden onset of repeated violent coughs without intervening respirations). FIRST 1–2 WEEKS: runny nose followed by shallow, irregular nonproductive coughing; changes into deep spasms of paroxysmal coughing; vomiting and inspiratory whooping.	Maintain strict isolation in hospital. Antibiotics. Corticosteroids. Fever management. Encourage fluids. Monitor respiratory status. Provide a quiet environment and reduced physical activity to prevent coughing episodes.

Figure 19–6   *continued*

COMMUNICABLE AND INFECTIOUS DISEASES OF CHILDHOOD

Disease	Signs and Symptoms	Treatment and Nursing Care
Poliomyelitis	Virus is introduced into mouth, where it replicates in the oropharyngeal mucosa and in the Peyer's patches in the ileum. Virus enters bloodstream and central nervous system (CNS), where it attacks the motor neurons of the spinal cord and occasionally the brain stem. Infection of these cells results in death of the lower motor neurons and flaccid paralysis of the muscles they innervate. In cases of limited CNS involvement, symptoms include fever, meningeal irritation (stiff neck and back), or fever, malaise, headache with nausea, vomiting, sore throat.	Maintain strict isolation in hospital.
Agent: Three serotypes of poliovirus		Monitor respiratory status. May need ventilation.
Transmission: Pharyngeal secretions and feces, primarily via oral-fecal route (where sanitation and personal hygiene are poor)		Fever management.
		Encourage fluids.
Incubation period: 7–24 days (range of 3–36 days)		Encourage food intake when patient is ready to eat.
Communicability period: Infectious for up to several weeks before symptoms develop; virus is excreted in pharyngeal secretions for a few days and in the stool for several weeks		Physical therapy, positioning, and range-of-motion exercises are important.
		Maintain bed rest.
		Sedatives, if indicated.
Prevention: Trivalent vaccine (live oral poliovirus vaccine [OPV] or inactivated poliovirus vaccine [IPV]) (see Chapter 9)		Hot, moist packs to muscles in spasm.
		Follow-up home care arrangements on discharge.

Figure 19–6   *continued*

COMMUNICABLE AND INFECTIOUS DISEASES OF CHILDHOOD

Disease

Rabies (acute viral infection of the CNS)

Agent: Rhabdoviridae; domestic, wild, and farm animals

Transmission: After inoculation, the virus enters the wound and travels along the nerves from the point of entry to the CNS

Incubation period: Highly variable (average of 6 weeks); determined by the location of the bite and the distance the virus must travel to the brain

Communicability period: Not communicable

Prevention: Human diploid cell vaccine (HDCV) and human rabies immune globulin (HRIG) should be given to all persons bitten by animals in whom rabies cannot be excluded and for nonbite exposures to animals suspected or proved to be rabid

Signs and Symptoms

Runs its course in 1 week. HYDROPHOBIA: Swallowing is difficult, produces painful contracture of the muscles of deglutition, leading to a reflex contraction at the sight of liquids. Periods of excitability (mania) and quiet. Usually results in death.

Treatment and Nursing Care

Follow guidelines for rabies prophylaxis:

DOMESTIC DOG AND CAT: (1) If healthy and available for 10 days of observation at time of attack: thoroughly clean bite with soap and water; no further treatment is needed, unless animal develops rabies. (2) Rabid or suspected rabid: administer HRIG.

WILD ANIMAL: Regard as rabid unless proved negative by laboratory test; administer HRIG.

LIVESTOCK, RODENTS, RABBITS: Consider individually; consult local and state public health officials. Bites of rodents or rabbits and hares almost never call for rabies prophylaxis.

Figure 19–6   *continued*

COMMUNICABLE AND INFECTIOUS DISEASES OF CHILDHOOD

Disease	Signs and Symptoms	Treatment and Nursing Care
Roseola infantum (exanthem subitum) *Agent*: Herpes virus type 6 *Transmission*: Unknown; disease of infants and toddlers (6 months–3 years) *Incubation period*: Unknown *Communicability period*: Unknown *Prevention*: None	Very high fever for 3–4 days followed by rash. Irritability. Macules and papules appear first on the trunk and spread to face, neck, and extremities. Rash can last from 24 to 48 hours.	Fever management. Reassure parents that rash will disappear in a few days.
Rubella (German or 3-day measles) *Agent*: RNA virus of the togavirus group *Transmission*: Direct contact; droplet *Incubation period*: 14–21 days *Communicability period*: Begins about 7 days before onset of rash and lasts for 4 days after *Prevention*: Primary rubella infection induces lifelong immunity; live attenuated virus vaccine (see Chapter 9)	Nonspecific maculopapular rash lasting 3 days or less. Appears on face; progresses to neck, trunk, and legs. GENERALIZED LYMPHADENOPATHY: Postauricular, suboccipital, and posterior cervical lymph nodes. Itching, occasionally low-grade fever, headache, malaise, coryza, sore throat, anorexia.	Fever management (antipyretics, tepid sponge bath). Pain management (acetaminophen). Isolate child from pregnant women. Encourage fluids (popsicles, soft drinks).

Figure 19–6   continued

Communicable and Infectious Diseases of Childhood

Disease

Scarlet fever (scarlatina)

Agent: Group A beta-streptococcal disease resulting from infection with strains of beta-hemolytic streptococci

Transmission: Respiratory secretions; caused primarily by intimate or direct contact

Incubation period: 24–48 hours

Communicability period: Not communicable

Prevention: None

Signs and Symptoms

Occurs primarily in children 2–18 years old, most often in winter and spring. Characterized by erythematous skin rash; blanches on pressure; most visible on the neck, chest, skinfolds; peeling of skin (tips of toes and fingers). Strep throat, fever, pain, swelling, beefy redness of pharynx with exudate and tender cervical nodes, strawberry tongue. If untreated, can cause acute rheumatic fever and glomerulonephritis.

Treatment and Nursing Care

Maintain fluid balance.

Antibiotics (penicillin is the drug of choice; erythromycin).

Fever management.

Maintain bed rest.

Advise parents of the importance of taking antibiotics for the full number of days prescribed.

Advise parents of the importance of follow-up throat cultures, if indicated.

Figure 19–6   *continued*

COMMUNICABLE AND INFECTIOUS DISEASES OF CHILDHOOD

Disease

Tetanus (lockjaw)

Agent: *Clostridium tetani* (anaerobic, gram-positive rod that exists in both vegetative and spore forms)

Occurrence: Not a communicable disease; occurs as a complication of puncture wounds, compound fractures, abrasions, burns, injections, surgery, animal bites, gastrointestinal infections, abortions, abscesses, and chronic skin ulceration

Etiology: Spores can survive for years; found in soil, dust, animal feces, and less commonly in human feces and on human skin; organisms thrive on necrotic tissue and lack of oxygen; exotoxin travels along motor neurons and is disseminated through bloodstream; fixes to gangliosides in skeletal muscle, spinal cord, brain, autonomic nervous system

Incubation period: From trauma to onset of symptoms, 2 days–3 weeks (usually 6–8 days)

Communicability period: Not communicable

Prevention: Active immunization with tetanus toxoid (see Chapter 9)

Signs and Symptoms

Clinical disease is a result of the effects of the neurotoxin on various receptors. EARLY SIGNS: Stiffness or cramps in muscles around wound; deep tendon hyperreflexia; stiffness of neck, jaw; facial pain. PROGRESSIVE DISEASE: Change of facial expression, sudden contractures of muscle groups (opisthotonos). Laryngeal, diaphragmatic, and intercostal muscle spasms may produce acute respiratory failure.

Treatment and Nursing Care

Antitoxin serum therapy.

Medications (sedatives, psychotherapeutics, anti-anxiety agents, muscle relaxants).

Monitor for breathing difficulties.

Maintain airway. Intubation and ventilation may be needed.

High fatality rate; teach parents the importance of child's receiving tetanus immunization and the importance of wound cleaning.

Figure 19–6   *continued*

Communicable and Infectious Diseases of Childhood

Disease	Signs and Symptoms	Treatment and Nursing Care
Typhoid fever (acute bacterial disease) *Agent*: *Salmonella typhi* (natural pathogen of humans only) *Transmission*: Most often traced to ingestion of food or water contaminated with human waste *Incubation period:* 7–21 days (average of 14 days) *Communicability period*: CARRIERS: Following treated or untreated infection; *S. typhi* is carried in the stool for 1–2 months *Prevention*: Killed-cell vaccine; enteric coated capsule now available (mutant strain); UNPLEASANT SIDE EFFECTS: fever, headache, myalgia, malaise, localized pain and swelling	Fever, malaise, chills, headache, generalized aches in muscles and joints. Enlarged spleen. Leukopenia and small discrete rose-colored spots (caused by bacterial emboli in the skin capillaries) may appear on the trunk. Abdominal distention and tenderness.	Antimicrobial therapy (chloramphenicol, trimethoprim-sulfamethoxazole, ampicillin, amoxicillin, cephalosporins). Maintain strict isolation; enteric precautions should be taken. Instruct parents and visitors to avoid use of child's toilet. Abdominal assessment. Fever management.

Figure 19–6   continued

In the pediatric age group, infection with HIV occurs:

- in infants of infected mothers (through blood, amniotic fluid, or breast milk)
- in children who received blood and blood products from HIV-infected donors before mandatory screening was instituted in March 1985
- in individuals who abuse intravenous (IV) drugs and participate in homosexual or heterosexual activities without precautions

Symptoms. The time between infection and illness can be as long as 10 years. Diagnosis is based on the clinical presentation of symptoms and is confirmed by serological tests or viral cultures or both. AIDS in children is primarily a disease of infants and presents with the following symptoms:

- hepatosplenomegaly
- lymphadenopathy
- oral candidiasis
- failure to thrive
- weight loss
- diarrhea
- chronic eczema
- fever of unknown origin

Treatment. AIDS is a chronic disease that affects many body systems, resulting in acute exacerbations. There is no cure. Treatment is supportive and focuses on preventing infection, maintaining good nutrition, and treating specific symptoms. Zidovudine (AZT) syrup has been authorized for use in children from 3 months to 12 years who have either HIV-associated symptoms or a T-lymphocyte cell count of less than 400 (Spratto and Woods 1993). DDI (dideoxyinosine) is also used to treat HIV infection in children over 6 months of age.

Nursing Care. Nurses should always follow universal precautions to minimize exposure to HIV (see earlier discussion). Nurses who care for children with AIDS should reassure parents that "extensive follow-up of household contacts of both adults and children with AIDS has failed to demonstrate any evidence of HIV transmission via shared living space, kitchens, or bathrooms or through casual contact" (Last 1992). Nurses can help educate the public to reduce fear, panic, prejudice, and discrimination related to the disease and its causes.

Because of the life-threatening nature of the disorder, psychosocial support to families of children with AIDS is an essential part of care. Depending on the progression of the disease, children may be relatively symptom-free or require supportive home care. Encourage parents to keep infected children in school as long as possible. Nurses can play an important role in providing information to school officials, teachers, schoolmates, and their parents to help them understand that HIV transmission does not occur through normal daily contact.

REVIEW QUESTIONS

A. Multiple choice. Select the best answer.

1. If you were trying to explain the difference between an infectious disease and a communicable disease to a patient, which of the following would be the best statement?
   a. Communicable diseases are more serious than infectious diseases.
   b. Communicable diseases spread, either directly or indirectly, between people; infectious diseases are caused by organisms invading a body directly, then multiplying to produce the disease.
   c. Many infectious diseases have to be reported to local health departments; communicable diseases do not.
   d. Disease is caused by damage to the cells, secretion of a toxin, or an antigen-antibody reaction in the host.

2. Which of the following stages of infection may occur simultaneously?
   a. latent period and incubation period
   b. latent period and communicability period
   c. incubation period and disease period
   d. latent period and disease period

3. Universal precautions are designed primarily to
   a. minimize the risk of exposure to patients with AIDS
   b. be used in high-risk clinical situations
   c. protect health care providers from terminally ill patients
   d. minimize the risk of exposure to blood and body fluids of all patients

4. Children are placed in isolation to interrupt the chain of infection by preventing the spread of microbes. Which of the following would *not* be a reason for placing a child in short-term isolation?
   a. infectious disease
   b. immunodeficiency disease
   c. an allergic reaction
   d. chemotherapy

5. Most children with acquired immunodeficiency syndrome (AIDS) are
   a. adolescents
   b. school-age children
   c. preschool children
   d. infants

6. Which of the following childhood diseases has the longest incubation period?
   a. diphtheria
   b. chickenpox
   c. hepatitis B
   d. measles

7. Parvovirus is the agent responsible for which disease?
   a. fifth disease
   b. measles
   c. mononucleosis
   d. mumps

8. Angela, 6 years old, has complained of a headache and queasiness for the past two days and now has developed a moderate fever and parotid gland swelling. These signs and symptoms are characteristic of
   a. fifth disease
   b. mumps
   c. Lyme disease
   d. rabies

9. Marco's mother brings him to the walk-in clinic. He has a low-grade fever and rash, with clear, fluid-filled vesicles. The nurse suspects that Marco has
   a. rubella
   b. chickenpox
   c. measles
   d. roseola

10. Which of the following diseases is usually transmitted by droplet?
    a. hepatitis
    b. poliomyelitis
    c. tetanus
    d. diphtheria

SUGGESTED ACTIVITIES

- Children in isolation can become lonely and depressed. Suggest three techniques that might be used to relieve loneliness for infants, children, or adolescents.

- If you work with children, you are apt to be asked many questions about communicable diseases. Develop a memory-assisting system for remembering five facts about a particular disease. Share your system with other students.

- Develop a poster display to teach adolescents about AIDS.

BIBLIOGRAPHY

Foster, R. L., M. M. Hunsberger, and J. J. Tackett Anderson. *Family-Centered Nursing Care of Children*. Philadelphia: W. B. Saunders, 1989.

Gershon, A. A. Herpesvirus. *Emergency Medicine* (November, 1991): 105–115.

Grimes, D. *Infectious Diseases*. St. Louis, MO: Mosby-Year Book, 1991.

Holcroft, C. Acyclovir approved for childhood chickenpox. *Nurse Practitioner* 17, no. 5 (1992).

Last, J. M., and R. B. Wallace. *Public Health and Preventive Medicine*, 13th ed. Norwalk, CT: Appleton & Lange, 1992.

Pilliteri, A. *Maternal and Child Health Nursing*. Philadelphia: J. B. Lippincott, 1992.

Rudolph, A. M. *Rudolph's Pediatrics*, 19th ed. Norwalk, CT: Appleton & Lange, 1991.

Sharts-Engel, N. C. An overview of maternal-child infectious diseases (1976–1990). *American Journal of Maternal-Child Nursing* 16 (1991): 58.

Spratto, G. R, and A. L. Woods. *RN's NDR '93*. Albany, NY: Delmar Publishers, 1993.

Weingarten, C. T., and S. M. Gomberg. Measles: Again an epidemic. *Pediatric Nursing* 18, no. 4 (1992): 369–371.

Wong, D. L. *Whaley & Wong's Essentials of Pediatric Nursing*, 4th ed. St. Louis, MO: Mosby-Year Book, 1993.

*I*ntegumentary Conditions

OBJECTIVES

AFTER STUDYING THIS CHAPTER, THE STUDENT SHOULD BE ABLE TO:

- NAME FIVE SKIN CONDITIONS THAT AFFECT INFANTS AND TODDLERS AND DESCRIBE THEIR CAUSES, SYMPTOMS, TREATMENT, AND NURSING CARE.
- NAME FOUR SKIN CONDITIONS THAT AFFECT PRESCHOOL AND SCHOOL-AGE CHILDREN AND DESCRIBE THEIR CAUSES, SYMPTOMS, TREATMENT, AND NURSING CARE.
- NAME TWO SKIN CONDITIONS THAT AFFECT ADOLESCENTS AND DESCRIBE THEIR CAUSES, SYMPTOMS, TREATMENT, AND NURSING CARE.
- NAME FOUR TYPES OF BURNS, AND IDENTIFY THE MOST COMMON.
- DESCRIBE ONE METHOD USED TO ASSESS THE EXTENT OF A BURN INJURY.
- IDENTIFY THE AMERICAN BURN ASSOCIATION CRITERIA FOR BURN SEVERITY.
- DISCUSS THE CARE OF CHILDREN WITH MINOR BURNS.
- IDENTIFY TWO GOALS OF BURN WOUND CARE AND DESCRIBE TREATMENT MEASURES FOR BURN WOUNDS.
- IDENTIFY NURSING CONSIDERATIONS IN CARE OF THE BURNED CHILD.

KEY TERMS

PRIMARY IRRITANT	KERION
ALLERGEN	COMEDONES
ANAPHYLAXIS	ESCHAR

*i*ntegumentary conditions occur frequently in children of all ages. The nurse needs to be able to accurately identify these conditions and understand their causes and treatment. Effective treatment of skin conditions often requires that children receive long-term care and follow-up or adhere to a specific treatment plan. For this reason, teaching the parents and child about the condition, its cause, and its treatment is an important aspect of nursing care for many skin conditions.

Burns are a common cause of injury in children, especially young children (see Chapter 10). Most burn injuries are minor and do not require hospital admission. Major burns, however, are serious injuries that require skilled medical and nursing care.

OVERVIEW OF THE SYSTEM

The skin and its accessory structures — hair, nails, and glands — make up the integumentary system. The skin performs several important functions: protection, body temperature regulation, excretion, sensation, and vitamin D production.

The two principal layers of the skin are the epidermis and dermis. The epidermis, which helps to protect the body against bacterial invasion, is the outermost nonvascular layer of the skin. The dermis — containing nerves, nerve endings, sebaceous and sweat glands, and hair follicles — is the thicker, inner layer of the skin that lies below the epidermis. Below the dermis is the subcutaneous fatty tissue (sometimes called the hypodermis), consisting of loose connective tissue (muscle and fat), Figure 20–1.

Lesions are common presenting signs of many integumentary conditions. Primary skin lesions are illustrated in Figure 20–2 (page 285).

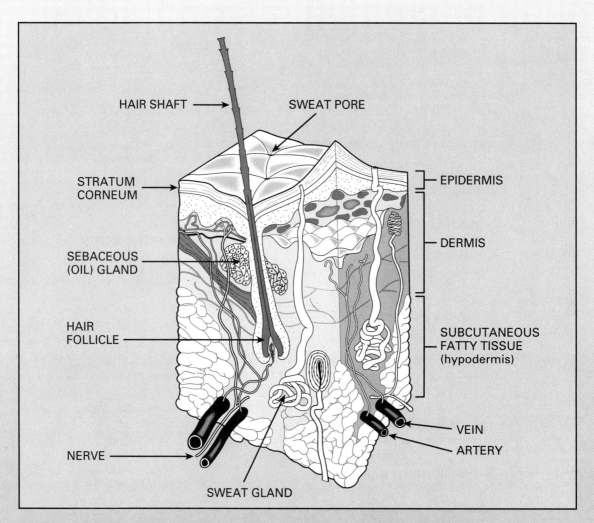

HAIR SHAFT

SWEAT PORE

STRATUM
CORNEUM

EPIDERMIS

DERMIS

SEBACEOUS
(OIL) GLAND

HAIR
FOLLICLE

SUBCUTANEOUS
FATTY TISSUE
(hypodermis)

VEIN
ARTERY

NERVE

SWEAT GLAND

Figure 20–1   *Cross section of the skin*

284

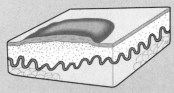

PLAQUE - Raised thickened portion of skin, well-defined edge and a flat or rough surface.
ex. psoriasis, eczema

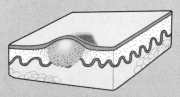

PUSTULE - Pus-filled raised area
ex. acne, impetigo

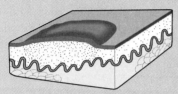

WHEAL - Elevated area, irregular shape formed as a result of localized skin edema
ex. hives, insect bites

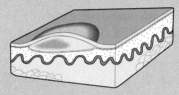

VESICLE - Fluid-filled raised area.
ex. blister, chickenpox, herpes simplex

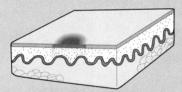

MACULE - A flat spot, flush with the skin surface, a different color.
ex. freckle, rash of measles, roseola

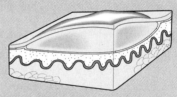

BULLA - Fluid-filled blister greater than 1 cm
ex. large blister

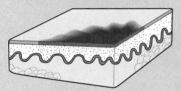

PATCH - Flat surface tissue that differs from surrounding area in color, texture
ex. port wine mark.

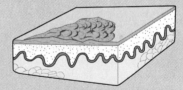

SCALE - Excess dead epidermal cells.
ex. Seborrheic dermatitis

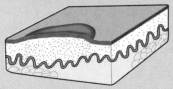

PAPULE - A raised spot on the surface of the skin
ex. flat wart, nevus

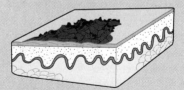

CRUST - A collection of dried serum and cellular debris
ex. eczema, impetigo

Figure 20–2   Primary skin lesions

Infant and Toddler

Miliaria Rubra

Miliaria rubra, also called prickly heat or heat rash, is caused by plugging of the sweat ducts. Sweat leaks into the surrounding skin when exposed to heat and high humidity, causing fine red papules or vesicles, inflammation, and a stinging or prickling sensation. The rash is most often found in areas prone to sweating, such as the neck, groin, and axillae, and underneath clothing. Lesions usually heal by themselves; however, an anti-inflammatory lotion may be prescribed. A cool environment and lightweight clothing should be encouraged.

Contact Dermatitis

Contact dermatitis is an inflammation of the skin caused by a **primary irritant** or **allergen** contact. Primary irritants are chemical substances such as bleaches, dyes, soaps, detergents, and gasoline. Common allergens are poison ivy, oak, and sumac; wool; fur; shoe leather; nickel; and rubber (latex). Recently, cases of reactions to latex have been reported, ranging from contact dermatitis to **anaphylaxis**, a hypersensitivity response to a previously encountered antigen (Fritsch and Fredrick Pilat 1993). Latex is found in gloves, catheters, airway equipment, monitors, intravenous equipment, plastic syringes, and adhesive tape.

A primary irritant contact dermatitis develops within a few hours after contact, peaks in 24 hours, and disappears. An allergic contact dermatitis can take as long as 18 hours to appear, peaks between 48 and 72 hours, and can last for two to three weeks. The basic features of the skin lesions are erythema, edema, and a papulovesicular rash in patches or streaks. Pain, pruritus, and burning may be present. Treatment includes avoiding further contact with the allergen, topical steroids, and antihistamines to reduce itching.

Diaper Dermatitis

Diaper dermatitis, or diaper rash, is the most common irritant contact dermatitis in infancy. It is usually caused by prolonged contact of the skin with urine and stool. It may also occur as a result of inadequate cleansing of the diaper area; contact with detergents, ointments, or soaps; or friction.

Symptoms can include erythema, edema, vesicles, and weeping involving the perineum, genitals, and buttocks, with extension to the inner thighs. *Candida albicans* (monilia) is the causative organism in 80% of diaper rashes that last longer than four days (Rosenstein and Fosarelli 1989). Figure 20–3 shows the typical lesions of a monilial diaper rash.

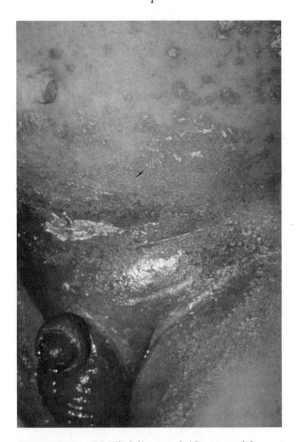

Figure 20–3 *Monilial diaper rash (Courtesy of the Centers for Disease Control and Prevention, Atlanta, GA)*

Treatment includes frequent diaper changes, avoidance of plastic pants, exposing the diaper area to the air, cleansing the diaper area at each diaper change, and applying protective ointment (Balmex, A&D, Desitin). Caution parents to avoid using commercially available baby wipes, because the alcohol in these products will further dry and irritate the inflamed area.

SEBORRHEIC DERMATITIS

Seborrheic dermatitis is a chronic, inflammatory skin disease. It consists of erythematous, scaling, crusting lesions that can be greasy or dry and yellow in appearance. Lesions occur in areas that are rich in sebaceous glands, such as the scalp, face, back, behind the ear and in creases. The eyebrows and eyelashes also can be involved.

This condition is commonly seen in newborns and infants (as cradle cap) and at puberty (as dandruff or flaking). Treatment consists of topical steroids (except for cradle cap), shampoos (such as Head & Shoulders or Sebulex), and antibiotics, when indicated.

ATOPIC DERMATITIS (ECZEMA)

Description. Atopic dermatitis (eczema) is a general term used to describe chronic superficial inflammation of the skin in different types of patients. Atopic dermatitis has been associated with allergy and is thought to have a hereditary tendency. It is one of the most common skin disorders in children (Zitelli and Davis 1991).

Symptoms. Atopic dermatitis can be divided into three clinical phases (infantile, childhood, and adolescent) based on the age of the child and the distribution of the lesions.

1. *Infantile*: Lesions, typically red, itchy papules and plaques, are followed by crusting. The face and scalp are usually involved first (Figure 20–4); later the rash may spread to the extensor aspects of the extremities, buttocks, thighs, anogenital region, and trunk.

2. *Childhood*: Lesions are typically dry, papular, more thickened, and pruritic. Areas involved are the wrists, ankles, antecubital and popliteal fossae, and the back and sides of the neck. Sometimes the soles of the feet are involved (atopic feet) and there is erythema, cracking, and pain.

3. *Adolescent*: Lesions are pruritic and have a thickened, hardened appearance with varying degrees of erythema and scaling. Areas involved are the hands (most often), eyelids, neck, feet, and flexor areas.

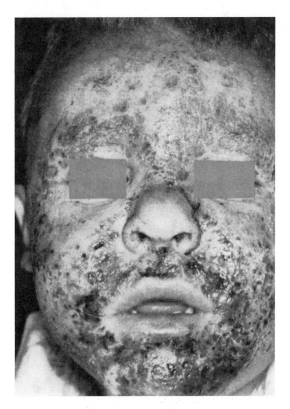

Figure 20–4 *Infantile eczema (From Stewart, Danto, and Maddin,* Dermatology, *4th ed. C. V. Mosby, St. Louis, 1978)*

Treatment. Treatment focuses on reducing inflammation and preventing secondary infection by hydrating the skin, which helps to relieve itching.

Acute Condition

- If weeping is present, wet compresses (cotton cloth soaked in aluminum acetate solution) are applied to the area.
- Systemic antibiotics are prescribed if superimposed infection is suspected.
- Topical steroids (triamcinolone) may be prescribed for maintenance therapy of mild dermatitis of the face and intertriginous areas.
- Apply emollients to dry, scaling, or fissured eruptions.
- Use oatmeal baths (Aveeno) to soothe inflammation.
- Antipruritics (Vistaril, Atarax) may be prescribed to relieve itching.

Chronic Condition

Parents should be taught the following measures:

- Dress the child in cotton clothes and avoid wool clothing and perfumed soaps.
- Wash the child with mild soap (Dove, Tone).
- Apply steroid cream or lotion in small amounts frequently.
- Use prescribed medications when needed to relieve pain.

Nursing Care. The nurse should teach the parents and child about the causes of atopic dermatitis and how to prevent frequent occurrences. Counsel parents about diet, clothing, and the use of soaps and lotions. Encourage compliance with the treatment plan. Treatment failures can be frustrating for both parents and child. Emphasize the importance of not scratching the lesions to avoid secondary infection. Keeping the nails clean and cutting fingernails and toenails short reduces the chance of infection. Advise parents of young children to have the child wear cotton gloves or socks on the hands to prevent scratching, especially at bedtime.

PRESCHOOL AND SCHOOL-AGE CHILD

IMPETIGO

Impetigo is a highly contagious, superficial infection of the skin caused by *Streptococcus* and *Staphylococcus* organisms. The most common sites are the face, extremities, hands, and neck.

In a group A streptococcal infection, the lesion begins as a papule that changes to form a small, thin-walled vesicle with an erythematous halo. At first, the vesicle is filled with clear fluid, which later becomes cloudy; the vesicle then ruptures, forming a superficial honey-colored crust. In staphylococcal infection, the initial macule may form small, thin-walled pustules or the larger flaccid bullae known as bullous impetigo. Lesions may coalesce over time, and satellite lesions may form.

Impetigo commonly causes pruritus, burning, and secondary enlargement and tenderness of the regional lymph nodes. Treatment involves the use of systemic antibiotics (penicillin, erythromycin), when indicated. Scrubbing lesions with hexachlorophene (pHisoHex) and applying topical antibiotics aid in control of lesions but do not cure the infection. Teach parents to keep the child's fingernails short and clean. Applying a topical bactericidal ointment (Bactoban) aids in reducing secondary infection.

RINGWORM

Ringworm refers to a group of fungal infections of the skin, hair, and nails. These highly contagious infections occur in all age groups and are usually spread from person to person or from animal to person. There are three common causative organisms: trichophyton, microsporum, and epidermophyton.

The most common types of infection (identified by the Latin word *tinea* and a word indicating the area affected) are:

- *Tinea capitis*: a fungal infection of the scalp and hair, characterized by scaling and patchy hair loss. Sometimes the short broken-off hairs result in inflammation with a boggy patch and pustules (called a **kerion**).
- *Tinea corporis*: a superficial fungal infection of the smooth hairless skin of the body, called "ringworm" because of the characteristic round lesions with central clearing and a scaly, annular border. More than one lesion may be present, Figure 20–5.
- *Tinea cruris* ("jock itch"): a fungal infection that occurs on the inner aspects of the thighs and scrotum.
- *Tinea pedis* ("athlete's foot"): a fungal infection of the foot and toes, characterized by fissuring and pinhead-sized lesions.

Diagnosis is made by observation; by using an ultraviolet light (Wood's lamp) to look at the lesions, which fluoresce if ringworm is present; by examining scrapings from the lesion in a potassium hydroxide (KOH) preparation under the microscope; and by fungal cultures.

Treatment is similar regardless of the causative organism, but differs with the site and extent of the infection. Topical therapy is used for localized skin infection; systemic therapy for widespread skin infection and infection of the scalp, hair, or nails (Rosenstein and Fosarelli 1989). If the hair or nails are involved, griseofulvin is the treatment of choice (Hathaway et al. 1993).

PEDICULOSIS CAPITIS (LICE)

Description. Pediculosis capitis is an infestation of the scalp by lice. The female louse,

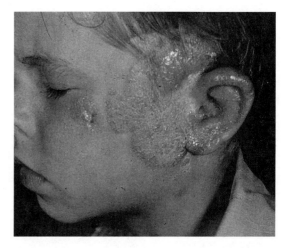

Figure 20–5 *Ringworm (tinea corporis) of the face and scalp (Courtesy of the Centers for Disease Control and Prevention, Atlanta, GA)*

Figure 20–6, lays eggs at the base of the hair shaft close to the skin, where the warmth of the scalp provides the heat necessary for incubation. The eggs (nits) can be seen as oval, white, 0.5-mm dots attached firmly to the hair shaft. They are usually located about 0.5–1 cm from the scalp but sometimes run the entire length of the hair shaft.

Symptoms. Itching is the primary symptom. Head lice can be found anywhere on the scalp,

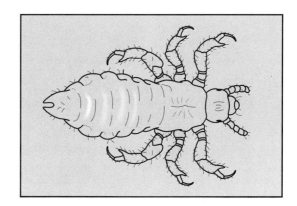

Figure 20–6 *The female head louse (enlarged)*

but are most often seen on the back of the head and neck and behind the ears. Scratching causes inflammation and secondary bacterial infection, with pustules, crusting, and cervical adenopathy. The eyelashes may be involved, causing redness and swelling. Although nits resemble dandruff, they are cemented to the hair rather than easily moved along the hair shaft, as is dandruff (Habif 1990).

Treatment. Treatment consists of washing the hair with a pediculicide, such as lindane (Kwell) shampoo. Parents should be told to use approximately 30 mL of the shampoo; work into a lather; rub for five minutes; then rinse and dry with a towel. The dead nits will remain attached to the hair until removed. To remove the nits, the hair should be combed with an extra-fine-toothed comb. Vinegar compresses applied to the hair for 15 minutes will help to remove the nit shells.

Nursing Care. Reassure the parents and child that anyone can become infested with lice. Notify the child's school, day-care center, babysitter, and parents of playmates, because lice are easily transmitted from child to child.

Teach parents how to prevent the spread of lice and reinfestation, Figure 20–7.

Scabies

Scabies is a contagious infestation caused by the mite *Sarcoptes scabiei*. Infestation begins when a fertilized female mite burrows into the stratum corneum (dead horny layer of the epidermis; see Figure 20–1) to bury her eggs. The burrow enlarges from several millimeters to a few centimeters in length during her 30-day life cycle (Habif 1990).

Symptoms include pruritic papules, vesicles, pustules, and linear burrows. An eczematous eruption caused by hypersensitivity to the mite is sometimes seen. Secondary infection can also occur.

The linear burrow is the diagnostic sign of scabies. It consists of a small, scaly, linear lesion with pinpoint vesicles at the end, in which the female mite lives (Zitelli and Davis 1991). Areas of involvement include the webs of the fingers, axillae, flexures of the arms and wrists, belt line, nipples, genitals, and lower buttocks. In infants, the palms, soles of the feet, head, and neck can be affected. Diagnosis is made by examining microscopically scrapings

---

Preventing Pediculosis (Lice)

- Soak combs, brushes, and hair accessories in pediculicide such as lindane (Kwell) for 1 hour or in boiling water for 10 minutes.

- Machine wash all washable clothing, towels, and bed linens in hot water and dry in a hot dryer for at least 20 minutes. Dry clean nonwashable items.

- Thoroughly vacuum carpets, car seats, pillows, stuffed animals, rugs, mattresses, and upholstered furniture.

- Seal nonwashable items in plastic bags for 14 days if unable to vacuum or dry clean.

- Instruct children not to share combs, hats, or scarves.

Figure 20–7   (*Adapted from Clore, Dispelling the common myths about pediculosis,* Journal of Pediatric Health Care, *1989*)

from a burrow or an unscratched papule and observing a mite, egg, or mite feces.

Treatment consists of applying a scabicide such as lindane (Kwell, Scabene), available as a cream, lotion, or shampoo. The scabicide is applied from the neck down and washed off after six to eight hours.

Because lindane becomes concentrated in the central nervous system, it is not recommended for use on infants. Eurax lotion is used, instead. Like lindane, Eurax is applied from the neck down, but it is applied nightly for two nights and washed off 24 hours after the second application. Infants sometimes need to be retreated in 7 to 10 days. To prevent the infant from touching the body and then putting the fingers in the mouth, keep the hands covered during treatment.

All family members should be treated at the same time as the affected child. In addition, advise parents to wash all clothing and bed linens to prevent reinfestation.

BITES AND STINGS

Bites. Children frequently are bitten by animals as well as other children. Animal bites include bites from dogs, cats, snakes, and arthropods. It is not unusual for a child to be bitten by the family pet while playing. Examples of common arthropod bites are those of spiders, ticks, scorpions, mites, and centipedes. Bites of the black widow and brown recluse spiders are the most dangerous. Tick bites can transmit Lyme disease (see Chapter 19) and Rocky Mountain spotted fever.

Human bites usually occur while children are fighting with one another. These bites easily become infected by organisms that are part of the normal flora of the mouth.

Stings. Children are most frequently stung by bees, wasps, and ants. Common symptoms include pain, redness, itching, and swelling.

Some children, however, may have severe allergic reactions, resulting in anaphylactic shock.

Treatment. Treatment usually consists of cool compresses, local cleansing of the affected area, and application of a disinfectant. Oral antihistamines can be given to control swelling and reduce itching.

ADOLESCENT

ACNE

Description. Acne, a disorder of the hair follicle and its oil gland, is a common problem for adolescent boys and girls. Acne occurs primarily in the sebaceous follicles of the face, neck, shoulders, upper chest, and back. The sebaceous glands secrete excessive oil or sebum, which is deposited at the openings of the glands. Obstruction of the sebaceous follicle openings produces the lesions of acne.

Symptoms. The three major types of acne are:

- *Comedomal acne*: characterized by open (white head) and closed (black head) **comedones**, which are caused by an accumulation of keratin and sebum within the opening of a hair follicle.
- *Papulopustular acne*: characterized by rupture of the follicular walls, producing papules and pustules.
- *Cystic acne*: characterized by nodules and cysts that are scattered over the face, chest, and back. This type of acne requires vigorous treatment and can lead to severe scar formation.

Treatment. It is important for the nurse to understand the psychosocial impact that acne can have on the developing adolescent. Parents should be encouraged to seek medical care for the teenager with acne and not dismiss the condition as simply a part of the growing process. Acne appears at a time when the adolescent is attempting to build a new identity and form close relationships with members of the opposite sex. Acne may affect adversely the teenager's body image and self-esteem. Encouraging the teenager to talk, listening to his or her concerns, and offering emotional support and reassurance that this condition will not last forever are important aspects of care (Habif 1990).

Treatment involves the use of topical and oral agents, alone or in combination. Topical agents such as vitamin A (retinoid) cream and benzoyl peroxide are frequently prescribed, along with oral antibiotics. Topical agents are applied to the entire affected area in order to treat existing lesions and prevent new lesions from developing.

Nursing Care. Patient education is an important component of nursing care. The nurse should explain the cause of acne and the treatment plan to the adolescent.

Dispel myths about diet and dirt as causative factors, for example, that eating chocolate or fried foods causes pimples. Adolescent girls who use cosmetics should be advised to use nongreasy lotions and water-based products. The psychosocial impact of acne must not be overlooked. Explain that no drug will prevent the adolescent from developing additional lesions and that the results of treatment will not be visible for four to eight weeks. Reinforce the importance of follow-up visits and of complying with the treatment plan. Caution adolescents who are using retinoid agents to avoid or minimize exposure to sunlight, as the skin is more susceptible to burning.

HERPES SIMPLEX INFECTIONS

Herpes simplex is a viral infection caused by two different herpes viruses. Type 1 herpes

causes most oral, skin, and cerebral infections. Type 2 herpes causes most genital and congenital infections (Hathaway et al. 1993). Herpes simplex type 1 infection is more commonly seen in children.

Individuals with primary infections shed the virus in saliva, urine, stool, or from skin lesions. Intimate contact, shared eating utensils, and respiratory droplets are major modes of spread. Parents frequently pass the virus on to their children (Zitelli and Davis 1991).

Most children with symptomatic type 1 herpes are under 5 years of age and have an illness characterized by fever, malaise, localized vesicular lesions, and regional adenopathy. Symptoms in infected infants include high fever, irritability, and drooling. Children may also develop primary gingivostomatitis, characterized by multiple oral ulcers on the gingiva, tongue, buccal mucosa, and lips. Pharyngeal ulcers may occur in older children.

Vesicular lesions, also called "cold sores" or "fever blisters," often begin with a tingling or burning sensation of the upper or lower lip, followed by the appearance of grouped vesicles on an erythematous base. Within 24 hours, the vesicles usually begin to scab and form a crust, and the lesions resolve completely within about a week.

Treatment is symptomatic and involves keeping the lesions clean and dry, and providing pain relief if indicated.

BURNS

Burns are the second leading cause of unintentional injury and death in children and annually claim the lives of 1,200 children in the United States. In all, 60,000 children are hospitalized each year for treatment of burns. Child abuse is suspected in approximately 16% of these cases (Eichelberger et al. 1993).

CAUSES

Burn injuries are caused by exposure to thermal, chemical, electrical, or radioactive agents.

• Thermal burns are the most common type of burn and result from direct contact with flame, flash (blow torch), hot liquids (coffee, tea, grease), and grills, Figure 20–8.

• Chemical burns result from contact with or ingestion of agents that burn or irritate the skin surface, mucous membranes, or intestinal organs.

• Electrical burns result from contact with electrical cords, wall sockets, and appliances such as blow dryers and curling irons, Figure 20–9.

• Radiation burns result from contact with radioactive substances that give off alpha, beta, and gamma rays, causing tissue damage. X-rays are gamma rays, and the damage they cause can be severe.

CLASSIFICATION

The classification and severity of the burn are assessed by evaluating the following:

• type of burn
• duration of contact
• depth of burn injury; that is, superficial (first-degree), partial thickness (second-degree), or full thickness (third-degree), Figure 20–10
• areas affected, expressed as a percentage of body surface area (BSA); the Lund and Browder formula, Figure 20–11, is widely used to estimate the extent of burn injuries in children
• age and health of the child
• preexisting illness or condition

Burns are further identified as minor, moderate, or severe according to the American Burn Association criteria for burn severity.

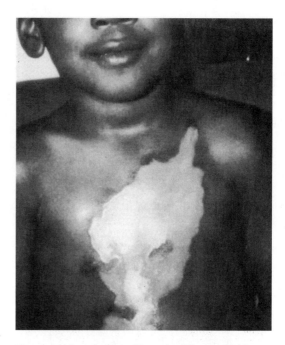

Figure 20–8 *A thermal burn (scald) caused by hot liquid decreases in width where the liquid drained down the chest to form an arrow point. (From Eichelberger, Ball, Pratsch, and Runion,* Pediatric Emergencies: A Manual for Prehospital Care Providers, *1992. Reprinted by permission of Prentice-Hall, Englewood Cliffs, NJ)*

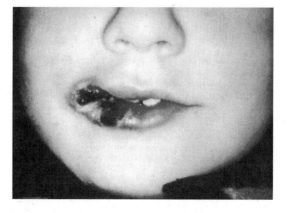

Figure 20–9 *Burn from biting an electrical cord (From Eichelberger, Ball, Pratsch, and Runion,* Pediatric Emergencies: A Manual for Prehospital Care Providers, *1992. Reprinted by permission of Prentice-Hall, Englewood Cliffs, NJ)*

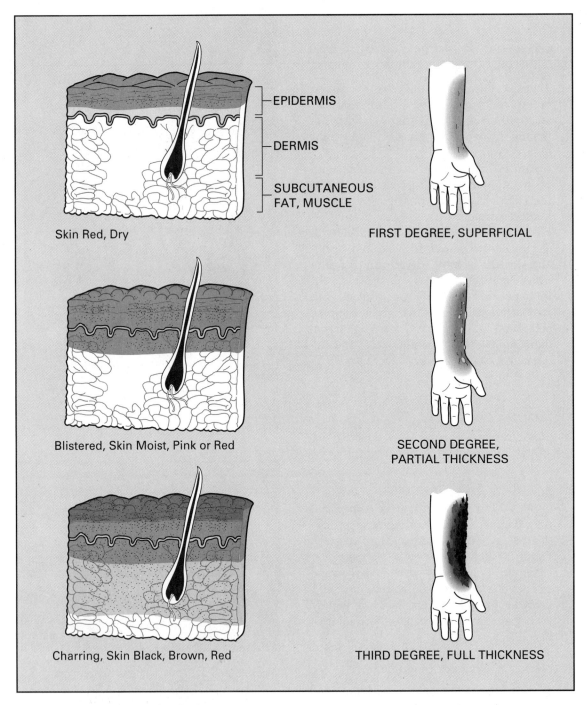

EPIDERMIS

DERMIS

SUBCUTANEOUS FAT, MUSCLE

Skin Red, Dry

FIRST DEGREE, SUPERFICIAL

Blistered, Skin Moist, Pink or Red

SECOND DEGREE, PARTIAL THICKNESS

Charring, Skin Black, Brown, Red

THIRD DEGREE, FULL THICKNESS

Figure 20–10   Burn depth classification

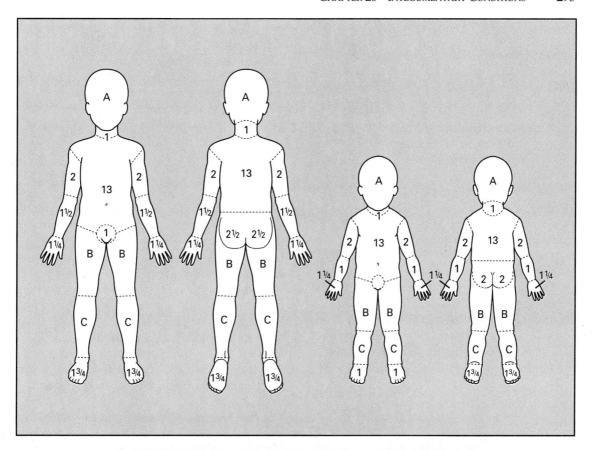

Area	Birth	1 yr	5 yrs	10 yrs	15 yrs	Adult
A (½ of head)	9½	8½	6½	5½	4½	3½
B (½ of one thigh)	2¾	3¼	4	4½	4½	4¾
C (½ of one leg)	2½	2½	2¾	3	3¼	3½

RELATIVE PERCENTAGES OF AREAS A, B, AND C, BY AGE

Figure 20–11   The extent of a child's burn is estimated using the Lund and Browder formula, which indicates relative percentages of areas affected. (Adapted from Artz and Moncrief, The Treatment of Burns, 2nd ed. W. B. Saunders, 1969)

Children with minor burns are usually treated in an out-patient facility. Children with moderate burns should be treated in a hospital that has a staff trained to deliver burn care. Children with burns involving the face, hands, feet, or genitalia usually require hospitalization so that they can be monitored for complications. Patients with major burns should be admitted to hospitals with specialized burn units (Budassi Sheehy 1990).

CARE OF MINOR BURNS

Nurses who work in clinics or other out-patient facilities are frequently called on to provide care to children with minor burns. Interventions include the following actions.

- Remove restrictive clothing and jewelry.
- Assess the extent of the burn.
- Soak the affected area in a mild antiseptic soap solution.
- Debride only open blisters; leave closed blisters intact.
- Cover the wound with an antimicrobial agent and a bulky dressing.
- Determine whether the child's tetanus immunization is up to date.
- Instruct parents in the use of antibiotics, if prescribed, and analgesia for pain relief.
- Instruct parents to keep the dressing clean and dry, to elevate the burned area or extremity for 24 hours, and to return to the facility in two days (Budassi Sheehy 1990).

CARE OF MAJOR BURNS

The child with a major burn injury who is admitted to a hospital requires immediate assessment and skilled medical and nursing care. Major burns cause significant disruption to essential body systems. Immediate care requires the following actions.

- Provide for the child's immediate survival from the burn incident.
- Monitor respiratory status and maintain a patent airway.
- Be aware of the signs of shock and monitor vital signs closely.
- Administer IV fluids as ordered; an intravenous line must be open at all times.
- Assess for bleeding.

During hospitalization, the child needs skilled and sensitive nursing care to provide pain relief, provide nutritional support, control infection, ensure adequate hydration, prevent electrolyte imbalances, and promote wound and tissue healing. Throughout the recovery period, the nurse acts to encourage physical mobility, promote normal growth and development, and provide emotional support for the child and family.

BURN WOUND CARE

Once the child has been stabilized, a treatment plan is established to care for the burn wound. Two primary goals of wound care are to protect the child from infection and promote healing of the wound. Burn wound care involves several procedures: cleansing the wound, hydrotherapy (whirlpool), application of burn dressings, surgical excision of **eschar** (the tough, leathery scab that forms over severely burned areas), debridement, and skin grafting. All of these procedures are frightening and painful, and emotional support of the child and family are important aspects of care.

Topical Treatment. Burns may be treated by open therapy or closed therapy. Open therapy involves exposing the burn to air and applying a topical medication directly to the wound. In closed therapy, the burn is covered first with a topical medication and then with a fine mesh gauze. Topical antibacterial agents reduce the number of bacteria present on the burn. The most common topical burn medications are Silvadeen, Sulfamylon, aqueous silver nitrate, Povidone-iodine, and bacitracin or triple antibiotic ointment.

Debridement. In second- and third-degree burns, debridement (the removal of foreign matter and dead, contaminated, or damaged tissue) is begun as soon as possible to reduce the chance of infection. Hydrotherapy, tub baths, soaks, or showers are used before debridement to soften and loosen eschar. Because debridement is very painful, pain medication is given before the procedure. Children need emotional support, understanding, and sensitive nursing care to cope with these difficult and painful treatment periods.

Skin Grafting.   Third-degree burns involve complete destruction of the epidermis and dermis. Because no epithelial cells remain, skin grafting is necessary. Grafts may be temporary or permanent.

There are three types of skin grafts:

- *Allograft*: fresh cadaver skin, which provides the best temporary skin graft. Allograft covering renders the burn pain-free and reduces the bacterial count on the burn surface.
- *Xenograft (heterograft)*: a temporary skin covering (usually pigskin) that is commercially available.
- *Autograft*: a layer of skin from the epidermis and part of the dermis (called a split-thickness graft) that is removed from an unburned portion of the child's body and then placed on the burn wound. Autograft provides a permanent skin covering.

Contractures and Scars.   Third-degree burns commonly heal with contractures and scars. Areas commonly affected by contractures are the hands, joints of the arms and legs, neck, face, calves, and legs. Preventive measures and treatment vary. Aggressive physical therapy should start as soon as the child can tolerate it.

NURSING CONSIDERATIONS IN CARE AND REHABILITATION OF THE BURNED CHILD

Care of the burned child is challenging. The child who has been burned is frightened, anxious, and in pain. Thus, the relationship that is established with the child is an integral part of the care that nurses provide.

The rehabilitative process begins at the time of hospital admission. Burns have a significant impact on the child, family, and nursing staff. It is important that each individual deal with his or her feelings about the injury and that open communication be encouraged throughout hospitalization and the rehabilitation phase.

Parents need to be encouraged to discuss the circumstances surrounding the burn injury. Feelings of guilt should be addressed so that the parents can become active participants in the child's care. Parents are encouraged to visit as often as possible, to provide emotional support to the child, and to assist with various aspects of physical care, such as dressing changes and baths. Most important, parents should not be afraid to touch and hold the child and to show love and affection no matter how badly disfigured the child initially appears. If indicated, social services, support groups, and pastoral care representatives can be recommended to families needing support.

Burned children experience intense pain during dressing changes, hydrotherapy, debridement, and positioning. The nurse helps the child through painful procedures by providing emotional support and understanding in addition to administering analgesics prior to procedures. The child should be kept as comfortable as possible. Diversionary activities should be provided during the recovery phase. Because major burns often require extended hospitalization with slow physical recovery, the nurse becomes a key member of the child's support group, along with parents and family.

How a child responds to the events that caused the burn, and to pain, treatments, and the possibility of disfigurement will depend on his or her age and developmental stage. Throughout the healing process, the nurse needs to keep in mind the child's developmental stage.

REVIEW QUESTIONS

A. Multiple choice. Select the best answer.

1. Which of the following disorders is apt to be seen in all age groups and is contagious?
   a. atopic dermatitis
   b. ringworm
   c. acne
   d. seborrheic dermatitis

2. A common presenting sign of impetigo is
   a. formation of a thin-walled lesion that ruptures, forming a honey-colored crust
   b. greasy or dry scaling lesions
   c. a widespread, erythematous rash
   d. papular lesions with a thickened, hardened appearance

3. Jamie, 9 years old, has recently developed tinea corporis. This infection is characterized by
   a. fungal infection of the head and scalp
   b. round lesions with central clearing and a scaly border
   c. vesicular lesions with weeping
   d. fissuring and pinhead-sized lesions

4. Which major type of acne is most likely to lead to severe scar formation?
   a. cystic acne
   b. papulopustular acne
   c. comedomal acne
   d. sebaceous acne

5. Symptomatic type 1 herpes is most commonly seen in
   a. children over 5 years of age
   b. adolescents who contract the infection through intimate contact
   c. children under 5 years of age
   d. school-age children who contract the infection from friends

6. The Lund and Browder formula is used to determine
   a. duration of contact
   b. depth of burn injury
   c. type of burn
   d. extent of burn

7. Which of the following might be used as a topical burn medication?
   a. betadine solution
   b. cortisone
   c. retinoid cream
   d. lindane

8. The most common types of burns are
   a. chemical
   b. electrical
   c. thermal
   d. radiation

B. Match the term in column I to the correct definition in column II.

Column I
1. atopic dermatitis
2. pediculosis capitis
3. xenograft
4. allograft
5. impetigo

Column II
a. a highly contagious bacterial infection of the skin, most commonly seen on face, limbs, hands, and neck
b. the best temporary skin graft; made of fresh cadaver skin
c. a chronic, inflammatory skin disease characterized by crusting lesions in areas rich in sebaceous glands
d. a commercially available temporary skin covering, usually pigskin
e. an infection caused by the laying of eggs or nits

SUGGESTED ACTIVITIES

- Make up teaching tools that can be used with parents of children in a particular age group (infants and toddlers, preschool and school-age, or adolescent) to help parents learn how to prevent, identify, and treat skin diseases common to the age group.

- Interview parents or children who have experienced one of the skin disorders discussed in the chapter. Find out about the feelings of the parent(s) or child, the reaction of others to the child, and the approaches to coping that were chosen by parent(s) or children.

- Interview a nurse who has worked on a burn unit. Find out about techniques that the nurse has used to make the experience less traumatic for burned children and their parents. Find out how the nurse deals with his or her own feelings and stress.

BIBLIOGRAPHY

Adamski, D. B. Assessment and treatment of allergic response to stinging insects. *Journal of Emergency Nursing* 16 (1990): 70–80.

Betz, C. L., and E. C. Poster. *Mosby's Pediatric Nursing Reference*, 2nd ed. St. Louis, MO: Mosby-Year Book, 1992.

Broadwell Jackson, D., and R. B. Saunders. *Child Health Nursing*. Philadelphia: J. B. Lippincott, 1993.

Budassi Sheehy, S. *Mosby's Manual of Emergency Care*, 3rd ed. St. Louis, MO: Mosby-Year Book, 1990.

Budassi Sheehy, S., J. A. Marvin, and C. D. Jimmerson. *Manual of Clinical Trauma Care: The First Hour*, St. Louis, MO: Mosby-Year Book, 1989.

Castiglia, P. T. Acne. *Journal of Pediatric Health Care* 3 (1989): 259–261.

Clore, E. R. Dispelling the common myths about pediculosis. *Journal of Pediatric Health Care* 3 (1989): 28–33.

Eichelberger, M. R., J. W. Ball, G. S. Pratsch, and E. Runion. *Pediatric Emergencies: A Manual for Prehospital Care Providers*. Englewood Cliffs, NJ: Brady/Prentice-Hall, 1992.

Fritsch, D. F., and D. M. Fredrick Pilat. Exposing latex allergies. *Nursing '93* 23, no. 8 (1993): 46–48.

Habif, T. *Clinical Dermatology: A Color Guide to Diagnosis and Therapy*, 2nd ed. St. Louis, MO: Mosby-Year Book, 1990.

Hathaway, W. E., W. W. Hay, Jr., J. R. Groothuis, and J. W. Paisley. *Current Pediatric Diagnosis and Treatment*, 11th ed. Norwalk, CT: Appleton & Lange, 1993.

Park, B. R., and D. Smith. Treatment of head lice and scabies in children. *Pediatric Nursing* 15 (1989): 522–524.

Rosenstein, B. J., and P. D. Fosarelli. *Pediatric Pearls: The Handbook of Practical Pediatrics*. St. Louis, MO: Mosby-Year Book, 1989.

Rudolph, A. M. *Rudolph's Pediatrics*, 19th ed. Norwalk, CT: Appleton & Lange, 1991.

Wong, D. L. *Whaley & Wong's Essentials of Pediatric Nursing*, 4th ed. St. Louis, MO: Mosby-Year Book, 1993.

Zitelli, B. J., and H. W. Davis. *Atlas of Pediatric Physical Diagnosis*, 2nd ed. St. Louis, MO: Mosby/Gower, 1991.

Conditions of the Eyes and Ears

OBJECTIVES

AFTER STUDYING THIS CHAPTER, THE STUDENT SHOULD BE ABLE TO:

- BRIEFLY DESCRIBE STRABISMUS AND DISCUSS ITS SYMPTOMS, TREATMENT, AND NURSING CARE.

- DESCRIBE THE CAUSE, SYMPTOMS, AND IMPLICATIONS OF SEVERAL COMMON CHILDHOOD EYE CONDITIONS.

- DESCRIBE SEVERAL TYPES OF TRAUMA TO THE EYE.

- DISCUSS THE IMPLICATIONS OF VISUAL IMPAIRMENT AND IDENTIFY METHODS OF VISION ASSESSMENT IN CHILDHOOD.

- BRIEFLY DESCRIBE OTITIS MEDIA AND DISCUSS ITS SYMPTOMS, TREATMENT, AND NURSING CARE.

- DESCRIBE SEVERAL TYPES OF TRAUMA TO THE EAR.

- DISCUSS THE IMPLICATIONS OF HEARING IMPAIRMENT AND IDENTIFY METHODS OF HEARING ASSESSMENT IN CHILDHOOD.

KEY TERMS

DIPLOPIA

PHOTOPHOBIA

VISUAL ACUITY

OCCLUSION THERAPY

VISUAL FIELD

TYMPANOMETRY

MYRINGOTOMY

*C*onditions of the eyes and ears are among the most common disorders affecting infants and young children. Because normal vision and hearing are essential for learning, assessment and treatment of eye and ear problems are important aspects of pediatric care. Vision and hearing screening are performed routinely throughout childhood. Problems such as strabismus, amblyopia, glaucoma, and cataracts should be diagnosed and treated promptly to prevent decrease or possible loss of vision. Children are also treated for infectious conditions, such as conjunctivitis or otitis media, and injuries to the eye and ear.

OVERVIEW OF THE EYE

The eye consists of external structures (eyelid, conjunctiva, lacrimal glands) that serve to protect and lubricate the globe of the eye, Figure 21–1a, and internal structures that make vision possible. Internal structures of the eye include the sclera, cornea, pupil, iris, lens, aqueous and vitreous humor, and retina, Figure 21–1b.

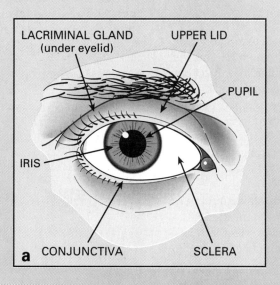

Figure 21–1 (a) External view of the eye. (b) Cross section of the eye.

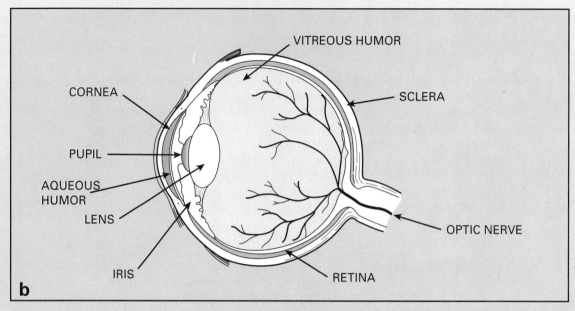

CORNEA

PUPIL

AQUEOUS
HUMOR

LENS

IRIS

VITREOUS HUMOR

SCLERA

OPTIC NERVE

RETINA

b

Figure 21–1   continued

CONDITIONS OF THE EYE

STRABISMUS

Description.   Strabismus refers to misalignment (crossing) of the eyes. Although commonly termed "cross-eye," the condition may affect one or both eyes, and it may involve eyes turning inward (esotropia), outward (exotropia), upward (hypertropia), or downward (hypotropia), Figure 21–2. Strabismus may occur as a result of muscle imbalance, poor vision, or a congenital defect (Hathaway et al. 1993).

Symptoms.   The child with strabismus may develop a squint or frown in an attempt to focus the eyes. Difficulty occurs when the child attempts to shift the focus from one distance to another. The child has trouble picking up objects and cannot see print or moving objects clearly. Common symptoms are double vision (**diplopia**), extreme sensitivity to light (**photophobia**), dizziness, and headache. Diagnosis is

often made by inspection of the child's eyes. The degree of fixation, angle of deviation, and the child's **visual acuity** (refractive ability) should be evaluated (Vaughan et al. 1992).

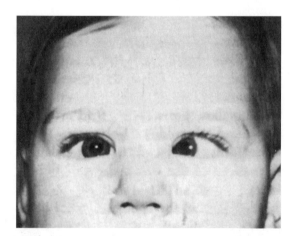

Figure 21–2   Strabismus (esotropia) (From Newell, Ophthalmology: Principles and Concepts, 7th ed. Mosby-Year Book, St. Louis, 1992)

302

Treatment. Treatment should begin as soon as the diagnosis is made. Treatment may involve wearing a patch over the stronger eye (**occlusion therapy**) to prevent amblyopia, performing eye exercises to help strengthen the weaker eye, or use of special prescription glasses or medications. If these approaches do not correct the deviation, surgery to align the eyes may be necessary.

Nursing Care. Once strabismus has been identified, the nurse can help ensure that the prescribed corrective treatment is carried out. If occlusion therapy or eye exercises have been ordered, the nurse should advise parents of the importance of having the child wear the eye patch or perform the exercises as prescribed.

AMBLYOPIA

Amblyopia, also known as "lazy eye," is a condition of reduced vision in one or both eyes. The most common cause is untreated strabismus, which causes the brain to suppress the visual image in the deviating eye. Amblyopia can also occur as a result of a refractive error. The child with amblyopia has reduced visual acuity in the affected eye. Treatment consists of patching, glasses, and visual exercises.

CATARACTS

A cataract is an opacity (or clouding) of the crystalline lens, which prevents the passage of light to the retina. Cataracts may occur in one or both eyes and may be congenital or acquired (the result of trauma or diseases). Children with cataracts have difficulty seeing objects clearly and may lose peripheral vision.

Early treatment is important to prevent long-term visual impairment. Treatment consists of surgery to remove the cloudy lens and fitting the child with removable contact lenses or glasses a few days after surgery.

GLAUCOMA

Glaucoma is a condition in which there is increased intraocular pressure within the eye. If untreated, this condition can eventually cause partial or complete loss of vision. Glaucoma is classified as primary (congenital) or secondary. Congenital glaucoma is rare. Symptoms can include corneal opacity, photophobia, and tearing. Secondary glaucoma occurs in children with congenital, metabolic, or inflammatory disorders of the eye (Rudolph 1991). Early surgery to reduce intraocular pressure is essential to prevent permanent blindness.

CONJUNCTIVITIS

Conjunctivitis, or "pink eye," is one of the most common eye conditions in children. It may result from bacterial, viral, or fungal infections; from allergic reactions; or from physical or chemical irritants (Hathaway et al. 1993). Symptoms include diffuse redness of the conjunctiva with a watery or purulent discharge from the eye. Vision is usually normal.

The treatment of conjunctivitis depends on the cause. Treatment of bacterial conjunctivitis involves identifying the causative organism, by smear or culture, and administering either a broad-spectrum antibiotic or ophthalmic drops or ointment. Conjunctivitis is extremely contagious. The nurse should instruct parents to wash hands after touching the child or giving eye drops or ointment and to keep the child's wash cloth and towels separate from those of other family members.

RETINOBLASTOMA

Retinoblastoma is a congenital, malignant tumor that occurs in the first two years of life. It is the most common retinal tumor occurring in childhood. The initial sign is the presence of a white reflex, or cat's eye reflex, in place of the normal red reflex. Early diagnosis and treatment are essential to prevent spread through the optic nerve and orbital tissues. Enucleation is the treatment of choice.

Trauma

Trauma to the eye may take many forms. The most common are foreign bodies, injury to the eyelid and cornea, burns, and child abuse.

Foreign Bodies. Foreign bodies are often found in the conjunctiva, cornea, and intraocular areas. A foreign body can usually be removed without difficulty from the conjunctiva using a moist cotton applicator or gauze pad. Before attempting to remove an object from the cornea, an anesthetic should be applied. More deeply imbedded foreign bodies are serious injuries that require ophthalmologic examination and prompt treatment (Hathaway et al. 1993). The nurse should instruct parents never to try to remove an object that has penetrated the eye.

Injuries to the Eyelids. Bruises to the eyelid should always be carefully assessed to determine whether there is any injury to the globe. Bruises can be treated initially using cold compresses to reduce bleeding and swelling. If the child sustains any type of laceration to the eyelid, referral should be made to an ophthalmologist.

Corneal Injuries. The cornea may be injured through abrasion or laceration. The child with a corneal abrasion is usually extremely uncomfortable. Treatment involves instillation of a mild paralyzing agent (cycloplegic) to the cornea, use of an antibiotic ointment, and patching of the eye for two to four days. The child with a corneal laceration should be referred to an ophthalmologist. Treatment involves suturing, observation for infection, and systemic antibiotics and tetanus toxoid, if laceration occurred with a contaminated object.

Burns. Burns that affect the external or internal structures of the eye are serious injuries. Burns to the eyelids should be treated like burns to any other part of the skin (see Chapter 20).

Chemical burns of the cornea and conjunctiva should be treated as an emergency, with tap water irrigations and topical anesthetics. The upper lid should be everted carefully and flushed thoroughly. Any child who suffers a severe chemical burn of the eye should be hospitalized and seen by an ophthalmologist.

Ultraviolet burns of the cornea can be caused by welders flash, exposure to snow on the ski slopes, or a treatment lamp or sunlamp. These burns cause severe pain and tearing and are treated using topical anesthetic, analgesics, antibiotic ointment, and eye patches.

Infrared burns, which can result from unfiltered observation of an eclipse or exposure to and penetration of x-rays, also require referral to an ophthalmologist. Infrared burns are serious injuries that can result in a permanent loss of vision.

Child Abuse. Injury to the eye may also be caused by child abuse. Common signs of such eye trauma include bruises of the eyelids, conjunctival bleeding, bleeding within the aqueous humor, and retinal hemorrhage. The nurse should refer a child with any of these symptoms to an ophthalmologist for a thorough examination. (Child abuse is discussed in more detail in Chapter 10.)

Visual Impairment

The function of the external and internal eye structures and related cranial nerves makes vision possible. Early diagnosis of a visual impairment is important, because vision is an essential sense for learning. Vision assessment should be a routine component of the child's physical examination. Evaluation should include screening children at risk because of heredity, maternal rubella infection, or prematurity; observing for behaviors that indicate a vision problem; and testing of visual acuity and **visual field** (area of vision).

It is recommended that routine eye examinations be performed shortly after birth, at 6 months, at 4 years, at 5 years, and then every two years until age 16. Color vision testing should be performed between the ages of 8 and 12 years (Vaughan et al. 1992). The Snellen alphabet chart and the "E" chart are commonly used to test distance vision, Figure 21–3a,b. The child with a visual acuity score of 20/200 or less in the good eye after correction or a visual field of no greater than 20 degrees in the better eye is termed legally blind.

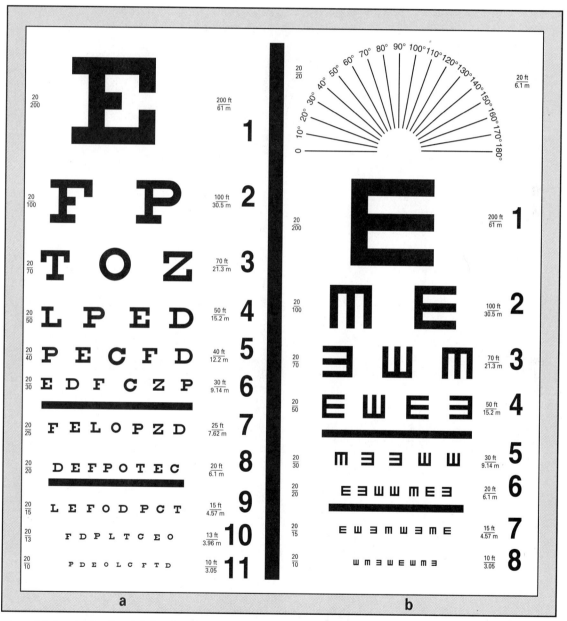

Figure 21–3 (a) Snellen alphabet chart for testing distance vision. (b) E test for testing distance vision in illiterate patients, particularly preschool children. (Courtesy of the National Society to Prevent Blindness)

OVERVIEW OF THE EAR

The ear is composed of three parts: the outer (or external) ear, the middle ear, and the inner ear, Figure 21–4a,b. The external auditory canal leads to the tympanic membrane, which separates the outer ear from the middle ear. The middle ear, made up of the ossicles (malleus, incus, and stapes), transmits sound from the tympanic membrane to the inner ear, composed of the cochlea and semicircular canals. The eustachian tube connects the middle ear to the pharynx and serves to equalize pressure inside the ear with that of the outside environment.

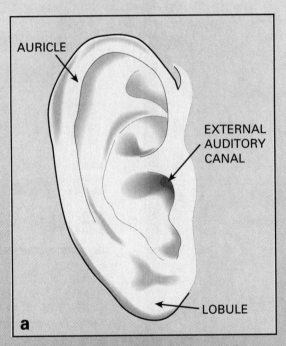

Figure 21–4   *(a) External view of the ear. (b) Cross section of the ear.*

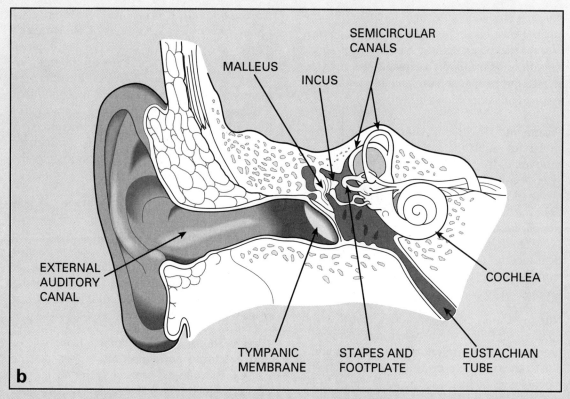

SEMICIRCULAR
CANALS

MALLEUS

INCUS

EXTERNAL
AUDITORY
CANAL

COCHLEA

b

TYMPANIC
MEMBRANE

STAPES AND
FOOTPLATE

EUSTACHIAN
TUBE

Figure 21–4   *continued*

CONDITIONS OF THE EAR

OTITIS MEDIA

Description.   Otitis media, an inflammation of
the middle ear, is a common disease in infants
and young children. Infection frequently occurs
during the winter months and is often caused
by *Streptococcus*, *Haemophilus*, or *Staphylococcus*
organisms.

Otitis media occurs as an acute or chronic
disorder. The acute form develops rapidly and
resolves within about three weeks. Chronic
otitis media is defined as an infection that lasts
more than three months.

Infants and children are prone to otitis
media because the eustachian tube is angled
more horizontally in children than in adults.
Impaired drainage in the tube causes secretions to pool in the middle ear, allowing bacteria to grow. This fluid causes pressure within
the tube, which is very painful.

Symptoms.   Acute otitis media frequently
occurs after an upper respiratory infection. Ear
pain, fever, crying, fussiness, irritability, pulling
at the affected ear, and loss of appetite are common symptoms. There may be visible drainage
from the ear.

Otoscopic examination reveals an immobile,
red tympanic membrane. Landmarks are either
poorly visible, absent, or distorted, depending
on whether fluid is present in the middle ear

space. **Tympanometry** (measurement of the internal ear pressure) is often performed to confirm the diagnosis. Because recurrence or persistence of otitis media places infants and children at risk for permanent ear damage or hearing loss, early identification is essential.

Treatment. Treatment consists of systemic antibiotics, antibiotic ear drops, analgesics, or antipyretic drugs to help reduce symptoms of fever and pain. Most children improve within two to four days. The child should be examined after the completion of antibiotic therapy for complications or residual hearing impairment. Some children may require **myringotomy** (surgical incision of the eardrum) and insertion of tympanostomy tubes to relieve symptoms of severe pain and to promote drainage.

Nursing Care. Nurses should be aware of the possibility of otitis media when caring for children with upper respiratory infections. In addition to the treatment measures outlined above, parents may be instructed to have the child lie on the affected side, to encourage drainage from the ear.

Parents should be advised of the possibility of temporary hearing loss (sometimes lasting several months), which may accompany acute otitis media. To help prevent future occurrences, the nurse should teach parents to place infants in an upright position for feedings, avoid propping bottles, and never allow the infant or young child to go to bed with a bottle. Parents should also teach small children how to blow their noses, as this clears out the eustachian tube, preventing pooling of secretions.

TRAUMA

Children frequently sustain trauma to the ear. Common forms of trauma are abrasions, lacerations, rupture of the tympanic membrane, and insertion of a foreign body.

Abrasions and Lacerations. Children may cause abrasions or lacerations of the ear canal by inserting sharp objects into the ear. Injuries can also be caused by parents' attempts to remove ear wax. In all cases, the tympanic membrane should be examined to ensure that it is free of injury. Abrasions and lacerations of the canal tend to heal readily; therefore, as long as the tympanic membrane is uninjured, no treatment is necessary. Lacerations to the outer ear require sutures.

Rupture of the Tympanic Membrane. A perforation of the tympanic membrane can occur as a result of a head injury, a blow to the side of the head and ear, or the insertion of a sharp, pointed object such as a stick, paper clip, bobby pin, or ballpoint pen into the ear canal. The child should be referred to an otolaryngologist, because these injuries do not heal spontaneously.

Foreign Bodies. Children may intentionally or unintentionally put almost any object into the ear. Objects that are frequently found include paper, wadded tissue, beads, earring parts, and insects. An initial attempt may be made to remove the foreign body by pulling on the earlobe to straighten the ear canal and then gently shaking the child's head. If this method fails, various other measures may be used to try to remove the object, including use of a cotton-tipped applicator coated with warmed wax, forceps, or irrigation. If the object is large or wedged in the ear canal, the child should be referred to an otolaryngologist for treatment (Hathaway et al. 1993).

HEARING IMPAIRMENT

Hearing is essential for normal speech development and learning. For this reason, hearing evaluation should be performed frequently in children from infancy through adolescence.

Each year, approximately 1,000 children are born deaf in the United States (Riley 1987).

Hearing loss may also occur during early childhood as the result of birth trauma, maternal rubella infection, chronic otitis media, meningitis, or antibiotics that damage cranial nerve VIII.

Screening is essential for early detection and diagnosis of hearing impairment. Attainment of hearing and speech milestones is used as an initial hearing screen. Sometimes hearing is assessed by watching the child's reaction to various auditory stimuli. Preschool children can be tested using earphones and pure tone audiometry.

REVIEW QUESTIONS

A. Multiple choice. Select the best answer.

1. Andrea, 8 years old, has diplopia and photophobia and complains to her mother of frequent headaches. These are symptoms of
    a. strabismus
    b. amblyopia
    c. glaucoma
    d. cataract

2. The white reflex is an initial sign of what disorder?
    a. glaucoma
    b. amblyopia
    c. retinoblastoma
    d. corneal laceration

3. Treatment for amblyopia might include all of the following except
    a. wearing a patch over the weak eye
    b. performing eye exercises to help strengthen the weaker eye
    c. surgery to align the eyes
    d. use of prescription glasses

4. A foreign body can usually be removed without difficulty from the
    a. conjunctiva
    b. cornea
    c. aqueous humor
    d. sclera

5. Color vision assessment is usually performed
    a. at birth, 6 months, and 4 years of age, and every 2 years thereafter
    b. at birth, 6 years, and 12 years of age
    c. between the ages of 8 and 12 years
    d. when a child enters school (5 to 6 years of age)

6. Michael, 5 years old, has acute otitis media. This condition
    a. requires surgical treatment using myringotomy
    b. is a congenital defect of the eustachian tube
    c. occurs frequently in summer months
    d. may be caused by *Haemophilus* organisms

7. The middle ear consists of the
    a. auricle, tympanic membrane, and ossicles
    b. ossicles, cochlea, and semicircular canals
    c. tympanic membrane and eustachian tube
    d. malleus, incus, and stapes

B. Match the term in column I to the correct description in column II.

Column I
1. amblyopia
2. glaucoma
3. cataract
4. retinoblastoma
5. conjunctivitis

Column II
a. increased pressure within the eye
b. a congenital, malignant tumor that occurs in the first two years of life
c. "lazy eye"; reduced vision in one or both eyes
d. clouding of the crystalline lens
e. redness and discharge caused by infection, allergic reaction, or physical irritant

SUGGESTED ACTIVITIES

- Make a poster or give a presentation on ways of preventing trauma to the eyes or ears.

- Discuss the importance of the eyes and ears in childhood development. Interview a special education teacher or a parent to find out how children with vision or hearing impairments compensate.

- There are a number of inspirational biographies of vision-, speech-, or hearing-impaired people. Read one of those biographies and demonstrate how the inspirational story can be used in a health care setting.

- Interview a health care worker who is involved with vision- or hearing-impaired clients. Ask what kind of differences exist between children who have been impaired since birth and those who develop an impairment later in life. Discuss the implications for you as a nurse dealing with those children or their families.

BIBLIOGRAPHY

Bluestone, C. D. Modern management of otitis media. *Pediatric Clinics of North America* 36 (1989): 1371–1387.

Broadwell Jackson, D., and R. B. Saunders. *Child Health Nursing*. Philadelphia: J. B. Lippincott, 1993.

Budassi Sheehy, S. *Mosby's Manual of Emergency Care*, 3rd ed. St. Louis, MO: Mosby-Year Book, 1990.

Fisher, M. C. Conjunctivitis in children. *Pediatric Clinics of North America* 34 (1987): 1447–1456.

Hathaway, W. E., W. W. Hay, Jr., J. R. Groothuis, and J. W. Paisley. *Current Pediatric Diagnosis and Treatment*, 11th ed. Norwalk, CT: Appleton & Lange, 1993.

Newell, F. W. *Ophthalmology: Principles and Concepts*, 7th ed. St. Louis, MO: Mosby-Year Book, 1992.

Riley, M. A. *Nursing Care of the Child with Ear, Nose, and Throat Disorders*. New York: Springer, 1987.

Rosenstein, B. J., and P. D. Fosarelli. *Pediatric Pearls: The Handbook of Practical Pediatrics*. St. Louis, MO: Mosby-Year Book, 1989.

Rudolph, A. M. *Rudolph's Pediatrics*, 19th ed. Norwalk, CT: Appleton & Lange, 1991.

Vaughan, D. G., T. Asbury, and P. Riordan-Eva. *General Ophthalmology*, 13th ed. Norwalk, CT: Appleton & Lange, 1992.

Wong, D. L. *Whaley & Wong's Essentials of Pediatric Nursing*, 4th ed. St. Louis, MO: Mosby-Year Book, 1993.

Cardiovascular Conditions

OBJECTIVES

AFTER STUDYING THIS CHAPTER, THE STUDENT SHOULD BE ABLE TO:

- DIFFERENTIATE BETWEEN CONGENITAL AND ACQUIRED HEART DISEASES AND GIVE AN EXAMPLE OF EACH.

- DESCRIBE THE CHANGES THAT TAKE PLACE IN THE CARDIOVASCULAR SYSTEM AT BIRTH.

- DIFFERENTIATE BETWEEN CYANOTIC AND ACYANOTIC HEART DEFECTS AND GIVE EXAMPLES OF EACH.

- DISCUSS COMMON DIAGNOSTIC PROCEDURES PERFORMED ON CHILDREN WITH CONGENITAL HEART DISEASE.

- DISCUSS THE CAUSES, SYMPTOMS, TREATMENT, AND NURSING CARE OF CONGESTIVE HEART FAILURE.

- DISCUSS THE CAUSES, SYMPTOMS, TREATMENT, AND NURSING CARE OF SYSTEMIC HYPERTENSION.

- DISCUSS THE CAUSES, SYMPTOMS, TREATMENT, AND NURSING CARE OF RHEUMATIC FEVER.

KEY TERMS

CONGENITAL HEART DISEASE

ACQUIRED HEART DISEASE

ACYANOTIC HEART DISEASE

CYANOTIC HEART DISEASE

BACTERIAL ENDOCARDITIS

CONGESTIVE HEART FAILURE

Cardiovascular conditions are some of the most serious illnesses that affect children. These conditions most often affect the child's heart and great vessels. A **congenital heart disease** develops during fetal development and is present at birth. The majority of these defects are diagnosed within the first month of life. An **acquired heart disease** occurs after birth as a result of complication of another disease.

Families of children diagnosed with congenital heart disease often experience anxiety, fear, and guilt because of their lack of understanding about their child's disease and its treatment (Kashani and Higgins 1986). The nurse can play an instrumental role by providing emotional support to parents. This support can include active listening, family referral to a counselor or therapist, teaching the family about their child's disease and its treatment, or referral to support groups in the community.

OVERVIEW OF THE SYSTEM

The cardiovascular system is composed of the heart (Figure 22–1), arteries, veins, and capillaries. The main function of the heart is to pump blood throughout the body and to the lungs, oxygenating and carrying nutrients to the cells and removing the waste products of metabolism. Arteries carry blood away from the heart. Veins carry blood to the heart. Capillaries provide available oxygen and nutrients to the cells.

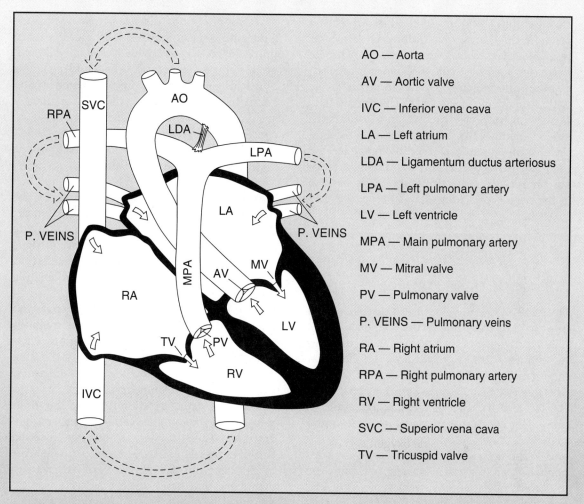

Figure 22–1   *Anatomy of the heart (Courtesy Ross Laboratories)*

Legend:

AO — Aorta

AV — Aortic valve

IVC — Inferior vena cava

LA — Left atrium

LDA — Ligamentum ductus arteriosus

LPA — Left pulmonary artery

LV — Left ventricle

MPA — Main pulmonary artery

MV — Mitral valve

PV — Pulmonary valve

P. VEINS — Pulmonary veins

RA — Right atrium

RPA — Right pulmonary artery

RV — Right ventricle

SVC — Superior vena cava

TV — Tricuspid valve

POSTNATAL CIRCULATION

At birth, the circulation of blood through the cardiovascular system changes. When an infant takes the first breath, the lungs fill with air. The lungs are now responsible for oxygenating the blood. The three fetal shunts — the ductus venosus, foramen ovale, and ductus arteriosus — that enabled the majority of blood to bypass the liver and the lungs are no longer needed and will, within days or weeks, cease to function.

The ductus venosus constricts at birth and

closes within 48 hours. As the infant breathes air into the lungs, the pulmonary vascular resistance (flow of blood into the lungs) decreases and systemic resistance increases, resulting in closure of the foramen ovale within several weeks of birth. The ductus arteriosus constricts at birth and, in most infants, closes anatomically within the first several days of life. It can take months, however, for total closure to occur, and the ductus arteriosus can reopen under stressful conditions such as hypoxemia or acidosis.

INFANT

CONGENITAL HEART DISEASE

Description. Congenital heart disease occurs in 8 to 10 of 1,000 live births (Hazinski 1992). Ninety percent of congenital heart diseases in children are a result of multifactorial inheritance (genetic or environmental factors). The most common causes are maternal alcoholism, rubella during the first trimester of pregnancy, insulin-dependent diabetes, and maternal trimethadione ingestion (Daberkow and Washington 1989). The majority of congenital heart diseases develop during the fourth through eighth weeks of fetal life, because it is during this time that the heart is developing from 2 tubes into a 4-chambered structure.

Classification. Congenital heart diseases are classified as either acyanotic or cyanotic. **Acyanotic heart disease** is usually associated with defects that increase the flow of blood to the lungs. Blood flows from the left to the right side of the heart, where the oxygenated blood mixes with the unoxygenated blood (a left to right shunt). No change in the infant's skin coloring is noted. The most common acyanotic heart defect is a ventricular septal defect.

Cyanotic heart disease is usually associated with defects that result in the mixing of unoxygenated blood with oxygenated blood, or a right to left shunt. The child's skin is bluish because of the unoxygenated blood circulating through the systemic circulatory system. Cyanotic heart defects may also be caused by an obstruction in the aorta or the left side of the heart. The most common cyanotic heart defect is tetralogy of Fallot.

Symptoms and Treatment. Several of the most common acyanotic and cyanotic heart defects of children are illustrated in Figure 22–2. Figure 22–3 (page 316) summarizes signs and symptoms and treatment for these defects. The defects can occur alone or in combination with each other.

Diagnosis is made by both invasive and noninvasive methods. Noninvasive methods include history, physical examination, chest x-ray, electrocardiogram (ECG), and echocardiogram. Invasive methods include cardiac catheterization and angiography.

Cardiac catheterization involves the insertion of a radiopaque catheter under fluoroscopy. The catheter is usually inserted through the femoral artery or vein into the heart, allowing visualization of the valves, chambers, and great vessels, as well as measurement of pressures and oxygen saturations within the heart. If angiography is performed at the same time, a contrast dye is injected through the catheter to observe blood flow through the heart. Nursing care for a child undergoing cardiac catheterization is summarized in Figure 22–4 (page 321).

Children with congenital heart defects are at risk for developing congestive heart failure and **bacterial endocarditis**. Congestive heart failure occurs when the heart fails to compensate for changes in blood flow and fails to pump blood efficiently through the heart (see Congestive Heart Failure, below). Bacterial endocarditis is a bacterial infection of the

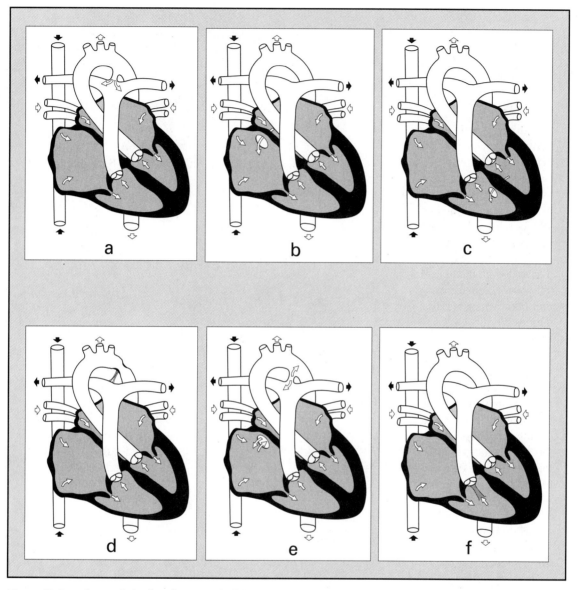

Figure 22–2   *Acyanotic (a–d) and cyanotic (e–f) heart defects (a) Patent ductus arteriosus (b) Atrial septal defects (c) Ventricular septal defect (d) Coarctation of the aorta (e) Complete transposition of the great vessels (f) Tetralogy of Fallot (Courtesy Ross Laboratories)*

valves or the inner lining of the heart. It occurs most often in children with valvular abnormalities, prosthetic valves, and heart defects that produce turbulent blood flow and after cardiac surgery in which a catheter was placed within the heart.

CONGENITAL HEART DEFECTS

ACYANOTIC DEFECTS
Patent Ductus Arteriosus

Description

The ductus arteriosus is a remnant of fetal circulation. It closes shortly after birth and becomes a ligament. Failure of the ductus to close results in a continued flow of blood from the aorta to the pulmonary artery (a left-to-right shunting of blood). Blood flow to the lungs is increased. Premature infants are most at risk Figure 22–2a.

Signs and Symptoms

Newborn:
Respiratory distress, congestive heart failure

Older Child:
Murmur, increased oxygen consumption, bounding pulses, widening pulse pressure, dyspnea

Atrial Septal Defect

An abnormal opening in the wall or septum between the atria. With the change in blood flow after birth, pressures are higher on the left side of the heart than on the right. Blood flows from the left atrium to the right atrium then to the right ventricle, pulmonary artery, and into the lungs. Blood flow is increased to the lungs, Figure 22–2b.

Most children with an atrial septal defect are asymptomatic. Symptoms include systolic murmur, increased number of respiratory infections, decrease in normal exercise tolerance, delayed physical growth, congestive heart failure (uncommon), and cardiac enlargement.

Figure 22–3 continued

CONGENITAL HEART DEFECTS

Ventricular Septal Defect

Description

An abnormal opening in the septum between the ventricles, causing blood to flow from the left ventricle to the right ventricle then to pulmonary artery and into the lungs, Figure 22–2c.

Signs and Symptoms

Symptoms vary with the size of the defect. Small or moderate-sized defects usually produce no symptoms and most close spontaneously, usually within the first year of life. Large defects usually are more serious. The child with a large ventricular septal defect has an increased amount of blood flow to the lungs. It may take 1 to 2 months before a child begins to have symptoms of congestive heart failure. Symptoms may include murmur, tachypnea, feeding difficulties, excessive perspiration, tachycardia, mild cyanosis, slow physical growth, splenomegaly, and irritability.

Treatment

ASYMPTOMATIC INFANT/CHILD SURGICAL MANAGEMENT: Defect is closed with synthetic patch.

SYMPTOMATIC INFANT/CHILD MEDICAL MANAGEMENT: Treatment of symptoms of congestive heart failure

Surgical management: Palliative surgery includes banding of pulmonary artery (a piece of prosthetic material is tied around the main pulmonary artery to constrict blood flow to the lungs). Complete repair involves closing the defect with a prosthetic patch.

Figure 22–3   *continued*

CONGENITAL HEART DEFECTS

Coarctation of the Aorta

Description

A narrowing in the lumen of the aorta that obstructs blood flow to the lower extremities and body, while blood flow to the head and upper extremities is increased, Figure 22–2d.

Signs and Symptoms

Symptoms depend on the severity of the defect, the anatomical location, and the presence of other heart defects.

Infant:
Congestive heart failure, failure to thrive

Older Child:
Systolic murmur, localized hypertension and hypotension, episodes of sudden or unexplained nosebleeds, frequent headaches, leg fatigue, full bounding pulses in upper extremities (hypertension), weak or absent pulses in lower extremities (hypotension), and visible pulsation

Treatment

Surgical management:
Removal of the narrowed segment. End-to-end anastomosis of the aortic segments or insertion of a graft between the two ends of the aorta

Pulmonary Stenosis

A narrowing at the entrance to the pulmonary artery that obstructs blood flow to the lungs, causing enlargement of the right ventricle (right ventricular hypertrophy) and decreased blood flow to the lungs.

Murmur, cardiomegaly, cyanosis (with severe stenosis), and right ventricular failure (with severe stenosis)

Surgical management:
Valvotomy (surgical valve replacement)

Nonsurgical management:
Balloon angioplasty during cardiac catheterization to dilate valve

Figure 22–3   *continued*

CONGENITAL HEART DEFECTS

CYANOTIC DEFECTS
Complete Transposition of the Great Vessels

Description	Signs and Symptoms	Treatment
Reversal of the anatomical positions of the pulmonary artery and aorta, establishing two separate circulatory systems. The aorta originating from the right ventricle is pumping unoxygenated blood throughout the body, and the pulmonary artery originating from the left ventricle is pumping oxygenated blood to the lungs, Figure 22–2e. Incompatible with life. Other defects must be present to allow oxygenated and unoxygenated blood to mix.	Cyanosis, tachypnea, full bounding arterial pulses, poor physical growth, clubbing of fingers and toes	*Nonsurgical management:* Prostaglandins are continuously given intravenously to keep ductus arteriosus open. During cardiac catheterization a balloon atrial septostomy (Rashkind procedure) is performed, which creates an opening between the atria. These two openings allow unoxygenated blood to mix with oxygenated blood, which then circulates throughout body. *Surgical management:* Arteries may be switched to their original position (Jalene procedure) using cardiopulmonary bypass, or a large, single atrium may be created (Mustard procedure), allowing diversion of systemic blood flow to left side of heart and to pulmonary artery. Also allows pulmonary blood flow to be diverted to right side of heart and to aorta.

Figure 22–3   continued

CONGENITAL HEART DEFECTS

Tetralogy of Fallot

Description

Consists of four heart defects: (1) ventricular septal defect, (2) right ventricular hypertrophy, (3) right ventricular outflow obstruction, and (4) overriding aorta, Figure 22–2f.

Signs and Symptoms

Cyanosis, poor physical growth, systolic murmur, hypoxic spells, polycythemia, activity intolerance, and squatting

Treatment

Surgical management: Palliative procedures are usually performed initially to increase blood flow to the lungs by an anastomosis between the subclavian artery and the pulmonary artery. Either a Blalock-Tussing shunt or a Modified Blalock-Tussing shunt is performed. Complete correction to close the ventricular septal defect and relieve right ventricular outflow obstruction will take place usually between the ages of 8 months and 3 years if infant or child is stable. Corrective surgery may take place sooner if the infant or child has severe hypoxemia, severe polycythemia, a decrease in exercise intolerance, or an increase in hypercyanotic spells (Hazinski 1992).

Figure 22–3   *continued*

NURSING CARE: CARDIAC CATHETERIZATION

Precatheterization

Nursing care before catheterization centers on support and teaching:

1. Teach the child and family about the procedure. Preparation of the child must be based on the child's cognitive and developmental level.

2. A visit to the catheterization laboratory is one of the most helpful ways to educate both the child and family.

3. If a visit is not possible, showing the child a picture book with photographs of the room and equipment can be helpful. Allow the child and family to ask questions to help relieve anxiety.

4. Obtain baseline vital signs.

Postcatheterization

1. Assess the child's vital signs.

2. Assess circulation to the extremity in which the catheter was introduced. For example, if the femoral vein is used (most common), the leg and foot are examined.

3. Compare both extremities for pulses, capillary filling time, color, temperature, edema, and sensation.

4. Keep the child on bed rest until at least 6 hours after the catheterization.

5. Assist the child to keep the extremity in which the catheter was inserted straight until ambulation is possible.

6. Assess the pressure dressing for signs of bleeding or hematoma. If blood is noted, notify the physician immediately.

Figure 22–4   Nursing care for the child undergoing cardiac catheterization

Nursing Care. Depending on the defect, nursing care may involve administration of medication, pre- and postsurgical care, and patient and family teaching about the defect and its treatment. Nursing care is directed toward improving cardiac output, reducing energy expenditure, promoting physical growth, and reducing the family's fears. Early identification of the signs and symptoms of congenital heart disease and identification of changes in the child's condition are important aspects of nursing care. Encourage the family to avoid overprotecting the child. Emphasize that the child should participate in normal age-appropriate activities and rest when he or she is tired. Figure 22–5 summarizes nursing care for the child with a congenital heart defect.

CONGESTIVE HEART FAILURE

Description. **Congestive heart failure** is not a disease, but rather a condition in which the blood supply to the body is insufficient to meet the body's metabolic demands. Congenital heart defects are the most common cause of congestive heart failure in children. Other causes include severe anemia, arrhythmias, and weak or damaged heart muscle.

Congestive heart failure can occur on either the left or the right side of the heart. Right-sided heart failure occurs when the right ventricle has difficulty pumping blood into the pulmonary artery. Blood then backs up on the right side of the heart and into the inferior and superior venae cavae.

NURSING CARE PLAN: Congenital Heart Disease

NURSING DIAGNOSIS	GOAL(S)
Failure to gain weight, respiratory difficulties with eating (tachypnea, retractions, nasal flaring)	The child will have an adequate intake of nutrients and calories.
Activity and exercise intolerance, fatigue on exertion, respiratory distress, tachycardia	The child will have reduced oxygen needs and reduced strain on the heart.

Figure 22–5   *Nursing care plan for congenital heart disease*

NURSING INTERVENTION	RATIONALE
Monitor caloric intake, daily weights, strict intake and output.	Daily weights enable monitoring of weight gain or loss.
Hold infant in a semi-upright position to feed.	Semi-upright position allows for better lung expansion and easier breathing.
Allow infant to rest after 15–30 mL of formula.	The more energy the child uses, the more oxygen is needed.
Feed at the first sign of hunger. Give small, frequent feedings every 2–3 hours. Alternate oral and gavage feedings. Provide a quiet environment with little stimulation during feeding.	Calories (energy) used for crying cannot be used to gain weight.
Educate family and child about diet therapy (high-calorie, high-carbohydrate, low-sodium, high-iron).	Helps ensure an adequate intake of nutrients.
Cluster nursing care to allow for periods of uninterrupted rest.	Rest gives the child energy to eat and play.
Attend to the child's crying or call light immediately. Place toys or personal items within easy reach. Position the child in semi-Fowler's position with loose unrestrictive clothing.	An increase in activity increases the body's need for oxygen.
Keep the temperature in the child's room neutral (not too hot or too cold).	An increase in the child's temperature increases metabolic rate, which in turn increases oxygen needs.

Figure 22–5   *continued*

Left-sided heart failure occurs when the left ventricle is unable to pump adequate amounts of blood into the aorta, causing blood to back up into the lungs. Because children's hearts are small, they frequently have both left- and right-sided heart failure.

Symptoms. Signs and symptoms of congestive heart failure include feeding difficulties, tachypnea, tachycardia, rales, hepatomegaly, splenomegaly, cardiomegaly, dyspnea, activity intolerance, decreased urine output, diaphoresis, slow growth pattern (failure to thrive), periorbital edema, poor peripheral circulation with cool extremities, and respiratory distress, Figure 22–6.

Treatment. Congestive heart failure is treated with medications. Digoxin is the drug of choice in children older than 1 month of age. Digoxin slows the child's heart rate, which increases the heart's force of contraction and the output of blood from the ventricles, Figure 22–7 (page 326). Diuretics such as furosemide (Lasix), spironolactone (Aldactone), and thiazides are given to reduce edema. Potassium supplements and potassium-rich diets may be used with diuretic therapy to reduce the chance of hypokalemia.

Nursing Care. The goal of nursing care is to limit the child's expenditure of energy. The nurse should cluster care so that the child has periods of uninterrupted rest. Try to meet the needs of the crying or fussy child as soon as possible. Encourage the child to take time to rest or take naps throughout the day. The child's room should be "neutral thermic," that is, neither too hot nor too cold. This temperature allows the child to use as little energy as possible for thermoregulation. Positioning the child in a semi-Fowler's position prevents pressure on the diaphragm, allowing gas exchange from increased lung expansion.

The child's intake and output should be strictly monitored often during each shift. Any significant difference between fluid that has been ingested and urine that has been excreted must be reported. Weigh the child at the same time every day to assess fluid status.

When feeding an infant with congestive heart failure, limit oral feedings to 20 to 30 minutes and burp infant after every 15 to 30 mL of formula. Many infants with congestive heart failure are given concentrated high-carbohydrate formulas containing 24 to 30 calories per ounce. Gavage feeding is sometimes necessary. Children should be encouraged to eat high-calorie, low-sodium, and high-nutrient foods. A nutritionist can be helpful in educating the family about the nutritional needs of the child.

Parent education is an important part of nursing care. Parents need to know about administration of medication as well as how to conserve the child's energy during feedings and activities.

School-Age Child and Adolescent

Systemic Hypertension

Hypertension refers to a consistent state of elevated blood pressure. Specifically, the systolic or the diastolic blood pressure is above the 95th percentile for the age and the sex of the child on more than three separate occasions (Broadwell Jackson and Saunders 1993).

Hypertension is categorized as either primary (essential) or secondary. Primary hypertension refers to a chronic increase in blood pressure that is not a result of any underlying disease or illness. Secondary hypertension results from another disease or illness.

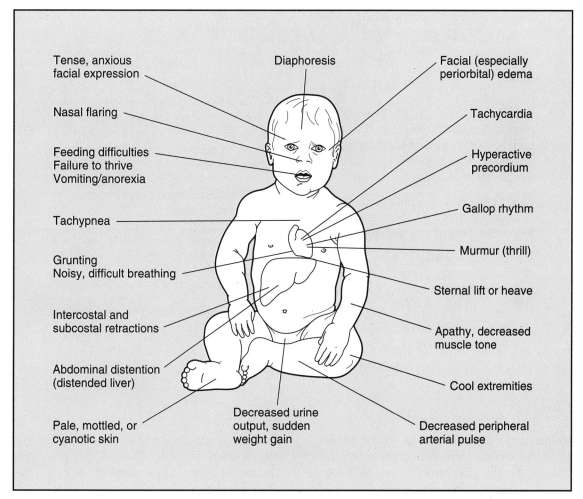

Figure 22–6   *Infant with congestive heart failure, physical assessment findings. (Adapted from* Critical Care Nurse 2, *no. 5, 1982, with permission from American Association of Critical-Care Nurses, Aliso Viejo, CA)*

In the United States, it is estimated that 1% to 2.5% of children between 3 and 18 years of age have hypertension. Genetics, race, sex, and environmental factors such as obesity, emotional stress, and excessive salt ingestion are thought to contribute to the development of hypertension. Treatment includes stress reduction, physical exercise, a salt-reduction diet, and medications (Broadwell Jackson and Saunders 1993).

RHEUMATIC FEVER

Description. Rheumatic fever is the most common acquired heart disease of young children and adolescents. It is a systemic inflammatory disease that affects primarily the heart, joints, brain, and skin. The damage to the heart usually involves the mitral valve and, as the disease progresses, the myocardium.

The disease usually develops about two to three weeks after an untreated group A beta-

DIGOXIN ADMINISTRATION TIPS

1. Check apical pulse for 1 full minute before administration.

2. Hold administration of digoxin if the pulse is less than 90 to 110 beats per minute (b.p.m.) for infants and less than 70 to 80 b.p.m. for older children or physician instructed limits; notify the physician.

3. Give digoxin on an empty stomach (1 hour before or 2 hours after eating) to increase absorption of medication.

4. If child vomits within 15 minutes after receiving digoxin, repeat the dose once. If child vomits again, notify the physician.

5. Check serum potassium levels before administering digoxin. Low potassium levels can enhance the toxic side effects of digoxin.

6. Observe child for signs and symptoms of digoxin toxicity such as nausea and vomiting, diarrhea, anorexia, tachycardia, bradycardia, arrhythmias, and hypotension.

7. Give medication at regular times 12 hours apart.

8. If two or more doses are missed, notify the physician.

9. Keep medication in locked cabinet.

10. Never double or increase dosage of medication.

Figure 22–7

streptococcal infection (strep throat pharyngitis). Antibodies formed to combat the toxin released by the streptococci react with tissue antigens, resulting in damage to various body organs. Young school-age children are often exposed to streptococcal infections, especially during the winter and early spring. However, only 3% or fewer children with strep throat infections develop rheumatic fever. This low incidence implies that hereditary or environmental factors play a role in increasing susceptibility to the disease.

Symptoms. Initial symptoms may include fatigue and joint tenderness. Symptoms can progress to include carditis, polyarthritis, erythema marginatum, subcutaneous nodules, and chorea. Carditis, the most serious clinical symptom, occurs in over 50% of children with rheumatic fever. Approximately 10% of children develop chorea, also known as St. Vitus dance, which is characterized by involuntary, rapid movements of the muscles of the face and limbs (Broadwell Jackson and Saunders 1993).

Treatment. The Jones criteria are used to differentiate rheumatic fever from other illnesses with similar symptoms, Figure 22–8. A throat culture is taken to identify the presence of group A beta-streptococci. A rising or elevated antistreptolysin-O (ASO) titer identifies the presence of antibodies to streptococci.

The goals of treatment are to eradicate the streptococcal infection, prevent permanent car-

JONES CRITERIA (UPDATED 1992)*

Major Manifestations

Carditis
Polyarthritis
Chorea
Erythema marginatum
Subcutaneous nodules

Minor Manifestations

Clinical Findings
Arthralgia
Fever
Laboratory Findings
Elevated acute phase reactants
Erythrocyte sedimentation rate
C-reactive protein
Prolonged PR interval

Supporting Evidence of Antecedent Group A Streptococcal Infection

Positive throat culture or rapid streptococcal antigen test

Elevated or rising streptococcal antibody titer

*If supported by evidence of preceding group A streptococcal infection, the presence of two major manifestations, or of one major and two minor manifestations indicates a high probability of acute rheumatic fever.

Figure 22–8 Guidelines for the diagnosis of initial attack of rheumatic fever. (Data from Committee on Rheumatic Fever, Endocarditis, and Kawasaki Disease of the Council on Cardiovascular Disease in the Young, American Heart Association, Dallas, 1982)

diac damage, reduce inflammation, and manage associated symptoms. Treatment includes administration of oral penicillin for 10 days. If the child is allergic to penicillin, erythromycin is prescribed. Aspirin or corticosteroids may be given to decrease the inflammatory process.

Nursing Care. Nursing care includes teaching the child and parents about the illness and its treatment and providing emotional support. Emphasize to the parents the importance of the child's receiving the complete 10-day course of antibiotics. Diversional activities should be provided for the child who may be on bed rest. These include books, tapes, puzzles, and art projects. Children with carditis are cautioned to avoid strenuous physical exercise for two to three months after the signs of cardiac inflammation have disappeared.

REVIEW QUESTIONS

A. Multiple choice. Select the best answer.

1. Bobby, age 4 months, is admitted for a cardiac catheterization that is to be performed tomorrow morning. Which of the following statements would best indicate that Bobby's mother understands about the procedure?
   a. "A cardiac catheterization takes only 10 minutes to perform, and Bobby will go home tomorrow afternoon."
   b. "Bobby's catheterization will be performed in his room by his pediatrician."
   c. "Bobby's catheterization will help his doctors to diagnose his heart problem."
   d. "The catheterization that the doctors are doing tomorrow will involve simply taking a picture of Bobby's heart."

2. Sally, 18 days old, is diagnosed with a heart defect. Her parents ask you what caused her heart problem. Your best response would be which of the following?
   a. "Sally's heart problem was caused by something you did wrong during your pregnancy."
   b. "Sally's heart problem developed during your last trimester from some type of virus you came in contact with."
   c. "I don't know. Maybe you should ask her doctor."
   d. "Sally's heart problem was probably caused by a combination of physical and environmental factors during your pregnancy."

3. Which of the following is a cyanotic heart defect?
   a. patent ductus arteriosus
   b. coarctation of the aorta
   c. tetralogy of Fallot
   d. atrial septal defect

4. Glenn, age 2 years, is diagnosed with coarctation of the aorta. Which of the following clinical symptoms would you expect to find?
   a. high blood pressure in the lower extremities and low blood pressure in the upper extremities
   b. low blood pressure in the lower extremities and high blood pressure in the upper extremities
   c. low blood pressure in the lower extremities and low blood pressure in the upper extremities
   d. high blood pressure in the lower extremities and high blood pressure in the upper extremities

5. Which of the following is a fetal shunt that can reopen under stressful conditions after total closure?
   a. foramen ovale
   b. ductus venosus
   c. ductus ovale
   d. ductus arteriosus

6. A child with congenital heart disease should be on what type of diet?
   a. High-calorie, high-carbohydrate, low-sodium
   b. High-calorie, high-carbohydrate, high-sodium
   c. Low-calorie, moderate-carbohydrate, low-sodium
   d. High-calorie, moderate-carbohydrate, low-sodium

7. The best position in which to place Molly, a 6-month-old infant with congestive heart failure, after feeding is
   a. prone, semi-Fowler's
   b. flat, prone
   c. Trendelenburg, prone
   d. supine, semi-Fowler's

8. Stephanie, 5 years old, will undergo a cardiac catheterization tomorrow morning. Which of the following approaches would best prepare Stephanie for the procedure?
   a. Tell Stephanie that the doctors will cut a small hole in her leg and thread a small catheter into her so the doctors can see her heart.
   b. Allow Stephanie and her family to visit the catheterization lab the evening before and provide masks, needles, syringes, gowns, and stethoscopes for a supervised play session after the tour.
   c. Show Stephanie pictures of her heart in a book and describe the procedure to her.
   d. Don't tell Stephanie anything until she is ready to go to her catheterization because preparing her the day before will upset her too much.

9. Common signs and symptoms of congestive heart failure include
   a. increased urine output
   b. erythema marginatum
   c. tachycardia
   d. increased peripheral arterial pulse

10. Sarah is a 4-month-old infant with congestive heart failure. Before giving Sarah her 8 A.M. dose of digoxin, you auscultate her heart rate. Her apical pulse is 84. What should you do?
    a. Give the medication first and then tell her physician.
    b. Hold the medication until her heart rate is greater than 110 b.p.m.
    c. Wait an hour and then give the medication.
    d. Hold her medication and notify her physician.

SUGGESTED ACTIVITIES

- Spend a few hours in a cardiac catheterization laboratory observing the procedure.

- Spend a day in a cardiology clinic. Interview children with congenital heart defects and their parents about what it is like to live with a heart disease.

- Attend a support group meeting for parents of children with congenital heart defects.

- Spend a day in the echocardiogram laboratory to observe diagnostic testing for heart disease.

- Visit the local offices of the American Heart Association and the March of Dimes to learn their purpose in relation to congenital heart disease. Assess parent teaching materials available from each organization.

BIBLIOGRAPHY

Adams, F., G. Emmanouilides, and T. Riemenschneider. *Moss' Heart Disease in Infants, Children, and Adolescents*, 4th ed. Baltimore: Williams and Wilkins, 1989.

Agamalian, B. Pediatric cardiac catheterization. *Journal of Pediatric Nursing* 1 (1986): 73–79.

Bowlen, J. Helping children and their families cope with congenital heart disease. *Critical Care Quarterly* 8 (1985): 65–74.

Broadwell Jackson, D., and R. B. Saunders. *Child Health Nursing*. Philadelphia: J. B. Lippincott, 1993.

Callow, L. A new beginning: Nursing care of the infant undergoing the arterial switch operation for transposition of the great arteries. *Heart & Lung* 18 (1989): 248–257.

Daberkow, E., and R. Washington. Cardiovascular diseases and surgical intervention. Pp. 427–465 in G. Merenstein and S. Gardner, eds. *Handbook of Neonatal Intensive Care*, 2nd ed. St Louis, MO: C. V. Mosby, 1989.

Foster, R. L. R., M. M. Hunsberger, and J. J. T. Anderson. *Family-Centered Nursing Care of Children*. Philadelphia: W. B. Saunders, 1989.

Garson, A., J. Bricker, and D. McNamara. *The Science and Practice of Pediatric Cardiology*, vol. 2, pp. 671–690. Philadelphia: Lea and Febiger, 1990.

Guyton, A. *Human Physiology and Mechanisms of Disease*, 5th ed. Philadelphia: W. B. Saunders, 1992.

Hagedorn, M., and S. Gardner. Physiologic sequelae of prematurity: The nurse practitioner's role. Part III. Congestive heart failure. *Journal of Pediatric Health Care* 4 (1990): 229–236.

Hazinski, M. *Nursing Care of the Critically Ill Child*, 2nd ed. St. Louis, MO: Mosby-Year Book, 1992.

Kashani, I., and S. Higgins. Counseling strategies for families of children with heart disease. *Pediatric Nursing* 12 (1986): 38–40.

Liebman, J., and M. Freed. Cardiovascular system. Pp. 445–491 in R. Behrman and R. Kliegman, eds. *Nelson's Essentials of Pediatrics*. Philadelphia: W. B. Saunders, 1990.

Moore, K. *The Developing Human: Clinically Oriented Embryology*, 4th ed. Philadelphia: W. B. Saunders, 1988.

Page, G. Tetralogy of Fallot. *Heart & Lung* 15 (1986): 390–399.

Wong, D. *Whaley & Wong's Essentials of Pediatric Nursing*, 4th ed. St. Louis, MO: Mosby-Year Book, 1993.

Respiratory Conditions

OBJECTIVES

AFTER STUDYING THIS CHAPTER, THE STUDENT SHOULD BE ABLE TO:

- NAME THREE RESPIRATORY CONDITIONS THAT AFFECT INFANTS AND DISCUSS THEIR CAUSES, SYMPTOMS, TREATMENT, AND NURSING CARE.

- NAME THREE RESPIRATORY CONDITIONS THAT AFFECT TODDLERS AND DESCRIBE THEIR CAUSES, SYMPTOMS, TREATMENT, AND NURSING CARE.

- IDENTIFY THE AGE GROUP MOST AT RISK FOR FOREIGN BODY ASPIRATION AND DESCRIBE APPROPRIATE NURSING ACTION FOR THIS EMERGENCY.

- DISCUSS THE CAUSES, SYMPTOMS, TREATMENT, AND NURSING CARE OF ASTHMA

- NAME SEVERAL OTHER RESPIRATORY CONDITIONS THAT AFFECT PRESCHOOL AND SCHOOL-AGE CHILDREN AND DISCUSS THEIR CAUSES, SYMPTOMS, TREATMENT, AND NURSING CARE.

Key Terms

RETRACTIONS

STEATORRHEA

INTUSSUSCEPTION

SWEAT TEST

LARYNGOSPASM

ALLERGIC SHINER

NASAL SALUTE

TRIGGER

spiratory illnesses are common throughout early childhood. In most children, these illnesses produce mild symptoms that can be managed at home. In chronic conditions, such as asthma, teaching the parents and child about the disease and its management is an important part of nursing care. Serious respiratory illnesses are potentially life-threatening and require skilled medical treatment and nursing care.

Overview of the System

The process of oxygenation and gas exchange is accomplished by the coordinated efforts of the neurological, cardiovascular, and respiratory systems. The respiratory system includes upper airway and lower airway structures, Figure 23–1.

The upper airway consists of the mouth, nose, pharynx, epiglottis, larynx, and trachea. Inspired air is normally warmed, moistened, and filtered before it enters the trachea and descends into the lower airway. Nasal cilia and mucus are the first line of defense against large, inhaled particles such as dust, pollen, and water. The palatine tonsils and adenoids fight harmful organisms by trapping and destroying them.

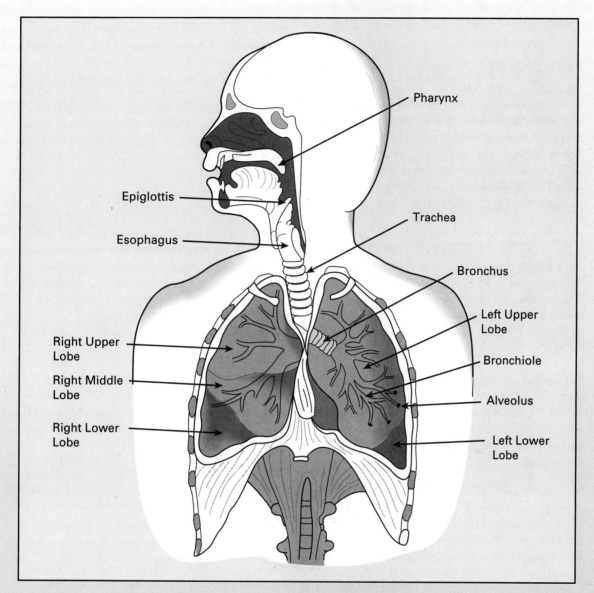

Pharynx

Epiglottis

Esophagus

Trachea

Bronchus

Left Upper Lobe

Bronchiole

Right Upper Lobe

Right Middle Lobe

Right Lower Lobe

Alveolus

Left Lower Lobe

Figure 23–1   *The respiratory system*

The lower airway consists of the two mainstem bronchi, one each on the right and left side, that further branch into bronchioles and alveoli throughout both lungs (DeJong and McCandless 1983).

INFANT

BRONCHIOLITIS

Description.   Bronchiolitis occurs when an infecting agent causes inflammation and obstruction of the bronchioles. It is a frequent cause of hospitalization of infants and children under 2 years of age. The respiratory syncytial virus (RSV) is the most common cause. RSV is transmitted through direct or close contact with respiratory secretions of infected individuals.

Symptoms.   The child has a history of rhinitis, a cough, and a low-grade fever for a few days before developing more frequent coughing, rales, wheezing, and labored breathing. Respirations are rapid, shallow, and accompanied by nasal flaring and **retractions** (a visible drawing in of the soft tissues of the chest), signs of severe distress.

Treatment.   Treatment includes oxygen, fluid therapy, airway support, and rest. Medications may be given by aerosol to open up the airways. Most children are managed at home unless underlying cardiac or pulmonary conditions exist.

Nursing Care.   If the child is hospitalized, nursing care consists of observation, administration of oxygen, hydration, and supportive airway measures. Observe the child frequently and watch for any worsening of respiratory symptoms. Grouping nursing tasks decreases stress and promotes rest.

Explain procedures to parents to help reduce their anxiety. Watching a child who is in respiratory difficulty is frightening for parents, and they need emotional support and reassurance that their child will get better.

Oxygen is administered using a mist tent, nasal cannula, or face mask (see Chapter 14). Holding the infant upright or elevating the head of the bed helps the child to breathe more easily and helps to drain mucus from the upper airways. Pulmonary hygiene and nebulized medications are usually administered by a respiratory therapist. The infant's nasal passages can be kept clear and open by using a bulb syringe (see Chapter 14). Acetaminophen may be given to control temperature. Adequate fluid intake is important to maintain fluid balance.

PNEUMONIA

Pneumonia is an inflammation of the lungs that occurs most often in infants and young children. It can involve a lobe of the lung or be spread throughout the lung and may be bacterial or viral in origin. Differentiating between viral and bacterial forms of pneumonia is important in order to establish an appropriate treatment plan.

Symptoms can include elevated temperature, cough, dyspnea, tachypnea, decreased breath sounds, pain on inspiration, and malaise.

Treatment is supportive and includes antibiotics, administration of oxygen if indicated, pulmonary care, hydration, and medication for pain (acetaminophen). The *Hemophilus influenzae* b (Hib) conjugate vaccine is recommended beginning at age 2 months as a preventive measure against *H. influenzae* pneumonia (Chapter 9). Nursing care is supportive and similar to that for the child with bronchiolitis.

CYSTIC FIBROSIS

Description.   Cystic fibrosis is inherited as an autosomal recessive disorder. It is primarily a disorder of the exocrine glands that affects many body systems. In 1989, chromosome 7 was identified as the cystic fibrosis gene (Collins 1992), making genetic counseling and prenatal diagnosis possible. The disorder occurs most often in Caucasian children.

Symptoms. Symptoms include a chronic cough and frequent respiratory infections.

Coughing occurs in an attempt to clear the lungs of thick, sticky mucus, which provides an environment conducive to bacterial growth, accounting for frequent respiratory infections.

Infants often present with meconium ileus. **Steatorrhea** (fatty stools) is a characteristic finding because blocked pancreatic ducts do not secrete the enzymes necessary to digest fats and proteins. Because essential nutrients are excreted in the stool, children with cystic fibrosis have difficulty maintaining and gaining weight. They may develop **intussusception** (telescoping of the bowel) or a prolapsed rectum because the large, bulky stools are difficult to pass.

Delayed bone growth, short stature, and a delayed onset of puberty are common. Metabolic function is altered as a result of imbalances created by excessive electrolytes lost in perspiration, saliva, and mucus.

Sterility in males is common because of blockage in or absence of the vas deferens. In females, increased mucus secretions block the passage of sperm, making conception difficult (George 1990, Landon and Rosenfeld 1984).

Treatment. Diagnosis is based on two positive sweat tests. The **sweat test** analyzes the sodium and chloride content of the child's sweat. Values greater than 60 mEq/L are diagnostic of cystic fibrosis. The goals of treatment are to maintain adequate respiratory function, prevent infection, and encourage exercise and good nutrition. Dornase alfa (recombinant DNase) may be administered to loosen secretions in an effort to decrease the incidence of respiratory tract infections. With improved treatment, children with cystic fibrosis now survive into adulthood. Overwhelming infection and multisystem changes, however, ultimately result in respiratory failure and death.

Nursing Care. Chest physiotherapy, consisting of postural drainage and chest percussion, is usually performed one to four times per day before eating and before bed to help drain mucus from the lungs, Figure 23–2. Aerosolized medications are frequently used before postural drainage to help loosen secretions.

Digestive problems resulting from malabsorption can be treated with pancreatic enzyme supplements and dietary modification. Pancreatic enzymes are taken orally with all meals and snacks, and they can be mixed in applesauce or strained fruits for young children. Enzyme replacement is important to reduce bulky stools and to promote adequate weight gain and absorption of nutrients. Water-soluble multivitamins and fat-soluble vitamins A, D, E, and K are recommended to prevent vitamin deficiency.

Children with cystic fibrosis lose a lot of salt in their sweat. Encourage parents to add extra salt to food and to offer salty snacks. Salt tablets should be taken only if prescribed by a physician.

The nurse can help parents understand and deal with issues related to body image, digestive problems, and the need for frequent hospitalizations. Encourage genetic counseling.

If it seems appropriate, the nurse should refer the family to social and other support services to assist them in dealing with the financial burdens from frequent hospitalizations, the purchase of medications and supplies, and the cost of medical follow-up. The Cystic Fibrosis Foundation, 6931 Arlington Rd., Suite 200, Bethesda, MD 20814, 800-FIGHTCF, is a source for information about cystic fibrosis.

Figure 23–3 summarizes nursing care for the child with cystic fibrosis.

TODDLER

BRONCHITIS

Bronchitis is an inflammation of the bronchi that usually occurs during a respiratory illness.

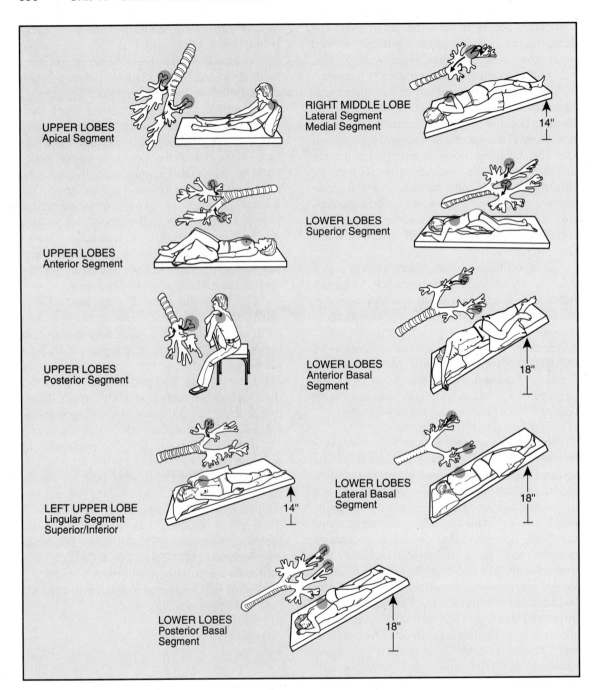

Figure 23–2   Postural drainage (From Datalizer Slide Charts, Addison, IL)

Bronchitis is caused most often by a virus, but it also can result from invasion of bacteria or in response to an allergen or irritant.

Symptoms include a coarse, hacking cough, which increases in severity at night, rhonchi, and wheezing. The child may complain of chest and rib pain because of the deep and frequent coughing.

Treatment consists of rest, humidification, and hydration to provide relief from coughing. Expectorants and cough suppressants are occasionally prescribed. Nursing care is primarily supportive.

CROUP

Description. *Croup* is a term used to describe acute inflammatory diseases such as laryngitis, bacterial tracheitis, and laryngotracheobronchitis (LTB) that result from swelling of the epiglottis, larynx, trachea, and bronchi. Acute viral LTB usually results from infection with one of the parainfluenza viruses that appear in the fall and early winter.

Symptoms. Croup usually has an acute onset after an upper respiratory infection. The child has inspiratory stridor (a high-pitched sound created by narrowing of the airway), a "barking" cough, a low-grade fever, and hoarseness. **Laryngospasms** (involuntary vibrating contractions of the muscles of the larynx) contribute to both increased hoarseness and stridor. If symptoms are not treated obstruction worsens and the child may develop air hunger, retractions, and respiratory distress.

Treatment. Children are treated at home unless they have expiratory stridor, respiratory difficulty, or dehydration. Treatment is supportive. Cool mist helps to moisturize

irritated airways and decreases mucosal swelling. Nebulized racemic epinephrine is given to relieve airway obstruction by reducing edema (Hathaway et al. 1993).

Nursing Care. Nursing care consists of good observation skills, keeping the child's airway open, encouraging fluids, rest, reducing stress, and providing emotional support. Intubation equipment should be kept at the bedside. Report any change in the child's respiratory status immediately. Encourage parents to help keep the child calm and quiet by holding the child on their lap or even sitting in the mist tent with the child. The parents and child are usually fearful, anxious, and apprehensive because of the child's respiratory difficulty. Reassure parents that the child will get better.

EPIGLOTTITIS

Description. Epiglottitis, an inflammation of the epiglottis, is most often caused by bacterial invasion of the soft tissue of the larynx by *Haemophilus influenzae* b. Diagnosis is usually made by lateral neck x-ray, which shows a narrowed airway and enlarged, rounded epiglottis. Epiglottitis requires immediate intervention to prevent possible respiratory arrest.

Symptoms. Symptoms include fever, sore throat, hoarseness or a muffled voice, difficulty swallowing, and inspiratory stridor. Throat pain, swelling, and difficulty swallowing cause the child to drool. The child typically sits up and leans forward to breathe. Epiglottitis can rapidly progress to a life-threatening condition. Edema can occur within minutes, obstructing the airway by blocking the trachea. A child who was noisily breathing will suddenly become wide-eyed, still, and

NURSING CARE PLAN: Cystic Fibrosis

NURSING DIAGNOSIS	GOAL(S)
Shortness of breath, thick respiratory secretions, chronic, productive cough	The child's respiratory status will improve and stabilize.
Inability to gain or retain weight	The child will maintain current body weight while hospitalized.
Foul, frequent, fatty stools	Stools will show firmer consistency and will decrease in frequency.

Figure 23–3

silent. A quiet child is the sign of a potentially dangerous situation.

Treatment. The goal of treatment is to maintain a patent airway. The airway is most often kept open by inserting an endotracheal tube, preferably in the operating room.

Nursing Care. Children are usually admitted to the intensive care unit when an endotracheal tube is in place. Intravenous antibiotics are given, and the child is placed in a mist tent. Suctioning may be necessary. Nursing care consists of keeping the child's airway open, maintaining adequate hydration, keeping the child in

NURSING INTERVENTION	RATIONALE
Assess respiratory status and vital signs as ordered.	Determines respiratory baseline.
Provide oxygen, nebulizer treatments, and pulmonary hygiene (postural drainage and chest percussion).	Pulmonary therapies thin and mobilize respiratory secretions.
Observe and support child during severe coughing episodes. Encourage rest.	During coughing spells, emotional support and respiratory assessment are essential.
Provide mouth care.	Mouth care removes foul taste.
Encourage appropriate handwashing and disposal of tissues.	Personal hygiene habits often need reinforcement.
Monitor daily weight using same scale at same time of day.	Establishes a baseline, enabling weight trends to be followed.
Administer pulmonary care before meals and evening snack.	Pulmonary care before meals improves respiratory effort and appetite.
Administer prescribed enzymes with all meals and snacks. Keep a record of quality and quantity of stools.	Appropriate enzyme therapy promotes firmer stools and reduced frequency.

Figure 23–3   *continued*

a quiet environment, and eliminating stress. The nurse needs to provide emotional support to the child and parents. Keeping parents informed of the child's condition helps to reduce their stress and fear. Reassure parents that prompt intervention usually results in rapid resolution of symptoms (Hathaway et al. 1993). Admin- istration of the Hib (*Haemophilus influenzae* b) vaccine reduces the incidence of epiglottitis.

FOREIGN BODY ASPIRATION

Infants and young children often explore objects by putting them in their mouths. For

NURSING DIAGNOSIS	GOAL(S)
Low self-esteem and feelings of powerlessness related to body changes and prolonged hospital stay	The child will have increased self-esteem and demonstrate independence through participation in own care before discharge.

Figure 23–3 *continued*

this reason, children between the ages of 6 months and 4 years are most at risk for aspiration of a foreign body. The child may have symptoms such as coughing, choking, gagging, and wheezing.

How severe the obstruction is depends on the size and consistency of the object and where it lodges in the respiratory tract. Common causes of airway obstruction include foods such as nuts, popcorn, hot dogs, and raw vegetables; small toy parts or objects such as beads, safety pins, coins, and buttons; and latex balloon pieces.

Foreign bodies lodged above the trachea usually can be coughed out easily. If the child is unable to cough out the object, chest and back thrusts or the Heimlich maneuver can be used (see Chapter 10). Objects that lodge in the trachea can be life-threatening.

Radiopaque objects can be seen on x-ray. Fluoroscopy and fiberoptic bronchoscopy are sometimes used to help with the location, identification, and removal of the foreign body.

The nurse needs to report any change in the child's respiratory status immediately. Parents need emotional support and understanding until the child is out of danger. Teach the parents and family how to child-proof their home. Recommend that parents learn cardiopulmonary resuscitation (CPR) and the Heimlich maneuver (see Chapter 10) for a child.

PRESCHOOL AND SCHOOL-AGE CHILD

EPISTAXIS (NOSEBLEED)

Epistaxis, or nosebleed, is common in childhood and occurs frequently in school-age children. The most common source of bleeding is from Kiesselbach's plexus, an area of plentiful veins located in the anterior nares. The most common causes of nosebleed are nosepicking, foreign bodies, trauma, and dryness.

NURSING INTERVENTION	RATIONALE
Encourage child to be involved in (and responsible for, if appropriate) own treatment plan. Offer choices for nutritious meals and allow preadolescent and adolescent to take enzymes on his or her own.	Preadolescents and adolescents need to have some control and independence related to activities of daily living. Choices improve feelings of self-worth.
Encourage child to dress in own clothes and continue school work. Encourage interaction with other children of same age and provide a means for child to contact peers. Obtain pass permission for out-of-hospital breaks (long hospital stay).	Age-related social needs should be recognized and promoted during hospitalization.
Encourage child to verbalize concerns about future.	Providing emotional support and active listening show concern.

Figure 23–3   *continued*

Children are frequently brought to the emergency room or clinic by a parent who has been unable to stop the nosebleed. The child and parent may be apprehensive and scared. The nurse should have the child sit upright with the head tilted forward to keep blood from dripping down the back of the throat.

A cotton ball or swab soaked with Neo-Synephrine, epinephrine, thrombin, or lidocaine may be inserted into the affected nostril to promote vasoconstriction if the bleeding does not stop. Sometimes the nostril has to be cauterized with silver nitrate after the bleeding has stopped.

The child is admitted to the hospital if the bleeding cannot be controlled. One or both nostrils are packed with petroleum jelly gauze, which usually remains in place between one and seven days. Hematocrit or hemoglobin is assessed if the bleeding has been significant. Blood pressure should be monitored.

Instruct parents that the child should avoid strenuous exercise, bending over and stooping for long periods of time, hot drinks, and hot baths or showers for the next three to four days. Elevate the child's head on pillows. The child who experiences frequent nosebleeds should be evaluated for underlying causes. A lack of household humidity should be addressed as a possible contributing factor.

ACUTE NASOPHARYNGITIS

Nasopharyngitis, better known as the "common cold," is caused most often by one of the rhinoviruses or coronaviruses but may also be caused by group A beta-streptococcus.

Symptoms include a red nasal mucosa and clear nasal discharge. The child may also have an infected throat with enlarged tonsils. Vesicles may be seen on the soft palate and in the pharynx. Symptoms can last up to 10 days or longer.

Treatment is supportive. Infants can be

treated with normal saline nose drops given every three to four hours, followed by suctioning with a bulb syringe (see Chapter 14). Suctioning is especially helpful before feeding. Normal saline nose drops, decongestants, or nasal sprays can be used for older children. Antihistamines may be helpful for children with profuse nasal drainage.

Instruct parents to use a cool mist vaporizer to help thin mucus secretions and decrease airway swelling. Give acetaminophen to reduce fever. Offer fluids to maintain hydration. Fluid intake can be encouraged by providing favorite noncitrus drinks, frozen pops, and ice chips.

STREPTOCOCCAL PHARYNGITIS (STREP THROAT)

Description. A "strep throat" is the result of an infection caused by group A beta-streptococcus. It affects the pharynx and tonsils and is seen most commonly in children 4 to 7 years of age.

Symptoms. Symptoms include a red throat, pain on swallowing, pharyngeal exudate, lymphadenopathy, and fever. A child who has difficulty swallowing, drools, or appears to be having respiratory distress should be seen by a physician immediately.

Treatment. Diagnosis is made by a positive throat culture. Children who are symptomatic are usually treated before the culture results are received. They are given oral penicillin for 10 days or an injection of long-acting penicillin G benzathine (Bicillin). Children who are allergic to penicillin are treated with erythromycin. Children should be treated within seven days of a positive throat culture. A follow-up throat culture after the medication therapy is complete is recommended to ensure that the strep bacteria have been eliminated completely. If a strep throat is not treated or the full course of antibiotics is not taken, complications

such as rheumatic fever, rheumatic arthritis, or acute glomerulonephritis can occur.

Nursing Care. Children are usually treated on an out-patient basis. Symptoms should begin to subside about 24 hours after the start of penicillin therapy. Emphasize to parents that the full course of antibiotic therapy should be completed as instructed. Acetaminophen reduces fever and helps relieve throat pain. Warm saline gargles may be indicated. Ice chips, frozen pops, and favorite beverages should be given frequently and in small amounts. Preventing dehydration is important. In children with repeated episodes of strep throat, removal of tonsils and adenoids is frequently recommended.

TONSILLITIS AND ADENOIDITIS

Description. Tonsillitis refers to chronic infection and enlargement of the palatine tonsils. Adenoiditis is a viral or bacterial infection causing enlargement of the pharyngeal tonsils.

Symptoms. Frequent throat infections, persistent redness of the anterior pillars, and enlargement of the cervical lymph nodes are common symptoms. The inflamed adenoids are associated with snoring and disrupted sleep patterns. Many children have associated ear infections and related hearing loss.

Treatment. Treatment for tonsillitis is the same as for pharyngitis. Children who have chronic tonsillitis are candidates for tonsillectomy. If the adenoids are enlarged, they may be removed at the same time. Both tonsillectomy and adenoidectomy continue to be controversial procedures and the end results need to be carefully evaluated against the potential for complications (Hathaway et al. 1993).

Nursing Care. The nursing care of children with tonsillitis is similar to that for children with pharyngitis (see preceding page). A soft or liquid diet eases swallowing. If surgery is indicated, prepare the child and parents through pre- and postoperative teaching (see Chapter 15). The greatest postoperative threat, after removal of the tonsils or adenoids, is bleeding. Good observation skills are essential during the first 24 hours after surgery. Watch for hemorrhage at the back of the throat. Oral fluids keep the pharynx moist and provide necessary hydration. Warn parents that 7 to 10 days after surgery, the suture scabs will loosen and that any bleeding from the nose or mouth at this time should be reported to the physician for prompt evaluation.

ALLERGIC RHINITIS

The most common cause of chronic nasal congestion in children is allergic rhinitis. Symptoms include sneezing, nasal congestion, watery discharge, mouth breathing, **allergic "shiners"** (dark circles under the eyes or discoloration more than normal), and a **nasal salute** (wiping the nose with the heel of the hand).

Treatment consists of minimizing or avoiding exposure to allergens; administering antihistamines, oral decongestants, or topical agents (cromolyn, steroids); and immunotherapy to identify and desensitize the child to known allergens.

ASTHMA

Description.   Asthma is a reactive airway disease that occurs in infants, children, and adolescents. It is a chronic condition with acute exacerbations. The stimulus (**trigger**) that precedes an asthmatic episode can be a substance or condition. Asthmatic triggers include exercise, infection, allergens, food additives, irritants, weather, and emotions.

During an asthma attack, increased mucus production, airway swelling, and mucus plugging of small airways occur in response to a trigger. Repeated episodes of muscle spasms, mucosal edema, and mucus plugging can cause the airway to become chronically scarred and irritated, resulting in air trapping.

Symptoms.   The child experiencing an asthma attack has rapid and labored respirations. Nasal flaring, retractions, audible expiratory wheezing, and a hacking or productive cough may be present. Because airways are narrowed and partially blocked, a state of hypoxia exists. The child may appear tired and anxious because of difficulty breathing.

Treatment.   The diagnosis of asthma is confirmed through pulmonary function studies such as spirometry and peak flow rates. A spirometer is used to measure the volume of air the lungs can move in and out. The use of a peak expiratory flow rate (PEFR) meter can assist in the management of asthma by helping to identify when obstruction occurs. This device measures the child's ability to forcefully push air out of the lungs. Skin testing may be done to identify allergens that act as asthma triggers. Other triggers also need to be identified, if possible.

The overall goal of treatment is to help the child achieve near-normal respiratory function while continuing normal growth and development. Pharmacological and supportive therapies are used to reverse the airway obstruction and promote respiratory function.

Nursing Care.   If the child is having difficulty breathing, oxygen may be required. Humidified oxygen can be given by nasal cannula or face mask. Having the child sit in a semi-Fowler's or upright position helps ease breathing.

Bronchodilators are often given by aerosol because they are absorbed quickly and response time is relatively short. Intravenous medications are also given. Drug levels should be monitored frequently. Keep the child in a quiet room and group tasks to avoid

NURSING CARE PLAN: Asthma

NURSING DIAGNOSIS	GOAL(S)
Rapid breathing, wheezing, retractions, and a cough	The child's respiratory status will improve and stabilize.
Dehydration	The child will be adequately hydrated before discharge.
Anxiety (parent) related to lack of knowledge about asthma management at home	Parents will be able to explain and provide asthma care before discharge.

Figure 23–4

NURSING INTERVENTION	RATIONALE
Assess respiratory status and vital signs as ordered and as necessary.	Determines respiratory baseline.
Provide humidified oxygen and elevate head of bed.	Oxygen and positioning improve oxygenation and ease breathing.
Provide aerosol treatment as ordered.	Promotes bronchodilation to ease breathing.
Encourage parents to stay with child and provide quiet, calm environment for rest and sleep.	Parents' presence usually reassures child and decreases anxiety in the unfamiliar hospital setting.
Provide reassurance and support.	Anxiety may increase symptoms.
Assess IV site and maintain IV fluid infusion.	Initially, the intravenous route will replenish fluids and allow the child to rest.
Check urine specific gravity and carefully monitor intake and output.	Hydration is evaluated by quality and quantity of urine output and vital sign stability.
Encourage fluids when child is able to take oral fluids.	Fluids provide hydration and thin secretions. Ability to tolerate fluids signals improvement.
Explain cause and symptoms of asthma.	Increased knowledge decreases anxiety.
Give parents written information about asthma and its treatment. Identify possible side effects of treatment.	Written information can be referred to later.
Refer parents to asthma support group and American Lung Association for further information.	Provides support and comfort.

Figure 23–4 *continued*

repeatedly disturbing the child. Monitor the child for any drug reaction.

Adequate hydration is essential to help thin mucus plugs trapped in the narrowed airways. Intake, output, and specific gravity should be monitored to evaluate the child's hydration status. Offer the child fruit-flavored juices, flavored ices, and favorite beverages when possible.

Supporting and educating the parents and child help them cope with and understand the disease, medication therapy, and the need for lifestyle changes. Parents need to be taught prevention and treatment of asthma and how to avoid frequent hospitalization. Refer parents to local support groups and to the American Lung Association.

Figure 23–4 (page 344) summarizes nursing care for the child with asthma.

Tuberculosis

Tuberculosis is an infectious disease caused by *Mycobacterium tuberculosis*. Transmission is through infectious particles called droplets. Symptoms include a chronic cough, anorexia, weight loss or failure to gain weight, and fever.

The child, immediate family, and suspected carriers should be skin tested for tuberculosis. Intradermal testing using purified protein derivative (PPD) (the Mantoux test) is considered the most accurate test. Active cases of pulmonary tuberculosis are required by law to be reported to public health agencies.

Treatment consists of antitubercular and corticosteroid medications, adequate nutrition, and rest. Parents need to be told about the importance of complying with drug therapy, since treatment may last 6 to 12 months.

Review Questions

A. Multiple choice. Select the best answer.

1. The structures most responsible for trapping and destroying harmful organisms in the respiratory tract are the
   a. bronchi
   b. tonsils and adenoids
   c. alveoli
   d. cilia

2. The infant with bronchiolitis is most likely to have which of the following clinical findings?
   a. retractions
   b. inspiratory stridor
   c. laryngospasm
   d. thick, tenacious mucus

3. Intussusception is a common finding in children who have
   a. pneumonia
   b. asthma
   c. cystic fibrosis
   d. tuberculosis

4. The treatment of choice for the child with croup to decrease mucosal swelling is
   a. immediate surgery
   b. suctioning of the airway
   c. positioning the child flat on the back
   d. cool humidified air via mist tent

5. A strep throat is a serious infection in children and requires prompt medical therapy because
   a. bleeding can occur without warning
   b. children cannot tolerate the severe throat pain
   c. left untreated, the heart and kidneys may be damaged
   d. the causative organism can cause sterility

6. Danielle, 5 years old, is brought to the emergency department by her parents. She is feverish and has a sore throat, difficulty swallowing, and inspiratory stridor. These are symptoms of
   a. croup
   b. epiglottitis
   c. bronchiolitis
   d. strep throat

7. The nasal salute is a symptom associated with
   a. allergic rhinitis
   b. bronchiolitis
   c. cystic fibrosis
   d. pneumonia

8. Which of the following respiratory conditions is frequently associated with ear infections and related hearing loss?
   a. allergic rhinitis
   b. strep throat
   c. tonsillitis and adenoiditis
   d. pneumonia

9. Pulmonary function studies and peak flow rates are used to diagnose which of the following respiratory conditions?
   a. pneumonia
   b. cystic fibrosis
   c. tuberculosis
   d. asthma

10. Which of the following is true concerning the medication therapy for a child with tuberculosis?
   a. There is no medication for the tuberculosis organism.
   b. The child must be hospitalized until the entire course of medication is completed.
   c. The medications have no side effects.
   d. The medication needs to be given for up to 12 months.

SUGGESTED ACTIVITIES

• Before caring for children with a respiratory disorder, review CPR and Heimlich maneuver procedures (Chapter 10). Ask parents if they know how to perform CPR. Encourage parents to learn CPR, and tell them where they can take classes.

• Contact the Cystic Fibrosis Foundation to obtain information on some aspect of care that interests you. Ask for professional and lay resources and compare the contents of all the booklets you obtain.

• Interview a child with asthma and his or her parents. Identify and compare the concerns that each one has about living with asthma. Which concerns are similar? Which ones are different? Can you make recommendations for alleviating any concerns they have?

Bibliography

Collins, F. S. Cystic fibrosis: Molecular biology and therapeutic implications. *Science* 256 (1992): 774–779.

DeJong, S., and S. McCandless. The respiratory system. Pp. 21–87 in J. B. Smith, ed. *Pediatric Critical Care.* New York: Wiley and Sons, 1983.

George, M. R. CF: Not just a pediatric problem anymore. *RN* 9 (1990): 60–65.

Hathaway, W. E., W. W. Way, Jr., J. R. Groothuis, and J. W. Paisley. *Current Pediatric Diagnosis and Treatment,* 11th ed. Norwalk, CT: Appleton and Lange, 1993.

Landon, C., and R. G. Rosenfeld. Short stature and pubertal delay in male adolescents with cystic fibrosis. *American Journal of Diseases in Children* 138, no. 4 (1984): 388–391.

National Asthma Education Program, Expert Panel Report. *Guidelines for the Diagnosis and Management of Asthma.* Bethesda, MD: U.S. Department of Health and Human Services, 1991.

Rosenstein, B. J, and P. D. Fosarelli. *Pediatric Pearls: The Handbook of Practical Pediatrics.* Chicaco: Year Book Medical Publishers, 1989.

Digestive and Metabolic Conditions

OBJECTIVES

AFTER STUDYING THIS CHAPTER, THE STUDENT SHOULD BE ABLE TO:

- NAME A COMMON ORAL INFECTION OF INFANCY AND DISCUSS ITS SYMPTOMS, TREATMENT, AND NURSING CARE.

- RECOGNIZE SYMPTOMS OF COLIC AND DISCUSS TREATMENT AND NURSING CARE OF THIS CONDITION.

- IDENTIFY COMMON CAUSES OF DIARRHEA IN INFANTS AND CHILDREN AND DISCUSS TREATMENT AND NURSING CARE OF THIS CONDITION.

- IDENTIFY THREE TYPES OF DEHYDRATION AND DISCUSS SYMPTOMS, TREATMENT, AND NURSING CARE OF THIS CONDITION.

- COMPARE AND CONTRAST THE SYMPTOMS, TREATMENT, AND NURSING CARE OF GASTROESOPHAGEAL REFLUX AND PYLORIC STENOSIS.

- DIFFERENTIATE BETWEEN TWO CONDITIONS CAUSING BOWEL OBSTRUCTION IN INFANTS AND CHILDREN.

- IDENTIFY THE TWO MOST COMMON TYPES OF HERNIAS IN INFANTS AND DISCUSS THEIR TREATMENT AND NURSING CARE.

- IDENTIFY TWO COMMON INTESTINAL PARASITES IN TODDLERS AND PRESCHOOL CHILDREN AND DISCUSS TREATMENT OF THESE DISEASES.

- IDENTIFY FACTORS THAT PLACE CHILDREN AT RISK FOR FOREIGN BODY INGESTION AND DISCUSS TREATMENT OF A CHILD WHO HAS INGESTED A FOREIGN BODY.

- DISCUSS THE SYMPTOMS, TREATMENT, AND NURSING CARE OF LEAD POISONING.

- NAME TWO CONDITIONS THAT AFFECT SCHOOL-AGE CHILDREN AND ADOLESCENTS, AND DISCUSS THEIR CAUSES, SYMPTOMS, TREATMENT, AND NURSING CARE.

KEY TERMS

FECALITH	POLYPHAGIA
POLYURIA	KETONURIA
POLYDIPSIA	KETOACIDOSIS

digestive and metabolic conditions involve alterations in functioning of the gastrointestinal and endocrine systems. These conditions have the potential to interfere with nutritional intake and fluid balance, resulting in symptoms ranging from electrolyte imbalances to impaired growth and even death. It is important for the nurse to be able to identify and recognize the presenting symptoms of these conditions in order to facilitate early intervention and prevent potentially life-threatening complications.

OVERVIEW OF THE SYSTEM

The gastrointestinal (GI) system consists of the structures of the oral cavity, pharynx, esophagus, stomach, small intestine, large intestine, liver, and gallbladder, Figure 24–1. The GI system enables the body to ingest, digest, and metabolize nutrients.

The endocrine system consists of glands and organs that secrete hormones that act on cells in other parts of the body. The pancreas functions to

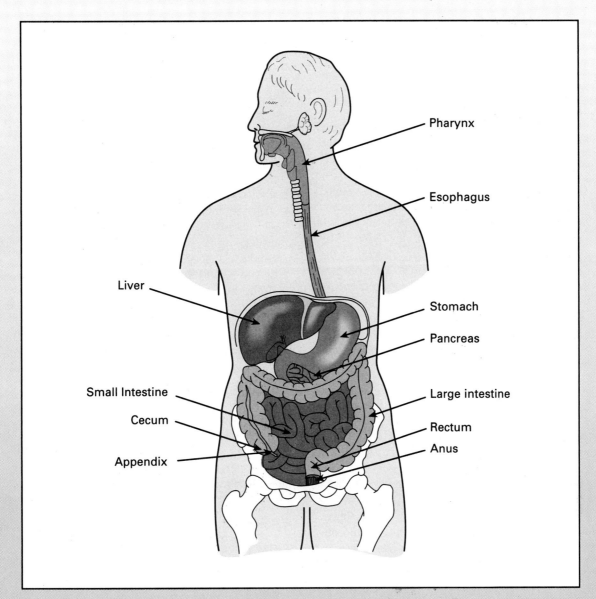

Figure 24–1 *The gastrointestinal system*

regulate blood glucose and meet the digestive needs of the body. The pancreatic hormones glucagon and insulin, produced in the beta cells of the islets of Langerhans, play an important role in glucose metabolism. When disease, infection, or trauma interferes with the functioning of the pancreas, both glucose metabolism and digestion can be impaired. This is the case in diabetes mellitus, discussed later in this chapter.

INFANT AND TODDLER

ORAL CANDIDIASIS

Oral candidiasis (thrush, moniliasis) is an infection of the oral cavity caused by the fungus *Candida albicans*. It appears on the tongue, palate, buccal mucosa, and gingiva as thick, cheesy white patches on an erythematous base. Oral candidiasis frequently occurs in infants who have a concurrent monilial diaper rash.

The child is treated with nystatin (Mycostatin) suspension for 7 to 10 days. Teach the parent to apply the suspension directly to the child's mouth with a cotton-tipped applicator or a finger after feedings. Nursing mothers are often instruc-ted to apply nystatin cream directly to the areola and nipple area and to wash the area before and after each feeding. Pacifiers, baby bottles, and nipples should be sterilized.

COLIC

Colic is a term used to describe certain behaviors of newborns — specifically, excessive crying and fussiness — sometimes associated with increased amounts of gas. Although crying and fussiness are normal, infants with colic have excessive, unexplained crying and fussiness. Brazelton (1962) conducted a study that concluded that newborns normally cry approximately two hours per day, increasing to three hours per day by 6 weeks of age. By the time the infant reaches 3 months of age, crying decreases to one hour per day. Crying usually occurs in the evening. Infants whose crying exceeds these parameters are said to have colic.

Colic usually begins during the first week after birth and diminishes by 3 to 4 months of age. Parents report that there is no apparent reason for the crying; the infant is not wet, has been fed, and is having no obvious distress. Colicky infants cannot be consoled and often have excessive gas, which causes them to draw their legs up to their chest. Despite many studies and much speculation, the true cause of colic is unknown and there is no definitive "cure."

The nurse can play an important role in teaching parents about the normal growth and development of infants and how to manage and cope with a colicky baby. Parents need understanding, emotional support, and constant reassurance that the colic will eventually resolve. Working with the parents, the nurse can suggest different techniques to reduce the infant's crying and fussiness, Figure 24–2.

Emphasize that colic is not a result of something that parents did wrong. Encourage them to take turns caring for the infant and to take "time out" away from the infant.

DIARRHEA

Description. Diarrhea is a gradual or sudden increase in the frequency and water content of

---

CALMING A COLICKY BABY

- Decrease stimulation
- Swaddle infant and place in a darkened room
- Rock, walk, or place infant in a swing
- Offer infant a pacifier
- Play soft music
- Hold infant close
- Take infant for a ride in a car

Figure 24–2

stools. It is a common occurrence in infants and children. Episodes of diarrhea can be acute, chronic, or recurrent.

Acute diarrhea can have a bacterial, viral, or noninfectious cause. The most common pathogens are *Shigella* (bacillary dysentery), *Salmonella*, and *Escherichia coli* ("traveler's diarrhea"). *Shigella* is frequently found in day-care centers and crowded living conditions. All three bacterial pathogens are transmitted via the fecal-oral route and invade, colonize, and reproduce in the child's intestinal tract (Grimes 1991).

The most common viruses causing diarrhea are rotavirus (also causes fever and vomiting; occurs in the winter and is usually the cause of diarrhea in hospital outbreaks and day-care centers), enterovirus (also causes vomiting and respiratory symptoms), and the Norwalk virus (lasts 24 to 48 hours and can occur in epidemic proportions).

Noninfectious causes of acute diarrhea include acute poisoning (lead and iron) and reactions to antibiotics (ampicillin).

Chronic diarrhea (lasting more than two weeks) can result from infectious and noninfectious conditions. Examples of infectious conditions are amebiasis and giardiasis. Examples of noninfectious conditions are ulcerative colitis, regional enteritis, Hirschsprung's disease, lactase deficiency, and malabsorption. Diarrhea is the most frequent cause of dehydration in infants and children. Its potential to cause a life-threatening medical emergency should not be underestimated (see later discussion).

Symptoms. The infant or child with diarrhea has frequent watery bowel movements with or without mucus or blood. The child may also have symptoms associated with gastroenteritis, such as vomiting, fever, and abdominal pain.

Treatment. Diagnosis is made on the basis of the history, physical examination, and laboratory data. The history helps to identify the duration, frequency, amount, and consistency of the stools as well as characteristics (e.g., pres-

ence of blood or mucus, color [black or pale], greasiness, and odor). A diet history is taken to assess for lactose intolerance as well as allergic reactions to medications (such as antibiotics). Ask parents about any recent travel and whether anyone else in the child's household has diarrhea (Rosenstein and Fosarelli 1989). A stool culture may be performed to identify the causative organism. Electrolytes are evaluated to assess the child's potential for dehydration.

The goals of treatment are to replace and correct any fluid and electrolyte imbalances and to maintain adequate nutrition. Children are usually managed as out patients and are not hospitalized unless they have moderate to severe dehydration. Lactose-containing formulas and milk are usually stopped. Breast-fed infants can continue to nurse. If the infant is not dehydrated and is tolerating oral feedings, a soy formula or an electrolyte solution (Pedialyte, Lytren) may be given. Older children are also given oral glucose and electrolyte solutions. IV fluids and electrolytes may be required. Medication may be indicated if a causative organism is identified.

Nursing Care. Care of the hospitalized child includes recording intake and output, monitoring IV fluids, encouraging oral fluids, weighing child daily, preventing skin breakdown, and providing emotional support. Teach parents how to care for the child after discharge.

The most important aspect of out-patient care is teaching the parents how to care for the child at home. Mothers who are breast feeding should be encouraged to continue and told that the infant may have a slight increase in stooling initially but that eventually the diarrhea will resolve. Teach parents never to dilute electrolyte solutions. Older children should be encouraged to drink fluids such as cola, ginger ale, and fruit-flavored juices or ices. The infant's diet can slowly be advanced from electrolyte solutions to a nonlactose formula (Isomil). Both infants and children can then slowly progress to the so-called BRATS diet (bananas, rice cereal, applesauce, toast, saltines). Encourage parents to call their health care provider if they have any questions about managing the child's condition.

Reinforce to parents the importance of good hygiene, especially thorough handwashing after bowel movements, after changing diapers, and before handling any food.

DEHYDRATION

Description. Dehydration occurs when the body loses excessive amounts of body fluids (especially water). At birth, total body weight is approximately 75% fluid; by adulthood, it is approximately 60% fluid. Thus, any sustained reduction in fluid intake or increase in fluid loss can place a child at risk for dehydration.

Normally, fluid loss occurs through the skin (evaporation), lungs, and urine. The body needs a certain amount of water every day to maintain normal fluid and electrolyte balance, Figure 24–3. This need is based on body weight.

Illness alters the child's metabolic status, increasing fluid requirements. Fever, sweating, vomiting, and diarrhea result in increased fluid losses. In addition, infants and children usually do not take in the same amounts of fluids when they are sick as when they are well.

When dehydration occurs, the child's extracellular volume decreases, causing decreased tissue perfusion and impaired renal function. This can result in acid-base imbalances, and electrolyte alterations such as potassium imbalances.

Fluid loss is expressed as a percentage of total body weight, as follows:

- Mild dehydration: fluid loss is less than 3% to 5% of body weight
- Moderate dehydration: fluid loss is less than 6% to 9% of body weight
- Severe dehydration: fluid loss is more than 10% of body weight

Dehydration is further described as isotonic, hypotonic, or hypertonic, depending on the electrolyte composition of the plasma. In isotonic dehydration, equal amounts of water and sodium are lost, but electrolytes are otherwise normal. In hypotonic dehydration, more electrolytes than water are lost. In hypertonic dehydration, more water than electrolytes is lost.

Symptoms. Symptoms depend on the degree of dehydration. Characteristic findings in mild or moderate dehydration can include lack of tears, dry mucous membranes, decreased skin turgor, pale or mottled color, decreased urinary output. Findings in severe dehydration include tachycardia, low blood pressure, and sunken sunken eyes. An infant should be assessed for a depressed anterior fontanelle.

Treatment. Diagnosis is based on history, physical examination, and laboratory data. Physical examination should include assessment of the infant's or child's weight, compared with previous weight, if possible, as well as vital signs, blood pressure, and intake and output.

The goals of treatment are to replace and restore normal fluid and electrolyte balance, correct any acid-base imbalance, and meet the child's nutritional requirements.

The child is treated with oral rehydration therapy or given intravenous fluids. Many

DAILY FLUID NEEDS	
Body Weight	**Fluid Need**
3–10 kg	100 mL/kg
11–20 kg	50 mL/kg
More than 20 kg	20 mL/kg

Figure 24–3

commercially prepared solutions are available to treat a child with mild or moderate dehydration. It is important that the child be given adequate amounts (concentrations) of water, sodium, chloride, potassium, and glucose to replace losses.

Nursing Care.   The child should be monitored frequently for a change in color, increased pulse, decreased urine output, and decreased or low blood pressure. These findings are signs of problems with perfusion that could lead to a medical emergency.

Teach parents how to recognize the signs and symptoms of dehydration and what to watch for during the rehydration period. Parents should offer the child 1 to 3 teaspoons (5 to 15 mL) of fluids every 10 to 15 minutes and then increase fluids slowly, as tolerated. Ice chips and frozen juice pops can also be offered to the child. Parents should weigh diapers and count the times that the child urinates or has a bowel movement, if indicated. Advise parents to call the health care provider if they have difficulty getting the child to take fluids.

GASTROESOPHAGEAL REFLUX

Gastroesophageal reflux (GER) is a spontaneous, effortless regurgitation that occurs when the lower esophageal sphincter relaxes, allowing gastric contents to flow backward into the esophagus. Although infants normally have some effortless spitting up of gastric contents, GER should be considered when an infant has recurrent regurgitation or vomiting associated with irritability.

Diagnosis is made in infants under 6 months of age by barium swallow (which shows the backflow of barium from the stomach to the esophagus), esophageal pH probe monitoring, and scintigraphy (DaDalt et al. 1989, Hathaway et al. 1993, Swischuk et al. 1988). In pH probe monitoring, a small catheter is inserted into the esophagus through the nose

and left in place for 18 to 24 hours. Measurement of pH indicates the number of reflux episodes. Scintigraphy involves radionuclide scanning to evaluate gastric emptying, gastroesophageal reflux, and lung aspiration.

Treatment focuses on techniques to reduce the reflux of feedings. Cimetadine or liquid antacids are sometimes given to reduce symptoms of colic. Metoclopramide (a smooth-muscle stimulant) given before meals has been found to be beneficial (Shannon 1993). Surgery may be required in the following cases: if the infant continues to have persistent vomiting resulting in failure to thrive after two to three months of treatment; if the infant develops severe esophagitis or esophageal strictures; or if the reflux causes the infant to have apneic spells (Hathaway et al. 1993, Shannon 1993).

Nursing care includes offering the infant small, frequent feedings thickened with rice cereal (2 to 3 teaspoons per ounce of formula). Breast-fed infants should continue nursing. After feeding, the infant should be placed in a prone position with the head elevated to 30 degrees to help reduce regurgitation.

PYLORIC STENOSIS

Description.   Pyloric stenosis is a congenital defect that results in an increase in the size of the circular muscle of the pylorus. This increase causes the pyloric sphincter to narrow at the outlet of the stomach. The resulting obstruction blocks the flow of food into the small intestine, Figure 24–4a.

Symptoms.   Initially, the infant has symptoms of regurgitation progressing to projectile vomiting after feedings, constipation, poor weight gain or weight loss, and dehydration. The infant is hungry and breast feeds well but develops failure to thrive, apathy, and fretfulness.

Treatment.   Diagnosis is made on the basis of the history, physical examination, and

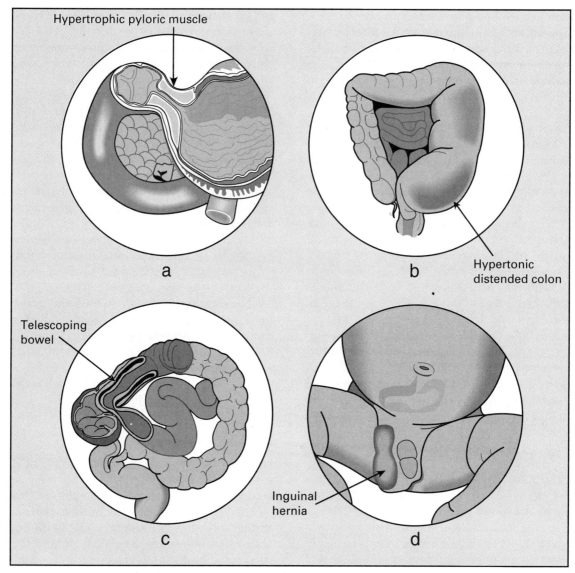

Figure 24–4 *Conditions that cause obstruction of the gastrointestinal tract. (a) Hypertrophic pyloric stenosis. (b) Hirsch-sprung's disease. (c) Intussusception. (d) Strangulated inguinal hernia. (Used with permission of Ross Products Division, Abbott Laboratories, Columbus, OH. From* Clinical Education Aid #4, © *Ross Products Division, Abbott Laboratories)*

radiological studies. Physical examination reveals a palpable olive-sized mass in the right upper quadrant of the abdomen. Gastric peristaltic waves can often be seen on the infant's distended abdomen. An upper GI series usually shows the classic "string sign" (an elongated, narrowed pyloric channel) and delayed gastric emptying. Treatment consists of surgery (pyloromyotomy) to release the constricting muscle fibers. The prognosis with surgical correction is excellent.

Nursing Care. Nursing care includes routine preoperative and postoperative care (Chapter 15).

Monitor the infant's fluid and electrolyte status and record intake and output. Monitor IV infusion rate and observe the infant for vomiting and dehydration. Provide emotional support to the parents and child.

HIRSCHSPRUNG'S DISEASE

Hirschsprung's disease is a condition that occurs when ganglion cells fail to develop in the mucosal and muscular layers of the colon during fetal development. Ganglion cells are needed to transmit peristaltic contractions, which pass stool through the bowel. The absence of peristalsis results in an accumulation of intestinal contents. The internal rectal sphincter is unable to relax and becomes hypertonic, resulting in obstruction, Figure 24–4b. A small segment or the entire colon can be involved, and obstruction can be partial or complete. Hirschsprung's disease may be life threatening.

In a newborn, the first clue is failure to pass meconium. Symptoms of poor feeding, irritability, vomiting, diarrhea, abdominal distention (which makes breathing difficult), and shock may develop if the condition remains undiagnosed. An older child may have symptoms of constipation, thin ribbonlike stools, abdominal distention, and failure to thrive.

Obstruction is usually diagnosed in a newborn within the first 24 to 48 hours after birth. Diagnosis is based on the history, physical examination, x-ray studies, barium enema, and biopsy.

Treatment usually involves performing a temporary colostomy. Generally, when the infant weighs about 20 lbs, the aganglionic sections of bowel are removed and corrective surgery is performed. The temporary colostomy is closed once the distended bowel has returned to normal function.

INTUSSUSCEPTION

Intussusception is the most frequent cause of intestinal obstruction during the first 2 years of life (Hathaway et al. 1993). It occurs when a proximal portion of intestine telescopes into an adjacent distal portion of intestine, Figure 24–4c. The most common site is the distal ileum, which pushes from the cecum into the colon (Rudolph et al. 1991). Swelling, bowel incarceration, vascular flow obstruction, bleeding from the mucosa, and hemorrhage can result. Partial obstruction can lead to complete obstruction, necrosis of the bowel, perforation, peritonitis, and (if untreated) death.

Characteristically, a seemingly normal infant or toddler, 5 to 18 months of age suddenly develops severe abdominal pain (Rudolph et al. 1991). The child screams, drawing up the legs, knees, and hips. Fever and vomiting may also occur. The pain stops and recurs. Initially the child has a normal bowel movement followed two to three days later by gelatinous, bright to dark red, bloody "currant jelly" stool. Examination reveals a tender distended abdomen, and a sausage-shaped mass is felt on palpation.

A barium enema is given, which serves as a contrast hydrostatic reduction and in most cases successfully restores the telescoped bowel to the proper position. If barium enema is unsuccessful, surgery is performed.

HERNIA

A hernia occurs when an organ protrudes through an abnormal opening in the muscle wall of the cavity that normally contains it. The most common types of hernias in children are inguinal and umbilical hernias, Figure 24–4d. The hernia consists of three parts: a sac or outpouching (peritoneum), the covering of the sac (derived from the abdominal wall), and the contents of the sac (bowel, ovary, or testis) (Foster et al. 1989).

Inguinal Hernia. If the processus vaginalis does not close during fetal development, an opening exists into the inguinal canal. Abdominal contents (bowel) can protrude through

COMMON PARASITIC CHILDHOOD DISEASES

Parasite	Symptoms	Treatment
Giardiasis (protozoan) *Causative organism: Giardia lamblia* (the most common parasite causing disease in the United States) *Transmission*: Person to person (especially children in day-care centers), animals (dogs, cats, beavers), food, water (contaminated reservoirs, lakes, streams)	Symptoms are variable, and children can be asymptomatic or develop severe life-threatening diarrhea, dehydration, and malabsorption (Rudolph et al. 1991). Symptoms include abdominal pain; vomiting; watery, foul-smelling diarrhea; anorexia; and fatigue.	Medications used to treat giardiasis are the anti-infective quinacrine hydrochloride (Atabrine) and the antibiotic furazolidone (Furoxone). (Metronidazole [Flagyl] is effective but not licensed in the United States to treat giardiasis.) Teach parents to use good personal hygiene. Wash hands after toileting and after changing an infant's diaper or touching stool. If a child is infected, wear gloves when handling soiled diapers or clothing. If there is any risk of contaminated water, boil water before drinking.

Figure 24–5

this opening, creating a painless inguinal swelling. An inguinal hernia frequently occurs in conjunction with a hydrocele (Chapter 26). Treatment consists of surgical repair to prevent incarceration.

Umbilical Hernia. Incomplete fascial closure of the umbilical ring during fetal development causes a hernial protrusion near the umbilicus. Intestine and omentum protrude through the weak abdominal wall. An umbilical hernia usually looks like a soft swelling or protrusion covered by skin. If closure does not occur by 5 years of age, surgical repair is performed to prevent strangulation of the bowel. Most umbilical hernias close spontaneously by the time a child is 2 to 3 years of age.

There are many "old wives' tales" about how to cure an umbilical hernia in infants. It is important for the nurse to dispel any myths, especially the use of belly bands and the taping of a silver or half dollar over the infant's umbilicus. Both of these measures increase the risk of strangulation of the herniated bowel and infection.

TODDLER AND PRESCHOOL CHILD

INTESTINAL PARASITES

Parasitic diseases are caused by helminths (worms), protozoans, and arthropods. Although it is more common to see these diseases in

COMMON PARASITIC CHILDHOOD DISEASES

Parasite

Pinworms (helminth)

Causative organism:
Enterobius vermicularis

Transmission: Inhaling or
ingesting freshly deposited
eggs. Hand to mouth transmission is common, espe-
cially when children
scratch the infected anal
area and then put their fingers in their mouth or bite
their nails. Frequently seen
in schools and day-care
centers.

Symptoms

The most common symp-
tom is intense perianal and
perineal pruritus (espe-
cially at night). Other
symptoms can include uri-
nary tract infection and
vulvovaginitis. Children
frequently wake at night
crying because of itching.
Tiny white worms can be
seen in the rectal area,
stool, or vagina.

Treatment

Cellophane tape test: The best
way to diagnose pinworms
is to take a tongue blade,
wrap cellophane around it,
and press it against the perianal area. The tape is put
over a drop of toluene on a
glass microscope slide and
examined for pinworms.

Commonly used medica-
tions to treat pinworms are
mebendazole (Vermox),
pyrantel pamoate
(Antiminth), and piperazine
citrate (Antepar). The child
and everyone in the household should be treated at
the same time. Treatment is
usually repeated in 2 to 3
weeks. All bed sheets, bed
clothing, and underwear
should be washed in hot
water, and the house vacu-
umed and damp mopped.

Reassure parents that pinworms are not a result of
uncleanliness.

Figure 24–5 *continued*

tropical and subtropical climates of the world where living conditions are poor, socioeconomic status is low, and diet is inadequate, they can occur anywhere. Children can acquire these diseases from contact with human or animal carriers (Hathaway et al. 1993, Rudolph et al. 1991). The most common parasitic diseases of childhood are giardiasis and pinworm infestation, Figure 24–5.

Children (especially toddlers and preschoolers) are more susceptible to parasitic infestations than are adults because of their poor hygiene, frequent hand to mouth activity, and habit of playing in dirt. Nursing care centers on teaching parents appropriate treatment measures (Figure 24–5) and prevention (e.g., good hygiene practices).

Foreign Body Ingestion

Foreign body ingestion is not uncommon in children (especially toddlers and preschoolers) because they frequently put a variety of objects in their mouths. Objects commonly ingested include coins, toy parts, safety pins, buttons, marbles, and button-type (disc) batteries.

If a child is suspected of having ingested a foreign body, an x-ray should be taken. An object that reaches the child's stomach has a very good chance of passing through the GI tract. Parents should be instructed to watch for the object in the child's stool. An object that does not pass and continues to be seen on x-ray may require endoscopic removal. Surgery is considered if the child develops abdominal pain, obstruction, or perforation.

If a foreign body lodges in the child's esophagus, the child can have symptoms of choking, gagging, drooling, coughing, pain, or respiratory distress. The object is removed by esophagoscopy. Of particular concern are button-type (disc) batteries, which can lodge in the esophagus and leak alkaline, causing necrosis and esophageal perforation. Prompt removal is necessary. Safety precautions should be discussed with parents to prevent future ingestions.

Lead Poisoning

Description. Lead poisoning is a preventable public health problem of children than can lead to psychological problems, mental retardation, and disorders of the neurologic, hematologic, and renal systems. Children are exposed every day to unhealthy levels of lead in the environment (Figure 24–6).

Lead enters the body through inhalation or ingestion. Children who have pica (ingestion of nonfood substances) commonly eat paint chips and are at extremely high risk for lead poisoning. Lead poisoning is most often seen in children under 5 years of age.

Lead is absorbed through the gastrointestinal tract and stored in bone, blood, and soft tissue. The tissues of the erythroid cells of the bone marrow, the nervous system, and the kidneys are most frequently affected. Lead in the body interferes with erythrocyte production and prevents hemoglobin formation, which can lead to anemia. Lead is excreted in the urine and may produce kidney damage.

Symptoms. Symptoms depend on the child's age and blood lead level. A child can be asymptomatic if levels are low. Common symptoms include lethargy, anorexia, vomiting, irritability, abdominal pain, headaches, and decrease in activity level. More severe symptoms include ataxia, clumsiness, encephalopathy, seizures, and mental retardation.

Treatment. Routine screening (fingerstick) of blood lead level is performed on children between 9 months and 6 years of age. The Centers for Disease Control and Prevention (CDC) has developed a classification system for lead poisoning based on the child's blood lead level concentration. This system enables health care providers to identify children with low, moderate, or high risk for lead poisoning and those requiring retesting.

Sources of Lead

- Lead-based paint
- Household dust
- Soil and water (contaminated from lead pipes and solder)
- Air near highways (from burning of leaded gasoline)
- Fruit tree sprays
- Ceramics made with leaded glass
- Folk remedies (e.g., powders that are used to treat fevers)

Figure 24–6

Diagnosis is based on elevated blood lead and free erythrocyte protoporphyrin (FEP) levels. If blood lead levels are elevated after fingerstick, confirmation should be made by venipuncture. X-ray studies of the long bones may be done to identify lead lines. Abdominal x-rays may reveal recently ingested lead.

Treatment focuses initially on identifying and removing lead sources from the child's environment, reducing the amount of lead ingested, providing dietary counseling to improve the child's diet and correct any nutritional imbalances, and encouraging a low-fat high-iron diet, which prevents lead from binding to body tissues. Children with high lead levels require chelation therapy. An agent is administered that binds with the lead to prevent its absorption by the body.

Nursing Care. Nursing care focuses on reinforcing dietary counseling, providing emotional support to parents, teaching parents to prevent further exposure, and providing referrals to social services or community resources for environmental clean-up. Monitor for seizures and renal function.

SCHOOL-AGE CHILD
AND ADOLESCENT

APPENDICITIS

Description. Appendicitis is an inflammation of the vermiform appendix (the blind sac at the end of the cecum). It is the most common cause of abdominal surgery in children.

Obstruction of the appendiceal lumen — which can occur as a result of a **fecalith** (a hard, impacted fecal mass), inflammatory changes, lymphoid tissue, parasitic infestations, or stenosis — blocks the flow of mucoid secretions, causing pressure to build up in the blood vessels of the lumen. Inflammation and ulceration of the appendiceal mucosa follow. Without treatment, necrosis and eventual rupture of the

appendix occur. Rupture of the appendix can result in peritonitis from fecal and bacterial contamination of the peritoneal cavity.

Symptoms. The child usually presents with a low-grade fever, generalized abdominal pain that localizes to the right lower quadrant, and abdominal tenderness. Vomiting, diarrhea, or constipation can also occur. The child has a decreased activity level and is most comfortable lying on the side with the knees flexed. If the appendix ruptures and peritonitis develops, the child will have a sudden relief of pain followed by severe pain, abdominal distention, tachycardia, rapid shallow respirations, and restlessness.

Treatment. Diagnosis is based on the history, physical examination, laboratory tests, and occasionally x-ray studies. On examination, the child has abdominal tenderness, pain, and guarding. An appendectomy is the treatment of choice. Before surgery, the child is kept NPO (given nothing by mouth) and an intravenous infusion is started to correct any fluid and electrolyte imbalances. If surgery is uncomplicated by perforation, the prognosis is excellent and the child is discharged within 5 days.

If the appendix ruptures before surgery, the child is started on intravenous antibiotics and nasogastric suctioning is begun. Postoperatively, the child requires a 7- to 10-day course of antibiotics, intravenous fluids, nasogastric suctioning, and dressing changes.

Nursing Care. Nursing care is the same as for any child undergoing surgery (Chapter 15). Before surgery, provide reassurance and emotional support. After surgery, check the abdominal dressing frequently for signs of increased drainage and infection. Monitor vital signs frequently, administer prescribed medications for pain and fever, and encourage the child to cough and deep breathe. It will be easier for the child to cough if a pillow is used to splint the surgical site. Provide emotional support. On discharge, instruct parents to watch for any redness or drainage from the incision. Tell parents to keep the incision clean and dry. The child should avoid contact sports and lifting any heavy objects.

DIABETES MELLITUS

Description. Insulin-dependent diabetes mellitus (IDDM), type I, previously called juvenile-onset diabetes mellitus, is a chronic metabolic condition that occurs in children as a result of a loss of pancreatic beta cell function, resulting in limited production of insulin. The deficiency of insulin leads to a decreased availability of glucose in the cells and to a buildup of glucose in the blood. Because carbohydrates are unavailable for energy, the body metabolizes fat, instead. The breakdown of fat, however, results in an excess of ketones, which are then excreted through the lungs and urine.

Several factors are thought to influence the development of IDDM. These factors include genetic predisposition, environment, and immunological mechanisms. A child inherits a susceptibility to IDDM, not the disease itself (Rudolph et al. 1991). A viral infection of the beta cells of the islets of Langerhans is then believed to trigger an immune response that results in destruction of the beta cells.

Symptoms. The cardinal sign of IDDM is **polyuria** (excessive urine output), especially at night. Other characteristic findings include nocturnal enuresis, **polydipsia** (excessive thirst), weight loss, **polyphagia** (markedly increased food intake), glycosuria (glucose in the urine) with or without **ketonuria** (loss of ketones in urine), and hyperglycemia (elevated blood glucose).

Treatment. Diagnosis is made on the basis of the history, physical examination, and blood and urine testing. Glucose tolerance tests are usually not required to diagnose IDDM

(Rudolph et al. 1991). It is not uncommon for a child with early symptoms of IDDM to be diagnosed during a routine urinalysis.

Treatment of the child with IDDM depends on the severity of the condition at the time of diagnosis. Children may be hospitalized initially or treated on an out-patient basis. Management includes restoring fluid balance, correcting electrolyte imbalances, regulating insulin dosage, monitoring and correcting acidosis and glucose levels, and diet therapy.

Insulin can be given as a single dose of intermediate-acting (Lente or NPH) insulin, as multiple doses of short-acting regular insulin at different times of the day, or as a twice-daily combined dose of intermediate- and short-acting insulin mixed and given in the same syringe (usually before breakfast and before supper). Insulin doses are regulated according to the child's levels of glucose and ketones. Blood glucose levels and urine glucose and ketones are monitored before meals and at bedtime. Diet, exercise, illness, and emotional stress may all affect insulin needs.

Injection sites are rotated in a consistent pattern to different areas of the body (e.g., upper arms, thighs, abdomen, buttocks), Figure 24–7. Rotation improves the absorption of insulin by preventing development of fat pads in the injection site area. Absorption occurs rapidly in the arm and is slowest in the thigh (Wong 1993).

An alternative to daily injections of insulin is the insulin pump, which mimics pancreatic insulin secretions by providing either a slow, steady infusion or a larger (bolus) amount of regular (short-acting) insulin when needed. The pump is a small, battery-operated device, the size of a calculator. It consists of a syringe with a mechanized plunger connected by a catheter to a needle inserted in the subcutaneous tissue, usually in the abdomen (Clark and Plotnick 1990).

Diet therapy is important in the overall management of the child with IDDM. A well-

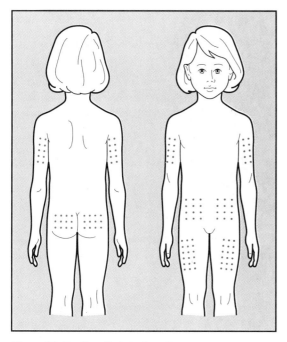

Figure 24–7   Insulin injection sites

balanced diet is required that meets the caloric needs of the child and supplies the necessary nutrients to promote growth, while avoiding concentrated sugars. The child's total caloric intake should be distributed over three meals and three snacks, consumed at consistent intervals throughout the day. The American Dietetic Association food exchange lists can be used to provide a carefully measured diet for the diabetic child. To ensure compliance, a dietician should help the child and family plan an exchange diet based on the foods that the child likes.

Long-term medical management of IDDM focuses on maintaining normal growth and development and preventing episodes of hypoglycemia and ketoacidosis. Hypoglycemia (low serum glucose concentration) can result from the administration of an excessive amount of insulin, a change in body requirements, or an inadequate intake of food. Symptoms include tachycardia, sweating, flushing, shakiness, drowsiness, headache,

weakness, anxiety, and behavioral changes. Children with these symptoms require immediate treatment with simple sugar. Untreated hypoglycemia may result in loss of consciousness, convulsions, brain damage, and death.

Diabetic **ketoacidosis** is a complication of IDDM that results from accumulations of ketones in the body. Signs and symptoms include acetone (fruity) odor to the breath, dyspnea, vomiting, polyuria, dehydration, weight loss, mental confusion, and, if untreated, coma. Without emergency treatment, ketoacidosis can be fatal. Treatment involves restoring fluids, administering normal saline and regular insulin (via injection or drip), and monitoring glucose level, acidosis, vital signs, serum ketones, electrolytes, and fluid intake and output.

Nursing Care. The nurse's role includes managing the child during the initial hospitalization and providing continuing education to the child and family. Nursing care of the hospitalized child depends on the child's condition at the time of admission. Initial care focuses on monitoring the child's fluid and electrolyte status, measuring intake and output, monitoring intravenous fluids, checking vital signs, checking urine and blood for glucose and ketones, and administering insulin. The child should be watched closely for signs of ketoacidosis or hypoglycemia.

The education of the child and family is as important as the medical management of the child (Rudolph et al. 1991). Teaching should include how to administer insulin, how to test the urine for ketones, how to measure blood glucose levels, how to recognize hypoglycemia and hyperglycemia, and how to manage diet. Parents should also know when to contact a health care provider (for example, if ketone levels are moderate to high). Emphasize the importance of having the child wear some type of medical identification (e.g., Medic-Alert bracelet).

NURSING CARE PLAN: Insulin-Dependent Diabetes Mellitus

Nursing Diagnosis	Goal(s)
Risk for injury: hypoglycemia or ketoacidosis	The child will maintain or regain normal blood glucose levels.
Inability to gain weight despite adequate caloric intake	The child will have appropriate weight gain.
	The child and parents will state understanding of diabetic diet.
Anxiety related to lack of knowledge about disease and its management	The child and parents will state knowledge of insulin therapy, dietary management, and symptoms to report to their health care provider.

Figure 24–8

NURSING INTERVENTION	RATIONALE
Monitor blood glucose and urine glucose and ketone levels.	Provides a guide to insulin needs. Low blood glucose levels are indicative of hypoglycemia; elevated glucose and ketones are indicative of ketoacidosis.
Administer insulin as prescribed.	Insulin promotes utilization of glucose.
Assess vital signs and level of consciousness (LOC).	Changes in vital signs and LOC indicate poorly regulated blood glucose.
Provide three meals per day and three snacks at the same time each day consisting of the appropriate amounts of calories, carbohydrates, proteins, and fats.	Regulating daily calories and eating food at consistent intervals help the child to gain weight.
Educate child and parents about diet therapy and relationship between diet, exercise, and insulin requirements.	Knowledge helps ensure compliance with treatment plan.
Provide information about exchange lists.	Exchange lists help regulate dietary intake.
Explain cause, symptoms, and treatment of IDDM.	Knowledge decreases anxiety.
Provide written materials for parents and child to take home.	Written materials reinforce teaching and can be referred to after discharge.
Teach parents and child: how to recognize and treat a hypoglycemic episode; to monitor ketone levels and call the child's health care provider if levels are elevated.	Early identification allows for prompt management.
Encourage school-age child or adolescent to take responsibility for self-care (glucose testing, insulin injections, and diet).	Self-management provides a sense of control and independence.
Encourage child and parents to verbalize concerns about disease and its management. Refer to peer support groups if indicated.	Provides child and family with an outlet and an opportunity to work through concerns.

Figure 24–8 continued

Dietary teaching should include the following points:

- The child should eat a well-balanced diet but avoid pure sugar foods.
- Meals and snacks should be eaten at about the same time every day. Snacks are necessary to prevent insulin reactions.
- The amount of fat and cholesterol in the diet should be decreased.
- Exercise is important to reduce stress and promote well-being. Vigorous exercise should be scheduled after meals to minimize the risk of a hypoglycemic episode.
- The child should always carry simple sugar (glucose tablets, sugar cubes, hard candy) to ingest in case a hypoglycemic episode occurs.

Emotional support is essential for both the child and parents to help them cope with the limitations of a chronic disease. Parents can be referred to organizations such as the American Diabetes Association, 1660 Duke Street, Alexandria, VA 22314 (800) 232-3472, for information and educational materials.

Self-management is an essential component of diabetes management. The school-age child can be encouraged to begin taking responsibility for aspects of daily care, such as testing blood glucose and injecting insulin. Self-care provides the child with a sense of control. Summer camps for children with diabetes also foster a sense of independence and responsibility. Adolescents are at particular risk for noncompliance with the daily management regimen. They may rebel against the limitations and regimentation imposed by the disease. Encouraging adolescents to discuss their feelings and helping them to learn more about the disease, how to adjust their diet so they do not feel different from peers, and how to manage reactions may be beneficial.

Nursing care of the child with IDDM is summarized in Figure 24–8 (page 364).

Review Questions

A. Multiple choice. Select the best answer.

1. All of the following are common causes of diarrhea in infants except
   a. rhinovirus
   b. *E. coli*
   c. *Salmonella*
   d. rotavirus

2. Recurrent regurgitation is a characteristic sign of which of the following conditions?
   a. colic
   b. gastroesophageal reflux
   c. intussusception
   d. Hirschsprung's disease

3. Jamie, 2 weeks old, has symptoms of projectile vomiting and poor weight gain. Which of the following conditions would you suspect?
   a. colic
   b. gastroesophageal reflux
   c. pyloric stenosis
   d. Hirschsprung's disease

4. All of the following are characteristic findings in children with IDDM except
   a. polyuria
   b. polydipsia
   c. polyphagia
   d. polycythemia

5. The "string sign" is a classic finding in which of the following disorders?
   a. pyloric stenosis
   b. intussusception
   c. gastroesophageal reflux
   d. Hirschsprung's disease

6. A child with moderate dehydration has a fluid loss of approximately
   a. 3% to 5% of body weight
   b. 6% to 9% of body weight
   c. 10% to 13% of body weight
   d. 13% to 15% of body weight

B. True or false. Write *T* for a true statement and *F* for a false statement.

1. ___ Colic usually resolves by the time an infant is 3 to 4 months of age.

2. ___ Fever is the most common cause of dehydration in infants and young children.

3. ___ Intussusception commonly occurs suddenly in a previously healthy child.

4. ___ Immediate surgical repair is essential for infants with umbilical hernias.

5. ___ Intestinal parasitic diseases are common in children of all ages.

6. ___ Foreign body ingestion is most common in young infants.

7. ___ The child with appendicitis usually assumes a semi-Fowler's position.

SUGGESTED ACTIVITIES

- Interview the parents of an infant with colic. Ask parents what strategies they have used to manage the infant's symptoms. Which strategies have been successful? Which have been unsuccessful?

- Write or call the American Diabetes Association (see information provided in the chapter) to request educational materials on IDDM. Assess these materials regarding their use in parent teaching.

BIBLIOGRAPHY

Boyle, J. T. Gastroesophageal reflux in the pediatric patient. *Gastroenterology Clinics of North America* 18 (1989): 315–337.

Brazelton, T. B. Crying in infancy. *Pediatrics* 29 (1962): 579–588.

Broadwell Jackson, D., and R. B. Saunders. *Child Health Nursing*. Philadelphia: J. B. Lippincott, 1993.

Cervisi, J., M. Chapman, B. Niklas, and C. Yamaoka. Office management of the infant with colic. *Journal of Pediatric Health Care* 5, no. 4 (1991): 184–190.

Clark, L. M., and L. P. Plotnick. Insulin pumps in children with diabetes. *Journal of Pediatric Health Care* 4 (1990): 3–10.

DaDalt, L., S. Mazzoleni, G. Montini, F. Donzelli, and F. Zacchello. Diagnostic accuracy of pH monitoring in gastroesophageal reflux. *Archives of Disease in Childhood* 64 (1989): 1421–1426.

Foster, R. L. R., M. M. H. Hunsberger, and J. T. Anderson. *Family-Centered Nursing Care of Children*. Philadelphia: W. B. Saunders, 1989.

Grimes, D. *Infectious Diseases*. St. Louis, MO: Mosby-Year Book, 1991.

Hathaway, W. E., W. W. Hay, J. R. Groothuis, and J. W. Paisley. *Current Pediatric Diagnosis and Treatment*, 11th ed. Norwalk, CT: Appleton and Lange, 1993.

Rosenstein, B. J., and P. D. Fosarelli. *Pediatric Pearls: The Handbook of Practical Pediatrics*. Chicago: Year Book Medical Publishers, 1989.

Rudolph, A. M., J. I. E. Hoffman, and C. D. Rudolph. *Rudolph's Pediatrics*, 19th ed. Norwalk, CT: Appleton and Lange, 1991.

Shannon, R. S. Gastroesophageal reflux in infancy: Review and update. *Journal of Pediatric Health Care* 7, no. 2 (1993): 71–76.

Swischuk, L. E., C. K. Hayden, D. H. Fawcet, and J. N. Isenberg. Gastroesophageal reflux: How much imaging is required? *Radiographics* 8 (1988): 1137–1145.

Tucker, J. A., and K. Sussman-Karten. Treating diarrhea and dehydration with an oral rehydration solution. *Pediatric Nursing* 13, no. 3 (1987): 169–174.

Wong, D. *Whaley & Wong's Essentials of Pediatric Nursing*, 4th ed. St. Louis, MO: Mosby-Year Book, 1993.

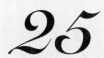

CHAPTER

25

Conditions of the Urinary System

OBJECTIVES

AFTER STUDYING THIS CHAPTER, THE STUDENT SHOULD BE ABLE TO:

- IDENTIFY FOUR STRUCTURAL DEFECTS OF THE GENITOURINARY SYSTEM AND DESCRIBE THEIR TREATMENT AND NURSING CARE.

- DESCRIBE THE SYMPTOMS, TREATMENT, AND NURSING CARE OF URINARY TRACT INFECTION AND IDENTIFY SEVERAL FACTORS PREDISPOSING A CHILD TO DEVELOP AN INFECTION.

- DESCRIBE THE SYMPTOMS, TREATMENT, AND NURSING CARE OF WILM'S TUMOR.

- COMPARE AND CONTRAST THE SYMPTOMS, TREATMENT, AND NURSING CARE OF NEPHROTIC SYNDROME, ACUTE GLOMERULO-NEPHRITIS, AND ACUTE AND CHRONIC RENAL FAILURE.

- DEFINE ENURESIS AND DESCRIBE ITS CAUSE, TREATMENT, AND NURSING CARE.

KEY TERMS

URINARY STASIS

VESICOURETERAL REFLUX

HYPOPROTEINEMIA

HYPOALBUMINEMIA

HYPERLIPIDEMIA

HYPOVOLEMIA

OLIGURIA

rinary conditions in children may be congenital or acquired (a result of infection, disease, or injury). Congenital conditions include structural defects such as hypospadias and epispadias. Acquired conditions include infection of the urinary tract and kidney disorders. Structural defects, if untreated, can have physical and psychological effects as the child matures. Acquired conditions, if untreated, can result in inflammation, tissue damage, and scarring. By assisting in early assessment and treatment of these conditions, the nurse can play an important role in preventing physiological and psychological complications.

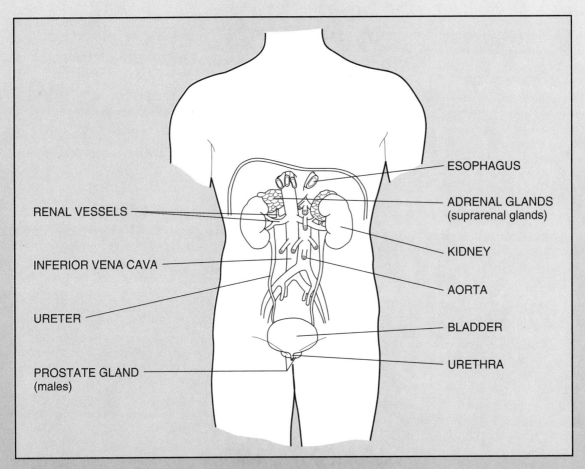

Figure 25–1   *The urinary system*

OVERVIEW OF THE SYSTEM

The urinary system is made up of the kidneys, ureters, urinary bladder, and urethra, Figure 25–1. The main function of this system is to excrete nitrogenous wastes, salts, and water from the body, thus preventing the buildup of toxic wastes. The kidneys also function to regulate fluid and electrolyte balance.

Each kidney consists of an outer layer (cortex) and an inner, striated layer (medulla). The nephron is the basic structural and functional unit of the kidney, Figure 25–2. Each kidney contains over 1 million nephrons (Fong et al. 1993).

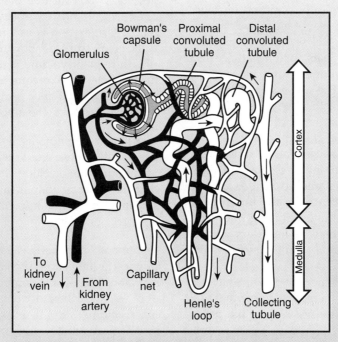

Figure 25–2   *Cross section of the nephron and tubules*

INFANT AND TODDLER

HYPOSPADIAS AND EPISPADIAS

Hypospadias is a congenital anomaly of males in which the urethral meatus is located on the ventral surface of the glans penis instead of at the tip. In epispadias, the meatus is located on the dorsal surface of the penis. Epispadias is usually associated with exstrophy of the bladder.

Diagnosis is made by observation at birth, and the defect is surgically corrected in stages beginning in the first year of life.

The goal of surgical repair is to give the child a penis that appears anatomically correct with a normal voiding stream and normal sexual functioning. The nurse should encourage parents to express their fears and concerns and provide emotional support.

Nursing care of the child with hypospadias or epispadias centers on monitoring vital signs; administering prescribed medications for pain, fever, and to reduce muscle spasms; preventing infection; and limiting the child's mobility. Restraints, although not usually recommended, may be necessary to prevent the young child from touching the surgical site.

Postoperatively, the child will have a bulky dressing over the perineal area that will compress the wound, dressings on the penis, and a catheter. Care should be taken to prevent bleeding. Observe for and report immediately any increased drainage. A tent should be made from the child's sheets to prevent bed linens from touching the surgical site, penis, catheters, or dressing.

The child is kept on complete bed rest with limited mobility for 48 to 72 hours after surgery. Bed rest is usually required for 7 to 10 days. Help the parents to provide age-appropriate diversional activities for the child on bed rest (such as videos, music, computer games, puzzles, paint, books).

URINARY TRACT INFECTION

Description. Urinary tract infections (UTIs) are the most common genitourinary disorders and the second most common infection of childhood. These infections can be bacterial, fungal, or viral in nature. *Escherichia coli (E. coli)* is the organism responsible for 90% of first-time UTIs (Tanagho and McAninch 1992). An infection can occur in the urethra, bladder, ureters, renal pelvis, or renal parenchyma.

Conditions that may predispose a child to develop a UTI include obstruction (functional or structural), urinary stasis, and vesicoureteral reflux. **Urinary stasis** occurs when the flow of urine is interrupted, allowing bacteria to multiply. Infrequent voiding is a common cause of urinary stasis. **Vesicoureteral reflux** occurs when there is an abnormal backflow of urine from the bladder to the ureters.

Symptoms. Symptoms are variable and depend on the cause and location of the infection. Symptoms can include frequency, urgency, dysuria, enuresis, abdominal pain, fever, strong-smelling urine, flank pain, and occasionally hemorrhagic cystitis.

Treatment. Diagnosis is based on the history, physical examination, presence of characteristic symptoms (flank or abdominal pain, masses, tenderness), and laboratory data (urinalysis including culture and sensitivity). Diagnostic radiological studies can include intravenous pyelography and voiding cystourethrogram [VCUG]). A urine culture should be performed on a midstream clean-catch specimen. If the child cannot cooperate, a suprapubic bladder tap may be performed. A UTI is present when a urine culture is found to have more than 100,000 colony-forming units of a single organism per milliliter.

When no functional or structural urinary tract abnormalities are found, other possible causes should be considered. These include infrequent or incomplete voiding, poor perineal hygiene, pinworms, or constipation.

Treatment depends on a multitude of variables including whether the child is symptomatic or asymptomatic, whether this is the child's first infection or a reinfection, and whether the child has a preexisting condition or a functional or structural abnormality. A 10-day course of antibiotics (sulfi-soxazole or ampicillin) is prescribed. The child should return within 48 hours of treatment for a follow-up urinalysis and culture, and again one to three weeks after treatment. In some cases, intravenous antibiotic therapy is required. Some authorities recommend follow-up cultures every one to three months for one year.

Nursing Care. It is important for the nurse to use good technique when obtaining a urine specimen from a child. Contamination frequently causes false positive results.

Teach parents to avoid putting tight nylon or silk underwear on the child. Tight underwear and synthetic materials trap moisture close to the body, providing an environment conducive to bacterial growth. Recommend the child wear cotton panties. Discourage the use of bubble bath, which can be irritating. Encourage fluids and have the parent take the child to the bathroom frequently. Teach parents the importance of good perineal hygiene. Reinforce that because the urethra is short in girls, contamination from rectal bacteria is common. Instruct parents and children to wipe the perineum from front to back. Teach sexually active teenage girls to void after intercourse.

Provide emotional support to parents and encourage them to ask questions. Reinforce to parents the importance of completing the prescribed course of medications and bringing the child back for follow-up cultures. Advise parents to call the health care provider if they have questions. Figure 25–3 summarizes nursing care for the child with a UTI.

WILM'S TUMOR

Description. Wilm's tumor, also known as nephroblastoma, is the most common solid malignant renal tumor in children. The tumor occurs in both boys and girls and usually presents as an abdominal mass during the third year of life. It can occur in either kidney and occurs bilaterally in 5% of cases (Tanagho and McAninch 1992). Although the cause of Wilm's tumor is unclear, the tumor is thought to originate during embryonic development and is frequently associated with other congenital anomalies (e.g., hypospadias, ambiguous genitalia, cryptorchidism).

Symptoms. An abdominal mass is usually discovered by parents while bathing or dressing the child or by the physician or nurse during a routine physical examination. The tumor is felt as a firm nontender flank mass (Foley et al. 1993). Once the mass is detected, no further palpation should be performed. Common symptoms include abdominal pain, hypertension, hematuria, vomiting, diarrhea, and fever. Children may, however, be asymptomatic.

Treatment. Diagnosis is made by physical examination, laboratory studies (urinalysis, blood studies), ultrasonography, computed axial tomographic (CAT) scanning, and magnetic resonance imaging (MRI). Treatment is multifaceted and consists of surgery, radiation therapy, and chemotherapy. The National Wilm's Tumor Study (NWTS) has developed a clinical staging classification system based on surgical and pathological findings that is used to develop a treatment plan for the child. Prognosis depends on early diagnosis, intervention, and staging of the tumor.

Nursing Care. Nursing care of the child with a Wilm's tumor involves preoperative, operative, and postoperative care. Throughout the child's care the family and child will

NURSING CARE PLAN: Urinary Tract Infection

NURSING DIAGNOSIS	GOAL(S)
Dysuria	The child will state and show relief from pain.
Risk for fluid and electrolyte imbalance (dehydration)	The child will maintain or regain normal fluid and electrolyte balance.
Knowledge deficit related to preventive strategies for UTIs	The child and parents will describe strategies for preventing UTIs.

Figure 25–3

Nursing Intervention	Rationale
Encourage frequent bladder emptying (every 3 to 4 hours).	Helps prevent urinary stasis, which encourages persistence of microorganisms.
Administer antibiotics as prescribed.	Antibiotics provide bactericidal action to kill bacteria that cause infection.
Measure pain using a pediatric pain scale (see Chapter 15).	Provides an objective measurement of a child's pain.
Provide comfort measures, such as warm baths.	Warm baths help to relieve symptoms of perineal irritation.
Encourage liberal intake of fluids. Avoid carbonated and caffeinated beverages.	Liberal fluid intake promotes normal hydration and helps prevent urinary stasis. Carbonated and caffeinated beverages may irritate the bladder mucosa in some children.
Maintain accurate intake and output records.	Enables monitoring of child's fluid status.
Administer intravenous fluids, as ordered.	IV fluids provide rapid rehydration.
Administer antipyretic medications, as indicated. Monitor vital signs frequently for evidence of recurrent fever.	Fever increases fluid loss.
Teach parents the importance of having the child: empty bladder frequently; drink adequate amount of fluids; avoid bubble baths; wear cotton underwear; perform good perineal hygiene.	These strategies help prevent recurrence of infection.
Teach girls to always wipe the perineum from front to back.	
Teach sexually active adolescent girls to void after intercourse.	

Figure 25–3   *continued*

need emotional support and understanding. Help-ing the parents cope with the diagnosis of their child's cancer requires compassion and sensitivity. Provide the family with opportunities to ask questions and discuss their feelings and fears.

Preoperative teaching using anatomically correct dolls and a visit to the surgical suite can help to reduce the child's and parents' anxiety (Chapter 15). Do not massage the abdomen as it may cause the tumor to rupture. Postoperatively, close monitoring of the surgical site, vital signs, and pain threshold is required (Chapter 15). Children require both radiation and chemotherapy and should be closely monitored for adverse reactions.

Preschool and School-Age Child

Nephrotic Syndrome

Description. Nephrotic syndrome is a disorder characterized by proteinuria, **hypoproteinemia** (a decreased amount of protein in the blood), **hypoalbuminemia** (abnormally low levels of albumin in the blood), **hyperlipidemia** (an excess of lipids in the plasma), and edema. It is most common in preschool children between 2 and 3 years of age, and it is more common in boys than in girls.

In this condition, large amounts of protein are produced and excreted in the urine. The exact cause of this proteinuria is unknown. Protein loss causes hypoalbuminemia, which in turn causes interstitial fluid to accumulate. Because the child has poor renal perfusion, increased amounts of sodium and water are reabsorbed by the renal tubules, resulting in edema.

Nephrotic syndrome can occur as a result of any type of glomerular disease or as a complication of other disorders such as lupus, diabetes, or sickle cell disease.

Symptoms. The cardinal sign of nephrotic syndrome is edema, which appears gradually and spreads slowly. The periorbital area is usually affected first followed by generalized pitting edema of the hands, ankles, and feet. The child may have a protuberant abdomen and abdominal discomfort because of fluid buildup. Urine may be dark and frothy. An increased susceptibility to infection may be evident.

Treatment. A combination of corticosteroid, diuretic, immunosuppressive, and antihypertensive medications is administered. It is important to prevent infection and restrict the amount of sodium in the child's diet during the acute phase of the disease.

The prognosis depends on the cause. Children who have a favorable response to corticosteroids usually have no significant problems. Other children can have frequent relapses and progressive renal disease.

Nursing Care. Nursing care includes providing emotional support to the parents and child, monitoring the child's fluid intake and output, checking urine for protein, preventing infection by keeping the child in reverse isolation, and administering medications as ordered.

On discharge from the hospital, the nurse should reinforce to parents the importance of completing the prescribed course of medications and of keeping follow-up appointments. Teach parents that the child can return to a normal diet without sodium restrictions except during edematous periods, if allowed by the physician.

Acute Glomerulonephritis

Description. Glomerulonephritis is a disease that causes inflammation of the glomerulus in the kidney. In most children, acute glomerulonephritis follows an infection of the pharynx, tonsils, or skin with group A beta-hemolytic streptococci. This form of the disease is referred to as poststreptococcal acute glomerulonephritis. Children between the ages of 3 and 10 years are most commonly affected.

In poststreptococcal acute glomerulonephritis, antigens localize in the kidney on the capillary wall. The kidney becomes edematous and enlarged. Inflammation, obstruction, and injury to the tissue occur, and glomerular filtration rate is impaired.

Symptoms. Approximately 50% of children are asymptomatic. The disease is usually discovered during routine urinalysis (Rudolph et al. 1991). In severe cases, which develop about 10 to 14 days after an acute streptococcal infection, the child can have a low-grade fever, headache, malaise, periorbital edema, proteinuria, decreased urine output, and hematuria. The urine is often brown or tea-colored. The child may also be hypertensive.

Treatment. Treatment involves administration of antihypertensive and diuretic medications and a low-sodium, low-protein diet. Bed rest is advised during the acute phase. Antibiotics may be prescribed if the streptococcal infection is still present.

Follow-up visits for blood pressure monitoring and urinalysis should occur for at least one year after treatment.

Nursing Care. Nursing care is similar to that provided for the child with nephrotic syndrome. Provide emotional support to the parents and child. Monitor fluid intake and output and help the child pick foods that he or she likes, while maintaining the low-sodium, low-protein diet. Test urine frequently for blood and protein. Provide diversional activities such as video tapes, games, puzzles, and audio books while the child is on bed rest.

RENAL FAILURE

Renal failure occurs when the kidneys are unable to excrete enough water, electrolytes, and waste products to maintain normal body fluid homeostasis (Rudolph et al. 1991). Renal failure can be either acute or chronic. Acute renal failure develops suddenly and can result from impaired renal perfusion, acute renal disease, or obstructive uropathy. Early recognition and treatment are important. Chronic renal failure is a progressive deterioration in renal function that develops as a result of an underlying kidney or urinary tract condition.

ACUTE RENAL FAILURE

Description. Acute renal failure is classified as prerenal, renal, or postrenal failure, depending on the underlying cause. Prerenal failure occurs when **hypovolemia** (diminished blood flow) develops, usually as a result of dehydration, blood loss, complications of surgery, hypotension, shock, burns, or trauma. Prerenal failure is generally reversible with treatment and prognosis is usually good. Renal failure occurs when the kidneys themselves are damaged by disease or toxins. Prognosis is poor. Postrenal failure occurs when an anatomical abnormality or functional barrier (congenital anomaly) obstructs urine flow from the kidneys to the urethral meatus. This obstruction is usually correctable and the prognosis, with surgery, is good.

Symptoms. The presenting symptoms are variable and depend on the cause of the renal failure. The classic and most common symptom is **oliguria** (decreased urine output). The urine may appear dark in color. Other symptoms include dehydration, edema, pallor, and hypertension.

Treatment. Diagnosis is made on the basis of the history, physical examination, and diagnostic studies (including blood studies, urinalysis, and x-rays of the chest and abdomen). Obstructions are frequently diagnosed by scan and biopsy (Broadwell Jackson and Saunders 1993).

Treatment is supportive until renal function returns and the kidneys are able to function normally. The underlying cause of the failure and any complications must be treated. Treatment includes preventing fluid overload and electrolyte imbalance (hyperkalemia, hypocalcemia, acidosis), preventing hypotension or hypertension, maintaining adequate caloric intake, and preventing infection (Rudolph et al. 1991). Dialysis is frequently required, Figure 25–4.

Nursing Care. Nursing care of a child in acute renal failure is multifaceted. The nurse must provide physical care and close monitoring of the child's condition while at the same time providing psychosocial support to the parents and child. Nursing care includes recording intake and output and weighing the child every day on the same scale. Monitor the child's blood pressure and administer antihypertensive drugs. Encourage adequate nutrition and help the child to choose a diet that is low in sodium, potassium, and protein and high in carbohydrate, fats, and vitamins. A dietician is frequently involved in diet planning.

If the child requires dialysis, the nurse will explain the procedure to the child and family,

---

INDICATIONS FOR DIALYSIS

- Severe hyperkalemia
- Metabolic acidosis
- Fluid overload with or without hypertension
- Uremia

Figure 25–4

---

monitor the child closely for any adverse effects, and provide emotional support to the child and family. (Refer to the discussion of chronic renal failure, following.)

Other nursing responsibilities include preventing infection, caring for the child if surgery is indicated, and educating the child and family about the disease, medications, diet and home care, and long-term management.

CHRONIC RENAL FAILURE/END-STAGE RENAL DISEASE

Description. Chronic renal failure occurs when a disease or abnormality of the kidneys or urinary tract results in a progressive destruction of nephrons, decreasing the ability of the kidneys to excrete metabolic wastes from the body. Causes of renal failure include developmental abnormalities of the kidney or urinary tract, inherited disorders, and acquired glomerular disease.

Chronic renal failure progresses through several stages. In the initial stages, the kidney is still able to compensate for the loss of nephrons. As more nephrons are destroyed, however, the decrease in renal function results in the buildup of metabolic wastes in the blood (Broadwell Jackson and Saunders 1993). End-stage renal disease occurs when the kidneys are no longer able to maintain fluid and electrolyte balance.

Symptoms. Symptoms depend on the stage of renal failure. Initial symptoms may be vague and nonspecific. With more advanced disease, symptoms can include fatigue, reduced exercise tolerance, decreased appetite, headache, anemia, electrolyte imbalance, metabolic acidosis, hypertension, and uremia.

Treatment. The goal of treatment is to help the child maintain the best quality of life possible by promoting normal growth and development and encouraging independence. Specific treatment centers on maintaining adequate nutrition by providing a diet with enough calories and protein for growth, limiting demands on the kidney, and preventing complications (bone disease, neurological abnormalities, and anemia). Antihypertensive, immunosuppressive, and antibiotic medications are frequently prescribed. Children with end-stage renal disease require dialysis or renal transplantation.

Nursing Care. Nursing care of the child with chronic renal failure is similar to care of the child with acute renal failure. However, the nurse needs to keep in mind the chronic nature of the disease, the effect of the disease on all body systems, and the psychological effects on the child and family of coping with a long-term and potentially terminal disease.

Specific nursing care includes monitoring fluid and electrolyte balance, recording intake and output, administering medications, helping the child and family with diet management, and providing psychosocial support.

Assist the family to arrange for home health care of the child by making referrals to appropriate agencies for visiting nurses, therapists, and equipment. Families should also be referred to social services, clergy, support groups, and for home teaching if appropriate.

ENURESIS

Enuresis is involuntary urination that occurs beyond the age when bladder control is expected to have been attained (usually 4 to 5 years of age), including either daytime or nighttime wetting. The condition is more common in boys than in girls.

Enuresis is classified as either primary or secondary. Children with primary enuresis have never been dry. Those with secondary enuresis have achieved control for months or years and then regress. Primary nighttime wetters represent the largest group of children.

Enuresis can be the result of a functional or structural problem, a symptom of an organic disease, or emotionally based. Common causes are urinary tract infections, small bladder capacity, diabetes, sexual abuse, and emotional problems. Before a treatment plan is devised, it is important that a detailed history, physical examination, and urinalysis (including culture) be performed to rule out any structural or organic causes.

Treatment involves counseling parents in the management of enuresis and providing emotional support to the parent and child, Figure 25–5. Occasionally children are treated with medications. Referral should be made for counseling if indicated.

GUIDELINES FOR PARENTS OF ENURETIC CHILDREN

- Restrict the child's fluids after dinner.
- Take the child to the toilet before he or she goes to bed, then again before the parent goes to bed, and once during the night hours.
- Work with the child to perform bladder-stretching exercises. For example, have the child drink large quantities of fluids and then hold the urine as long as possible.
- Use enuresis alarms that ring when the child has a full bladder but has not wet.
- Devise reward systems in which the child receives a sticker, star, or small favor when he or she is dry.

Figure 25–5

Review Questions

A. Multiple choice. Select the best answer.

1. Placement of the urethral meatus on the dorsal surface of the penis is characteristic of which of the following conditions?
   a. hypospadias
   b. epispadias
   c. vesicoureteral reflux
   d. nephrotic syndrome

2. Roberto, 7 years old, complains to his mother of urgency, enuresis, dysuria, and abdominal pain, and has a mild fever. These are characteristic signs and symptoms of
   a. urinary tract infection
   b. nephrotic syndrome
   c. acute renal failure
   d. acute glomerulonephritis

3. Ultrasonography, CAT scanning, and MRI may be used to diagnose which of the following conditions?
   a. hypovolemia
   b. urinary tract infection
   c. Wilm's tumor
   d. acute glomerulonephritis

4. A child with acute glomerulonephritis should be on what type of diet?
   a. low-sodium
   b. low-sodium, low-fat
   c. low-sodium, low-protein
   d. low-protein

5. A child with nephrotic syndrome is most likely to have which of the following clinical findings?
   a. vesicoureteral reflux
   b. vomiting and diarrhea
   c. low-grade fever
   d. periorbital edema

6. Brown urine is a common finding in children who have
   a. urinary tract infection
   b. nephrotic syndrome
   c. acute glomerulonephritis
   d. enuresis

B. True or false. Write *T* for a true statement and *F* for a false statement.

1. ___ A UTI is present when a urine culture reveals less than 100,000 colony-forming units of a single organism per milliliter.

2. ___ Wilm's tumor usually presents in children during the third year of life.

3. ___ Hyperproteinemia is a characteristic finding in children with nephrotic syndrome.

4. ___ Acute glomerulonephritis is most common in toddlers between the ages of 1 and 3 years.

5. ___ Acute renal failure involves a progressive destruction of the nephrons of the kidney.

6. ___ Initial symptoms in chronic renal failure are often nonspecific.

SUGGESTED ACTIVITIES

- Make a poster or other teaching tool identifying strategies to prevent UTIs in children and adolescents.

- Interview a child with nephrotic syndrome and his or her parents. Identify concerns that each one has about the condition. What strategies would you use to address their concerns?

- Visit a dialysis center that provides treatment to children with chronic renal failure. Discuss with nursing staff and parents the impact of this disease on the child's and family's lifestyle.

- Interview parents of an enuretic child. What problems or concerns did they experience related to their child's condition? What strategies did they use to manage the condition in their child?

BIBLIOGRAPHY

Bondi, E. E., B. V. Jegasothy, and G. S. Lazarus. *Dermatology*. Norwalk, CT: Appleton and Lange, 1991.

Broadwell Jackson, D., and R. B. Saunders. *Child Health Nursing*. Philadelphia: J. B. Lippincott, 1993.

Foley, G. V., D. Fochtman, and K. Hardin Mooney. *Nursing Care of the Child with Cancer*, 2nd ed. Philadelphia: W. B. Saunders, 1993.

Fong, E., A. S. Scott, E. Ferris, and E. G. Skelley. *Body Structures and Functions*, 8th ed. Albany, NY: Delmar Publishers, 1993.

Grimes, D. *Infectious Diseases*. St. Louis, MO: Mosby-Year Book, 1991.

Habif, T. P. *Clinical Dermatology: A Color Guide to Diagnosis and Therapy*, 2nd ed. St. Louis, MO: Mosby-Year Book, 1990.

Hathaway, W. E., W. W. Hay, J. R. Groothuis, and J. W. Paisley. *Current Pediatric Diagnosis and Treatment*, 11th ed. Norwalk, CT: Appleton and Lange, 1993.

Kutz, M., C. Rudy, and S. Walsh. Daytime incontinence. *Journal of Pediatric Health Care* 7, no. 2 (1993): 92, 99–100.

Last, J. M., and R. B. Wallace. *Public Health and Preventive Medicine*, 13th ed. Norwalk, CT: Appleton and Lange, 1992.

McGuire, P., and K. Moore. Recent advances in childhood cancer, advances in oncology nursing. *Nursing Clinics of North America* 25, no. 2 (1990): 447–460.

Rosenstein, B. J., and P. D. Fosarelli. *Pediatric Pearls: The Handbook of Practical Pediatrics*. Chicago: Year Book Medical Publishers, 1989.

Rudolph, A. M., J. I. E. Hoffman, and C. D. Rudolph. *Rudolph's Pediatrics*, 19th ed. Norwalk, CT: Appleton and Lange, 1991.

Tanagho, E. A., and J. W. McAninch. *Smith's General Urology*, 13th ed. Norwalk, CT: Appleton and Lange, 1992.

Wong, D. *Whaley & Wong's Essentials of Pediatric Nursing*, 4th ed. St. Louis, MO: Mosby-Year Book, 1993.

CHAPTER

26

*C*onditions of the Reproductive System

OBJECTIVES

AFTER STUDYING THIS CHAPTER, THE STUDENT SHOULD BE ABLE TO:

- NAME THE MAIN INTERNAL AND EXTERNAL MALE AND FEMALE REPRODUCTIVE ORGANS.

- DISCUSS COMMON BIRTH CONTROL METHODS, INCLUDING THEIR RISKS AND BENEFITS.

- EXPLAIN SAFER SEX PRACTICES AND THEIR IMPORTANCE.

- DESCRIBE COMMON SEXUALLY TRANSMITTED DISEASES AND HOW THEY ARE TREATED.

- EXPLAIN THE ROLE THE NURSE PLAYS IN HELPING ADOLESCENTS WHO ARE TRYING TO COPE WITH PUBERTY, SEXUAL MATURITY, OR PREGNANCY.

KEY TERMS

PUBERTY

HYDROCELE

MENARCHE

MENSTRUATION

AMENORRHEA

MENORRHAGIA

METRORRHAGIA

DYSMENORRHEA

ANOVULATORY MENSTRUATION

onditions of the reproductive system play only a small part in the health of infants and young children. However, the reproductive system plays a major role in the health of adolescents. **Puberty**, beginning about age nine, marks the start of hormonal changes that culminate in the mature functioning of the male or female reproductive system. With these physical developments come changes in sexuality and behavior that can have far-reaching health consequences. The onset of sexual activity puts the teenage girl at risk for pregnancy. Both sexes are at increased risk for acquiring sexually transmitted diseases such as gonorrhea, herpes, hepatitis, and AIDS.

Most adolescents feel uncomfortable with the physical and emotional changes that accompany puberty. They may remain ignorant of basic health information because of embarrassment. Regardless of the nurse's own beliefs and values, an environment must be created where the adolescent feels supported and at ease. Confidentiality and privacy are of major concern to teenagers. In caring for the adolescent, the nurse must provide age-appropriate information on reproductive maturation, sexually transmitted diseases, birth control, and pregnancy options in a nonjudgmental way.

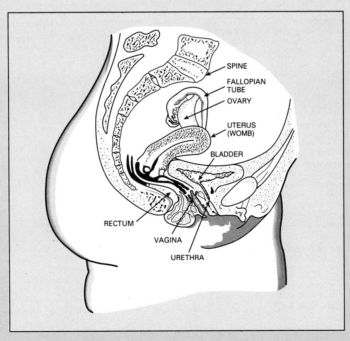

Figure 26–1   *Side view of female pelvic organs*

Overview of the System

The mature female reproductive system consists of the internal organs that make reproduction possible. These include two ovaries containing immature ova, two fallopian tubes, the vagina, and the uterus, a muscular organ that holds the fetus during pregnancy. Figure 26–1 shows the female reproductive organs in position relative to the other female pelvic organs. The female external genitals (the vulva) surround the opening of the vagina and include the mons pubis, labia minora, labia majora, prepuce, clitoris, urinary meatus, hymen, Skene's ducts, and Bartholin's glands.

The mature male internal reproductive organs include the sperm-producing testes, the seminal ducts for transporting sperm from the testes, the seminal vesicles, the prostate gland, and the bulbourethral (Cowper's) glands. The external male organs are the penis and the scrotum, which carry sperm and accompanying secretions to the outside. The male reproductive organs are shown in Figure 26–2.

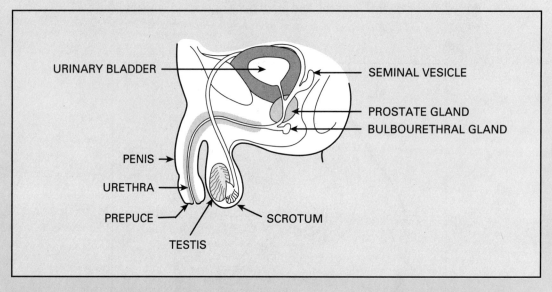

Figure 26–2   *Male reproductive organs*

INFANT AND TODDLER

HYDROCELE

A **hydrocele** is a condition in which fluid accumulates in a saclike cavity, especially in the tunica vaginalis (membrane encasing the testicle). It occurs when the processus vaginalis fails to close during fetal development, which enables fluid from the peritoneal cavity to enter the scrotum.

Diagnosis is made by physical examination. Palpation of the scrotum reveals a round, smooth, nontender mass. The mass is translucent on transillumination (passage of light through the walls of a cavity or an organ for inspection).

A hydrocele is often associated with inguinal hernia. Most communicating hydroceles close by the time the infant is one year of age. The fluid is then reabsorbed into the body. If the hydrocele is large, bowel may slip into the sac. Surgical intervention is necessary in these cases. Reassure parents that the condition often resolves itself without intervention and that the prognosis with surgery (if necessary) is excellent.

CRYPTORCHIDISM

Cryptorchidism refers to the failure of one or both testicles to descend into the scrotal sac. The testis can be located in the abdominal cavity, in the inguinal canal, or near the external ring where the ring enters the scrotum. The cause is unclear.

Diagnosis is made by examination and x-ray findings. Cryptorchidism should be differentiated from a retractile testis, which can be manually brought back down into the scrotum.

Treatment can include hormone therapy (intramuscular injections of the hormone human chorionic gonadotropin [HCG] to stimulate descent) or surgery. Surgery, if it is performed, usually takes place before the child is 5 years of age. The longer an undescended testicle remains out of the scrotal sac, the greater the risk of infertility. Other complications of untreated cryptorchidism include malignancy, hernia, torsion, and the psychological effect of an "empty" scrotum.

Teach parents about the surgical procedure, and discuss their concerns and fears related to their child's possible infertility. Because of the risk of testicular malignancy later in life, the importance of testicular self-examination and regular follow-up should be emphasized.

ADOLESCENT

ABNORMAL CONDITIONS RELATED TO MENSTRUATION

The first menstrual period, or **menarche**, normally occurs between the ages of 9 and 16. **Menstruation** is the process of shedding the unnecessary uterine lining when conception does not occur. The menstrual cycle begins with the first day of menstruation and is usually repeated every 28 days. This approximate cycle, however, varies with the individual. Abnormalities in the menstrual cycle may be caused by stress, endocrine dysfunction, overwork, change of climate, chronic disease, or other pathological conditions. Amenorrhea, menorrhagia, metrorrhagia, dysmenorrhea, and anovulatory menstruation are some common abnormalities.

- **Amenorrhea** is a permanent or temporary suppression of menstruation. It occurs as a normal condition before puberty, during pregnancy, between periods, and sometimes during lactation. The absence of menstruation may be congenital. It may also be caused by an obstruction of the cervix or vagina, which prevents external flow. A debilitating disease, severe anemia, thyroid imbalance, severe emotional distress, anorexia nervosa, and excessive exercise can also cause amenorrhea. A gynecologic examination is necessary to help determine the cause.

- **Menorrhagia** is menstrual bleeding that is excessive, prolonged, or both.
- **Metrorrhagia** is bleeding from the uterus that is not related to the menstrual period.
- **Dysmenorrhea** is painful menstruation. Primary dysmenorrhea refers to dysmenorrhea that is not caused by pelvic disease. Symptoms, which include cramping, abdominal pain, leg pain, backache, nausea, and headache, are related to an increased secretion of prostaglandins. They can be treated with nonsteroidal anti-inflammatory drugs, such as ibuprofen, which inhibit prostaglandin production. Secondary dysmenorrhea is caused by pelvic inflammatory disease (PID), ovarian cysts, endometriosis, or congenital abnormalities. Young women experiencing dysmenorrhea need to be examined by a physician to determine if any of these underlying conditions are present.
- **Anovulatory menstruation** is menstruation that takes place even though the ovary has failed to expel or discharge the egg. Without ovulation, fertilization cannot occur; failure to ovulate is one cause of infertility.

SEXUALLY TRANSMITTED DISEASES

Adolescents represent a population at risk for developing sexually transmitted diseases (STDs) because sexually active adolescents tend to have multiple sexual partners, fail to protect themselves against STDs, wait to seek medical attention, and do not tell their partners when they develop symptoms (Rudolph et al. 1991). The most common sexually transmitted diseases seen in younger children and adolescents are syphilis, gonorrhea, chlamydia, and genital herpes. Figure 26–3 outlines these diseases, their symptoms, and treatments. HIV (human immunodeficiency virus), which leads to AIDS (acquired immunodeficiency syndrome), is also transmitted through unprotected sexual intercourse. It is discussed in Chapter 19.

The nurse can play an important role in the prevention and treatment of STDs by educating teenagers. During routine history taking or assessment, be sure to ask about sexual activity and knowledge of STDs. If a teenager is diagnosed with an STD, discuss not only the treatment of the disease but also the importance of prevention. Explain the possible complications of STDs, which include infertility, ectopic pregnancy, and transmission of the disease to a fetus. Discuss methods of protection against STDs and the importance of informing sexual partners who might have been exposed to an STD about obtaining medical advice and possible treatment to avoid reinfection and the spread of the disease.

Always consider the possibility of molestation or sexual abuse by an infected adult or adolescent when a preadolescent child is diagnosed with an STD. Nurses have a legal responsibility to report cases of STDs in young children to local authorities.

SAFER SEX

Sexually transmitted diseases, including AIDS, are spread through sexual contact with an infected person. The only sure way to avoid STDs is to abstain from sexual activity. When the choice is made to be sexually active, safer sex practices reduce the risk of acquiring an STD. Safer sex guidelines are based on the concept of avoiding the exchange of body fluids. Figure 26–4 lists ways to reduce the risk of contracting an STD.

COMMON SEXUALLY TRANSMITTED DISEASES

Disease	Symptoms	Treatment
Syphilis *Causative organism: Treponema pallidum* *Incubation period:* 3 weeks	Primary syphilis manifests as a single lesion (chancre) at the site of contact. The characteristic chancre is a painless ulcer with a smooth base and indurated borders. The ulcer can appear in the genital area on the glans penis, labia, within the vagina, or in the perineal or rectal area. Painless, firm, enlarged inguinal lymph nodes can develop 1 to 2 weeks after the chancre appears. The chancre heals spontaneously in 1 to 5 weeks. (Bondi et al. 1991; Grimes 1991; and Habif 1990). Secondary syphilis appears as the primary lesion resolves. A diffuse, nonpruritic rash develops. Macular, papular, papulosquamous, or bullous lesions may be present. Mucous patches appear on mucosal surfaces. Broad-based, flat mucoid lesions (condylomata) appear on the genitals. The child develops flulike symptoms: sore throat, fever, malaise, lymphadenopathy.	Benzathine penicillin G or doxycycline is the antibiotic of choice. For children allergic to penicillin, erythromycin or tetracycline is given. Topical lesions can be treated with saline compresses followed by the application of a topical antibiotic (Polysporin) (Bondi et al. 1991).

Figure 26–3

COMMON SEXUALLY TRANSMITTED DISEASES

Disease	Symptoms	Treatment
Gonorrhea *Causative organism: Neisseria gonorrhoeae* *Incubation period:* 3 to 5 days	Symptoms associated with gonorrheal infections usually appear within 1 week of infection. Symptoms are varied and can include vulvovaginitis, urethritis, pharyngeal infections, anorectal gonorrhea, and pelvic inflammatory disease (PID). Preadolescent girls have a vaginal discharge that is thick, green, or creamy. Preadolescent and adolescent boys will have a yellow puslike urethral discharge associated with frequency, dysuria, and an erythematous meatus. Teenage girls frequently develop cervicitis, purulent vaginal discharge, and PID.	Antimicrobial therapy is the treatment of choice. Drugs recommended are ceftriaxone or cefotaxime given IV or IM. Children under the age of 8 years of age should also be given doxycycline.
Chlamydia *Causative organism: Chlamydia trachomatis* *Incubation period:* unknown	*C. trachomatis* is the most common cause of nongonococcal urethritis. Symptoms in adolescent girls include endocervicitis, mucopurulent yellow-green endocervical discharge, and PID. Adolescent boys can develop dysuria, urethritis, discharge, epididymitis, and proctitis.	Recommended medications include doxycycline or tetracycline, erythromycin, or sulfisoxazole.

Figure 26–3 continued

COMMON SEXUALLY TRANSMITTED DISEASES

Disease	Symptoms	Treatment
Genital Herpes *Causative organism:* Herpes simplex virus (HSV-2) *Incubation period:* unknown	Manifestations of herpes are varied and range from no symptoms to systemic involvement. Systemic symptoms include headache, fever, malaise, and myalgia. Small clusters of papules appear that develop into vesicles, pustules, and then ulcers. The lesions itch initially but when the ulcers break, there is pain. Ulcerations can appear on the external genitalia, between the vaginal folds and posterior cervix, or on the anus, buttocks, and thighs. Enlarged lymph nodes usually accompany the lesions.	Acyclovir is the drug of choice given orally and also applied topically to lesions. It is important to tell teenagers to wear a glove when applying ointment to lesions to prevent infecting other areas of the body and other people (Rosenstein and Fosarelli 1989).

Figure 26–3   continued

PREVENTIVE TEACHING: STDs

- Abstain from intercourse completely.
- Maintain a monogamous relationship.
- Limit the number of sexual partners.
- Use condoms for vaginal and anal intercourse.
- Do not have oral sex if partner has mouth sores or sores on the penis or vagina.

Figure 26–4

Consistently using a latex condom is the most effective way sexually active adolescents can protect themselves from STDs. Condoms lubricated with a spermicide such as nonoxynol-9 may provide greater protection than a condom alone. The correct use of condoms also prevents pregnancy.

BIRTH CONTROL

Sexually active adolescents have a poor record of using birth control. Many are embarrassed to seek the medical care necessary to obtain prescription birth control (e.g., oral contraceptives, Norplant implants, the cervical cap, the diaphragm). Others fail to use condoms, sponges, and spermicides, which are sold without a prescription, because they are reluctant to bring up the topic of birth control with their partner. Figures 26–5 and 26–6 show how to use two forms of nonprescription birth control.

Figure 26–7 shows some birth control methods and their effectiveness. When birth control is used, oral contraceptives and condoms are the birth control methods most frequently chosen by adolescents. Sterilization and intrauterine devices (IUDs) are not appropriate for teenagers. The rhythm method has a high rate of failure because it requires a great

deal of knowledge about fertility as well as repeated monitoring of body temperature. Figure 26–8 highlights the risks and benefits of different birth control methods.

ADOLESCENT PREGNANCY

More than one million adolescents become pregnant in the United States each year. About half of these pregnancies result in births. Most of the babies are born to single mothers.

A young woman may become pregnant for many reasons, including the desire to prove her womanhood, the need to have someone to love and care for, or ignorance about reproduction. Becoming pregnant may also be an act of self-assertion or hostility toward parental authority. Teenage girls are often not aware of the underlying reasons why they become pregnant. The vast majority consider their pregnancies accidents. Low self-esteem increases the risk that a girl will become pregnant.

When an adolescent becomes pregnant, she must decide whether to continue the pregnancy or to terminate it by elective abortion.

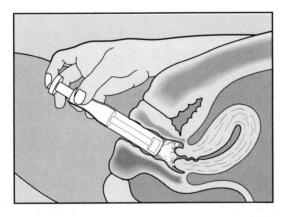

Figure 26–5   *Spermicides*

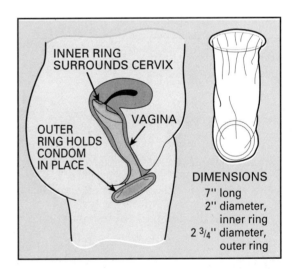

Figure 26–6   *The female condom*

METHODS OF CONTRACEPTION

Method	Percentage of Couples Using Method	Percentage of Women Who Avoid Pregnancy in a Given Year	Percentage of Women Experiencing Accidental Pregnancy during 1st Year of Use
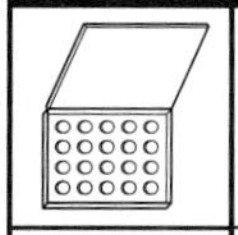 Oral contraceptives	18.5	97	3
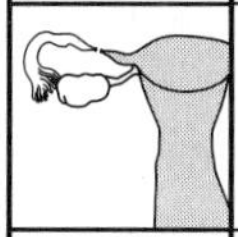 Female sterilization	16.6	99.6	0.4
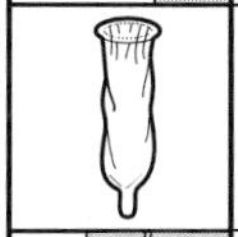 Male condom	8.8	86	12
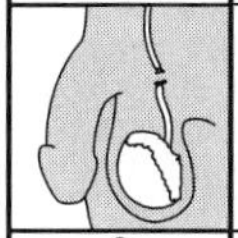 Male sterilization	7	99.8	0.15
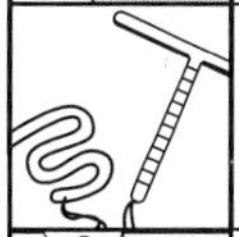 IUD	1.2	94	3
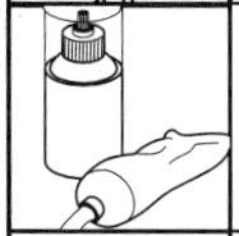 Spermicide	0.6	79	21
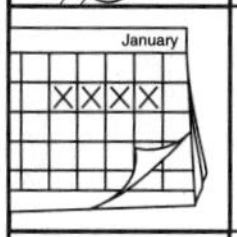 Rhythm/chance	1.8	80	85
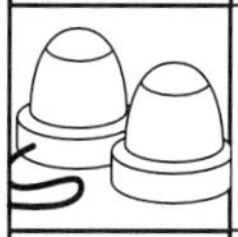 Cervical cap	1	73 – 92	18
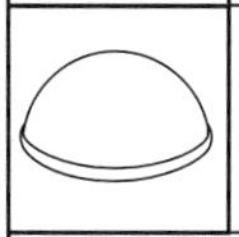 Diaphragm	1	84	18
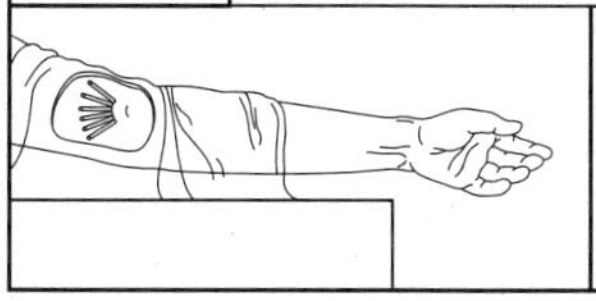 Implants Norplant capsules	Statistics unavailable		0.04

Figure 26–7   *Birth control options and their effectiveness rates*

CONTRACEPTION METHODS AND CONCERNS

Method	Risks	Side Effects	Noncontraceptive Benefits
Oral contraceptives	Cardiovascular complications such as stroke, blood clots, high blood pressure, and heart attacks with the higher-dose combined oral contraceptive	Possible nausea, headaches, dizziness, spotting, weight gain, breast tenderness, chloasma, cramping	Protects against PID, decreases risk of ovarian and endometrial cancer, decreases menstrual blood loss and dysmenorrhea (cramps), decreases benign breast disease, regulates irregular menses, protects bone density, decreases risk of atherosclerosis, lessens the risk of rheumatoid arthritis, decreases uterine fibroids, and decreases ovarian cysts
IUD	Pelvic inflammatory disease, uterine perforation, anemia	Menstrual cramping, spotting, increased bleeding	None known except progestin-releasing IUD, which may decrease menstrual pain and blood loss
Condoms	None known	Decreased sensation, allergy to latex, less spontaneity in love-making	Protects against sexually transmitted disease, including AIDS; delays premature ejaculation
Norplant implants	Infection at implant site	Menstrual changes, weight gain, headaches	May protect against PID, may decrease menstrual cramps, and blood loss
Sterilization	Infection	Pain at surgical site, psychological reaction with subsequent regret	None known
Abstinence	None known	Psychological reactions	Prevents infections including AIDS
Barriers (diaphragm, caps, sponges)	Mechanical irritation, vaginal infections, toxic shock syndrome	Pelvic pressure, cervical erosion, vaginal discharges if left in too long	Protects to some degree against sexually transmitted diseases

Figure 26–8   Major methods of contraception and some related concerns

This is a complex and emotionally difficult decision, especially for a teenager who may receive little support from her family or the father of the child.

In this situation, the role of the nurse is to provide information on pregnancy options and when possible to steer the pregnant adolescent to social workers and counselors who can help her understand and cope with the emotional, financial, social, and educational implications of her choice.

The nurse may have strong personal feelings about the issues of teenage pregnancy and abortion. As a professional, the nurse has a responsibility to see that the pregnant teen receives access to information about her options. If the nurse cannot comfortably discuss all the options available, the teen should be referred to a health professional or counselor who can provide a supportive nonjudgmental environment in which the teen can explore her feelings and choices. Whether the teen decides to continue the pregnancy to term or to end it with an abortion, she should receive appropriate health care as well as birth control counseling to discourage another accidental pregnancy.

Pregnant teenagers who decide to continue their pregnancies need prenatal health care and health care information. They need counseling about what to expect during and after the birth of the child. In addition, they must decide whether to keep their babies or to make plans for adoption. Today, most teenage girls choose to keep their babies.

Pregnant teenagers should be encouraged to continue attending school. Some schools have programs designed especially for them.

Adolescence is a very difficult time for pregnancy and motherhood. A teenage girl, who is already coping with the physical and emotional changes of adolescence, must simultaneously cope with the physical and emotional demands of pregnancy and motherhood. Counseling and support are especially important during this time. Regular prenatal health care can help ensure that pregnant adolescents remain healthy and give birth to healthy babies.

REVIEW QUESTIONS

A. Multiple choice. Select the best answer.

1. Roberto, age 3, has an undescended testicle. It is recommended that he
   a. wait until puberty to see if it descends
   b. receive injections of growth hormone to encourage the testicle to descend
   c. undergo surgery promptly to correct the condition
   d. receive psychological counseling to help him accept his condition

2. Amenorrhea is a normal condition during
   a. pregnancy
   b. periods of emotional stress
   c. weight gain
   d. exercise

3. Dysmenorrhea refers to
   a. failure to begin menstruation at an appropriate age
   b. painful menstruation
   c. vaginal bleeding between periods
   d. excessively heavy menstrual bleeding

4. Alicia, age 16, has contracted gonorrhea. She should be advised to
   a. inform her sexual partners
   b. practice the rhythm method
   c. receive a monthly gynecological examination
   d. report the case to the local authorities

5. Which of the following is a possible complication of a sexually transmitted disease?
   a. tunica vaginalis
   b. menarche
   c. sexual reproduction
   d. infertility

6. Safer sex practices include
   a. using a condom during intercourse
   b. knowing your partner
   c. having only oral sex
   d. using oral contraceptives

7. Which of the following is an advantage of condom use?
   a. protects against ovarian and endometrial cancer
   b. increases spontaneity
   c. protects against AIDS transmission
   d. can be about 97% effective in preventing pregnancy

8. One role of the nurse in counseling a pregnant teen is to
   a. determine the best pregnancy option available for the teen
   b. encourage the teen to name the father of her child so that he can help support the family
   c. enlist the teen in a self-help group
   d. provide a supportive environment in which the teen can explore her pregnancy choices

---

B. True or false. Write *T* for a true statement and *F* for a false statement.

1. ___ Cryptorchidism increases the chance of testicular cancer later in life.

2. ___ Secondary dysmenorrhea may be caused by pelvic inflammatory disease.

3. ___ Teens are at high risk for contracting STDs because their partners frequently fail to tell them when they have been infected.

4. ___ An early sign of syphilis is a lesion or painless ulcer at the site of contact.

5. ___ Symptoms of genital herpes include a thick, creamy discharge.

6. ___ An STD infection in a preadolescent child may be a sign of sexual abuse.

7. ___ Oral contraceptives are statistically the most effective appropriate method for a sexually active teenager to use to avoid pregnancy.

8. ___ The rhythm method is an effective method of preventing pregnancy in adolescents.

9. ___ A noncontraceptive benefit of using birth control pills is that they protect against pelvic inflammatory disease.

10. ___ High self-esteem increases the risk that a girl will become pregnant.

SUGGESTED ACTIVITIES

- Invite a nurse or counselor from an adolescent pregnancy prevention program to speak to the class.
- Interview a teenage mother about the type of information and support she received from medical professionals during her pregnancy.

- Make a display of the various types of birth control available, listing their advantages and disadvantages to teens.
- Discuss the issues surrounding abortion, and role play a counseling session with a pregnant teen requesting an abortion.

BIBLIOGRAPHY

Bondi, E. E., B. V. Jegasothy, and G. S. Lazarus. *Dermatology.* Norwalk, CT: Appleton and Lange, 1991.

Grimes, D. *Infectious Diseases.* St. Louis, MO: Mosby–Year Book, 1991.

Habif, T. P. *Clinical Dermatology: A Color Guide to Diagnosis and Therapy,* 2nd ed. St. Louis, MO: Mosby–Year Book, 1990.

Marks, M. G. *Broadribb's Introductory Pediatric Nursing,* 4th ed. Philadelphia: J. B. Lippincott, 1994.

Rosenstein, B. J. and P. D. Forsarelli. *Pediatric Pearls: The Handbook of Practical Pediatrics.* Chicago: Year Book Medical Publishers, 1989.

Rudolph, A. M., J. I. E. Hoffman, and C. D. Rudolph. *Rudolph's Pediatrics,* 19th ed. Norwalk, CT: Appleton and Lange, 1991.

Shapiro, P. J. *Basic Maternal/Pediatric Nursing.* Albany, NY: Delmar, 1995.

Thompson, E. D. and J. W. Ashwill. *Pediatric Nursing: An Introductory Text,* 6th ed. Philadelphia: W. B. Saunders, 1992.

Wong, D. L. *Whaley & Wong's Essentials of Pediatric Nursing,* 5th ed. St Louis, MO: Mosby–Year Book, 1995.

CHAPTER

27

*M*usculoskeletal Conditions

OBJECTIVES

AFTER STUDYING THIS CHAPTER, THE STUDENT SHOULD BE ABLE TO:

- NAME FOUR MUSCULOSKELETAL CONDITIONS THAT AFFECT INFANTS AND TODDLERS AND DESCRIBE THEIR CAUSES, SYMPTOMS, TREATMENT, AND NURSING CARE.

- NAME FOUR MUSCULOSKELETAL CONDITIONS THAT AFFECT PRESCHOOL AND SCHOOL-AGE CHILDREN AND DESCRIBE THEIR CAUSES, SYMPTOMS, TREATMENT, AND NURSING CARE.

- IDENTIFY THREE COMMON SPORTS INJURIES OF CHILDREN.

- IDENTIFY THE MOST COMMON TYPE OF CHILDHOOD FRACTURE REQUIRING HOSPITALIZATION.

- DESCRIBE NURSING CARE FOR THE CHILD IN A CAST, TRACTION, OR BRACE.

- NAME TWO MUSCULOSKELETAL CONDITIONS THAT AFFECT ADOLESCENTS AND DESCRIBE THEIR CAUSES, SYMPTOMS, TREATMENT, AND NURSING CARE.

KEY TERMS

PSEUDOHYPERTROPHY	STRESS FRACTURE
LORDOSIS	FRACTURE
GOWER'S SIGN	TRACTION
STRAINS	SCOLIOSIS
SPRAINS	LIMB SALVAGE

*m*usculoskeletal conditions of children may be congenital or a result of disease or injury. These conditions can have a significant impact on growth and development, resulting in altered motor function and impaired mobility. Through accurate assessment, nurses can help ensure early diagnosis and treatment of these conditions, thus maintaining mobility and preventing complications.

OVERVIEW OF THE SYSTEM

The skeletal system is composed of more than 200 bones. Along with the musculoskeletal system, it protects and supports the body and facilitates coordinated movements.

There are four classifications of bones, based on their form and shape: long, short, flat, and irregular, Figure 27–1. Both the diameter and length of the bone change as it grows. Growth in diameter occurs on the external surface of the bone as new bone is created. Growth in length occurs at the epiphyseal plates, located at the ends of the long bones. Injury to this area in a growing child is always potentially serious, because it may stop or alter the child's growth (Scoles 1988).

Joints connect the bones of the skeleton, permitting movement and flexibility. Joints are classified as fibrous, cartilaginous, or synovial, Figure 27–2. Skeletal muscles provide contour and shape over bones and are directly responsible for movement.

TYPES OF BONES		
Type of Bone	**Example**	**Function**
Long	Femur	Provide support to the body
Short	Tarsals, metatarsals	Facilitate motion within parts of the body
Flat	Sternum, skull	Provide protection to the internal organs
Irregular	Vertebrae	Vary in size and shape and accommodate other structures

Figure 27–1

TYPES OF JOINTS		
Type of Joint	**Example**	**Movement**
Fibrous	Bones of the skull in childhood	Very limited
Cartilaginous	Epiphyseal plates, symphysis pubis	Slightly movable
Synovial	Elbow, shoulder, fingers	The most movable type of joint

Figure 27–2

INFANT AND TODDLER

CONGENITAL HIP DYSPLASIA

Congenital hip dysplasia, also called congenital dislocated hip, is one of the most common congenital anomalies. It occurs in about 1 in 500 to 1,000 births. The degree of dysplasia varies from acetabular dysplasia to subluxation to complete dislocation. In acetabular dysplasia, the acetabulum is shallow, but the femoral head remains in place in the acetabulum. In subluxation, incomplete dislocation occurs. The head of the femur stays in contact with the acetabulum but is partially displaced. The most severe form of dysplasia is complete dislocation, in which the femoral head loses contact with the acetabulum and is displaced.

Assessment of the hips is performed as part of the routine newborn assessment. In an infant under 3 weeks of age, hip stability can be assessed by placing the infant supine with hips and knees flexed while abducting and lifting the femurs. If a click is heard or felt as the femur enters the acetabulum, the infant is said to have a positive Ortolani's sign. Other indicators of hip dysplasia include uneven gluteal folds and uneven knee height (Schaming et al. 1990).

Treatment should begin as soon as possible after diagnosis. On an infant or toddler, three or more cloth diapers pinned front to back or some type of abduction device, such as the Pavlik harness, may be used to abduct the hip area. This treatment may be all that is needed to maintain proper alignment until the hip is stabilized, usually within about three to six months. The older child may need to be placed in traction for gradual reduction of hip and flexor muscles, and then placed into a hip spica cast for approximately four to six months.

Parent education is an important part of the treatment plan. Explain to parents using drawings and demonstration how the hips must be kept abducted and flexed. If the child is in a hip spica cast, a thorough explanation must be given regarding cast care, positioning, and handling, as well as proper diapering and skin care.

CLUBFOOT

Clubfoot, or talipes, is a congenital deformity in which the foot is twisted out of its normal position. Specific deformities are differentiated depending on the specific malposition of the ankle and foot. Unilateral clubfoot is more common than bilateral, and the condition occurs twice as often in boys as in girls.

Treatment involves manipulation and casting to reposition the foot and ankle. Casting is performed in a series of steps to gradually stretch and contract structures around the foot. Casts are changed every few days for one to two weeks and then every one to two weeks. Correction usually occurs by six to eight weeks. Corrective shoes and nightly splinting are used for an additional three months. Surgical correction may be necessary if manipulation is ineffective. Follow-up and reevaluation are necessary to prevent recurrence (Kyzer 1991).

Teach parents how to care for the infant in a cast and how to identify potential problems. The developing infant needs stimulation and comfort while in the cast. Parents are encouraged to hold and cuddle the infant.

TORTICOLLIS

Torticollis, a disorder that occurs as a result of a shortened sternocleidomastoid muscle, is usually diagnosed in the newborn period. The infant's head is tilted to the affected side, with the neck flexed and the chin rotated toward the opposite shoulder.

When diagnosed early, torticollis is treated with passive stretching exercises. If the child has sufficient normal muscle, the muscle will stretch as the child grows (Brewer 1990). An operation to release the muscle may be performed if exercises are unsuccessful. Nursing care includes observing the newborn for normal range of motion of the neck and teaching parents how to perform exercises and activities that stimulate the infant to turn the head.

RICKETS

Rickets is a disorder of bone formation resulting from a deficiency of vitamin D, calcium, or phosphorus. It may be caused by inadequate dietary intake, poor absorption of nutrients, or lack of exposure to sunlight. The bones of the legs and skull are commonly affected. Bones are weakened and bent out of shape, so bowlegs and knock knees are often seen. The child may have deformed bone shaping, delayed calcification of teeth, and vague symptoms of apathy, irritability, shortened attention span, and pain.

Rickets can be treated by exposure to sunlight and by a diet with milk and milk products, enriched cereals and breads, and fish products (cod liver oil, herring, mackerel, salmon, tuna, and sardines). Nursing care includes teaching parents about the importance of dietary intake of vitamin D, calcium, and phosphorus.

PRESCHOOL AND SCHOOL-AGE CHILD

DUCHENNE'S MUSCULAR DYSTROPHY

Description. Duchenne's muscular dystrophy is an X-linked recessive genetic disorder that causes a progressive degeneration and weakening of skeletal muscles, eventually leading to death. It is the most common form of muscular dystrophy and affects boys almost exclusively.

Symptoms. Indications of muscle weakness are usually seen in the preschool child between the ages of 3 and 5 years. The child may have a history of delays in motor development, especially in beginning to walk. Initial symptoms include frequent falls and difficulty in climbing stairs, running, or riding a bicycle.

One of the classic signs of Duchenne's muscular dystrophy is **pseudohypertrophy** (seeming enlargement) of the muscles, particularly those of the calf. The muscles appear large, but the muscle fibers are replaced by fatty deposits, leaving nonfunctioning tissue. As the disorder continues, the child becomes progressively weaker. Signs of increasing muscle weakness include a waddling gait, **lordosis** (abnormal forward curvature of the lumbar spine), and **Gower's sign**, a characteristic self-climbing movement in which the child uses the arm muscles to compensate for weak hip extensor muscles in rising to an upright position.

Treatment. The disorder is incurable and most children die of respiratory complications, usually during adolescence. The goal is to maintain muscle function for as long as possible. Range of motion is maintained through exercises that are performed several times a day and by activities of daily living. Bracing and surgery to release contractures may help maintain muscle functioning.

Nursing Care. Nursing care involves helping the child and family to cope with a progressive, fatal disease; intervening to delay and reduce disabilities; maximizing the child's potential; and assisting the family to deal with the effects of the disease on all family members.

JUVENILE RHEUMATOID ARTHRITIS

Description. Juvenile rheumatoid arthritis (JRA) is a chronic inflammatory disease that affects primarily the joints but may also occur in a systemic form, affecting internal organs. The disease usually occurs in children under the age of 16 and gradually subsides by adulthood. Inflammation of the joint muscle leads to destruction of cartilage and bone in the joints.

Symptoms. The child with JRA has periods of exacerbation and remission of symptoms. Common symptoms include morning stiffness, swollen joints, a limp, increased fatigue, fever, irritability, anorexia, and failure to grow at expected rates (if the epiphyseal plates of the long bones are damaged). The knee, ankle, wrist, and finger joints are most often affected (Page-Goertz 1989).

Treatment. Treatment consists of anti-inflammatory drugs, splinting to prevent flexion contractures, and physical therapy. Nonsteroidal anti-inflammatory drugs are prescribed to decrease inflammation and relieve pain. Immunosuppressive drugs and corticosteroids may be prescribed for children with severe disease (Mosca and Sherry 1990, Reilly 1992).

Physical therapy is important to maintain maximum strength and range of motion and to prevent deformities. Activities performed in water are more easily tolerated, so pool activities are encouraged. Heat (from tub baths, showers, heating pads, or electric blankets) may help to decrease stiffness in the joints.

Nursing Care. Nursing care includes helping the child maintain as many normal activities as possible. The nurse promotes the general well-being of the child by encouraging good posture and body mechanics, weight control to prevent undue strain on the joints, and school attendance to maintain contact with friends. The nurse also provides the child and family with information about ways to relieve inflammation, exercises to maintain joint functioning and strength, methods to relieve pain, and support groups that provide help in coping with a chronic illness.

LEGG-CALVÉ-PERTHES DISEASE

Description. Legg-Calvé-Perthes disease is a disorder that occurs when circulation to the femoral head is disrupted, resulting in necrosis of the femoral head. The disease is most often diagnosed in children between the ages of 4 and 9 years and affects boys more often than girls (Hensiger and Fielding 1990).

Symptoms. Symptoms may develop over a period of weeks to months. The child may complain of pain in the hip or other areas of the leg, such as the groin, thigh, or knee. Movement of the hip increases the pain and rest decreases it. The child may limp occasionally on the affected side and have limited motion in the affected hip.

Treatment. The goal of treatment is to decrease or prevent deformity of the femoral head by keeping it within the acetabulum. Initial treatment is rest to decrease inflammation and restore motion. Traction may be used to stretch the hip muscles and increase the range of motion of the hip. Other treatment measures include use of nonweight-bearing devices (such as abduction braces, leg casts, and harness slings) or surgical reconstruction of the hip joint. Early diagnosis and treatment improve the child's prognosis (Dunst 1990, Thompson and Salter 1987).

Nursing Care. Nursing care involves teaching family members about the use and care of nonweight-bearing devices and how to carry out activities of daily living with these devices. Children on initial bed rest can be encouraged in activities or hobbies that do not require movement (coloring, puzzles, reading, and drawing, among others).

OSTEOMYELITIS

Description. Osteomyelitis is an infection of the bone, usually caused by *Staphylococcus* organisms. The long bones of the legs are the most common sites of infection. Bacteria may migrate to the bone through the bloodstream or enter the bone directly through a lesion or open fracture.

Within the closed space of the bone, edema and inflammation cause severe and constant pain in the affected area. An abscess may form, increasing pressure within the bone and causing the death of bone tissue. Without treatment, the infection may spread throughout the body.

Symptoms. The child may be irritable, anorexic, and weak, with a fever and localized edema and warmth in the extremity. Severe, localized pain is common with movement of the extremity. The child may avoid moving the extremity, holding it in a semiflexed position.

Treatment. Blood cultures are obtained, and intravenous antibiotics prescribed. Initially the child requires comfort measures such as bed rest, analgesics, and immobilization of the extremity with splints or casts. If the child does not improve, surgery may be required to remove areas of dead bone. Early diagnosis and treatment can help to prevent permanent damage to the bone and extremity.

Nursing Care. Nursing care includes giving analgesics for pain and positioning the extremity to maintain comfort. Assess circulation in the extremities and monitor vital signs at least every four hours. Encourage sedentary play and diversional activities to help the child deal with immobilization. A diet high in calories, protein, vitamin C, and calcium helps to promote bone healing. Figure 27–3 summarizes nursing care for the child with osteomyelitis.

SPORTS INJURIES

Contact sports often produce acute musculoskeletal injuries, such as tears in ligaments and tendons or bone fractures. Injuries to the knee are common among children of all age groups. A blow to the side of the knee can result in ligament injury or long bone fracture. Because the epiphyseal plates of young athletes have not closed, the plates are more easily injured than are the surrounding ligaments. These injuries have the potential to affect the child's overall growth.

Overuse may produce **strains** (pulling of a ligament) and **sprains** (muscle injury caused by overstretching). Early treatment for sprains and strains depends on the extent and type of injury and consists of rest, ice, compression, and elevation for 24 to 36 hours after the injury occurs. Complete tears require surgical intervention (Mourad and Droste 1993).

NURSING CARE PLAN: Osteomyelitis

NURSING DIAGNOSIS	GOAL(S)
Pain	Child states and shows relief of pain.
Lack of diversional activities	Child participates in play appropriate to age.
Risk for infection	By discharge, the child maintains vital signs within normal limits, and wound is free from purulent discharge.

Figure 27–3 *Nursing care plan for the child with osteomyelitis*

NURSING INTERVENTION	RATIONALE
Observe for crying, statements of pain, and guarding behavior.	Information is needed for baseline data.
Assess pain using a pain scale (see Chapter 31).	Provides an objective measurement.
Administer prescribed analgesics and monitor effectiveness.	Analgesics help control pain.
Support and maintain proper body alignment.	Reduces stress on the limb and prevents trauma.
Avoid unnecessary handling of the extremity.	Moving the limb can cause increased pain.
Provide toys and activity appropriate to child's age.	Play is a child's way of expressing him- or herself.
Encourage visits by parents and siblings and parental involvement in the child's care.	Helps prevent disruption of the family structure.
Encourage the child to maintain contact with peers.	Maintaining contact is important to prevent isolation.
Monitor vital signs every 4 hours and as needed.	Changes in vital signs are signs of infection.
Assess for pain, redness, swelling, or drainage at the site every 4 hours.	Any change may indicate further infection.
Maintain good handwashing technique.	Prevents the spread of bacteria.
When indicated, change dressing according to hospital policy.	Proper skin care is the key to preventing infection.
Administer antibiotics as ordered.	Antibiotics provide bacteriocidal action.
Maintain nutrition with a diet high in protein, calories, and vitamin C.	Diet helps promote bone healing.

Figure 27–3   *continued*

Stress fractures are fractures caused by repeated, prolonged stress on a bone. They rarely occur in very young children, but are more frequent in children 10 years of age or older. Most stress fractures can be prevented by proper conditioning and preseason training. Stress fractures usually occur after a rapid increase in a training activity over a short period of time. The pain of a stress fracture is usually worse during and immediately after activity but eventually becomes constant. In most cases, stress fractures are treated with immobilization and restricted activity until symptoms decrease and x-rays show evidence of new bone formation (Smrcina 1992).

FRACTURES OF THE EXTREMITIES

A **fracture** is a break that occurs in a bone, usually as a result of injury. Fractures are a common injury at any age but are more likely to occur in children as a result of traumatic injury from everyday activities. Most fractures are the result of a forceful blow. Fractures that occur in a bone weakened by disease processes are called pathological or spontaneous fractures (Campbell and Campbell 1991).

Because children's bones are still growing, they heal much more quickly than adults' bones. A fracture of the femur in a newborn heals completely in three to four weeks. In an adult, the same fracture would take six to eight weeks or longer to heal (Scoles 1988).

Types of Fractures. Fractures are described as open or closed, depending on whether a break also occurs in the skin (Barrett and Bryant 1990). Fractures may be further classified in terms of appearance:

greenstick: incomplete
complete: skin broken, fragments separated
bend: deformed, bent
buckle: raised
comminuted: fragmented
spiral: curved, twisting

Fracture of the Femur. A fracture of the femur is the most common type of childhood fracture treated in the hospital. Children who are involved in automobile accidents or fall from substantial heights may suffer a fractured femur. A fractured femur in an infant is uncommon and may be the result of child abuse (Cunningham 1991).

When the femur is fractured, strong tendon spasms occur, causing poor alignment of the fragments. Casting at this time is not possible. The child under 2 years of age and 40 pounds (18 kg) is placed in Bryant's traction for 7 to 14 days to restore alignment, Figure 27–6. A young child is then placed in a cast for three to four weeks. The child is positioned with hips flexed and both knees extended in a vertical position. The child's buttocks should be raised far enough off the bed that a nurse's hand can be placed beneath them. An older child is placed in 90-90 traction for four to six weeks and then casted for three to four weeks. In 90-90 traction, the lower leg is placed in a boot cast, and a skeletal pin or wire is placed through the distal fragment of the femur, Figure 27–7. Traction is maintained so that the femur is at a 90-degree angle to the bed. Buck's or Russell's traction may also be used.

Casting. A simple fracture of the limb may be treated by setting the bone and applying a cast. Casts are made from plaster of paris or, more commonly, from synthetic, lighter-weight, water-resistant materials such as fiberglass. A plaster of paris cast takes several hours to days to dry. Synthetic casts dry in a few hours and come in colors and designs.

A wet cast must be handled gently and supported with the flat of the hand or on pillows to avoid indentations that may cause pressure on the skin and lead to altered circulation and skin impairment. Turning the child frequently aids in the drying process.

Use of cool-air dryers and regular fans to circulate air may help dry the cast. Heated dryers are not used because they cause the cast to dry from the outside in, weakening the cast.

A protective barrier must be formed over the rough cast edges to prevent abrasion of the underlying skin. After the cast is dry, the raw edges can be protected by a "petaled" edge. "Petals" can be made from adhesive tape or mole skin cut approximately 1½ inches wide. These are placed over the edge of the cast, with each petal overlapping the next to form a smooth edge, Figure 27–4 (Skale 1992).

Swelling of the extremity may continue in the first few hours after cast application. If

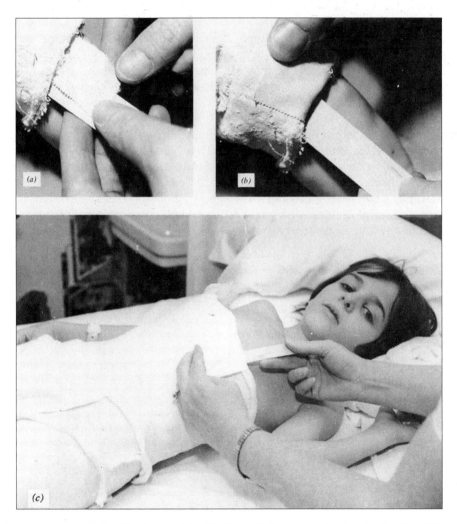

Figure 27–4   *Petaling a cast after it is clean and dry (a) Strips of adhesive are placed under the edge of the cast. (b, c) Adhesive strips are held in place with a tongue blade, and the upper edge is folded over the cast edge. After the edges are covered, the outer edges of the adhesive are covered with an encircling piece of adhesive to keep them in place.*

pressure is not relieved, the cast may become a tourniquet, reducing circulation and causing neurovascular damage. Keeping the extremity elevated helps prevent further swelling. Signs of impaired neurocirculatory function include blueness or coldness of a distal part, lack of a peripheral pulse, edema that does not improve with elevation, uncontrolled pain, and numbness or tingling of the affected extremity. Any of these symptoms requires immediate follow-up.

Nursing Care. Several nursing interventions may be implemented to help keep the cast dry and clean. If the cast surrounds the perineal area, cover the cast with plastic in order to prevent urine saturation. Occasionally, the child may be placed in a Bradford frame, a canvas-covered turning frame, to help keep urine and feces away from the cast (Schaming et al. 1990). Diapers can be folded narrowly and tucked under the edges of the cast. Diapers need to be changed immediately, before they become saturated with urine. A urine collection bag may be used for the infant. Plastic pants tend to hold

moisture and should not be used. Keeping the child in a semi-Fowler's position helps prevent soaking of the back of the cast. Educating parents about home cast care is essential. Figure 27–5 provides an example of home cast care instructions for parents.

Traction. Traction involves the use of weights and pulleys to realign bone fragments, reduce dislocations, immobilize fractures, provide rest for an extremity, help prevent contracture deformities, and allow preoperative and postoperative positioning and alignment. Significant pull is needed to restore alignment and overcome muscle spasms. There are two forms of traction: skin and skeletal.

Skin traction is applied to the skin surfaces. Examples of skin traction are Bryant's, Buck's, Russell's, and cervical halter traction, Figure 27–6. Nurses may assist with the application of skin traction and may remove and reapply skin traction according to physician's orders and institutional policies, provided that someone manually maintains the traction during the rewrapping process (Morris et al. 1988a).

Home Cast Care Instructions

- Keep the casted extremity elevated on pillows as directed by the physician.
- *Do not* allow the child to put anything inside the cast. Small items that might be placed inside the cast should be kept away from the child.
- If desired, clean the cast with a damp cloth and a dry, nonchlorine bleach cleanser if it becomes soiled.
- Contact your physician *immediately* if you note any of the following in or around the cast:

  - Pain, numbness, burning, or tingling
  - Foul odor
  - Discoloration of skin (darker or lighter than a comparable extremity)
  - Swelling (fingers or toes)
  - Cold fingers or toes not relieved by application of socks or mittens
  - A change in the ability to move the fingers or toes
- Notify the physician if the cast becomes loose and allows movement.

Figure 27–5 (*Adapted from* Information Sheet: Cast Care. *Sioux Valley Hospital, Sioux Falls, SD*)

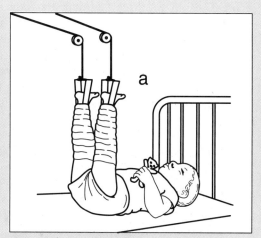

Bryant's Traction

Used for fractured femur in children under 2 years of age and under 18 kg (40 pounds). Also used as preparation for surgical repair of congenital hip deformities.

The child is positioned with hips flexed and both knees extended in a vertical position. The child's buttocks should be raised far enough off the bed that a nurse's hand can be placed beneath them.

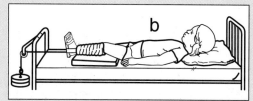

Buck's Traction

Used for arthritic conditions and as a temporary measure to provide support to a fracture before surgery.

A foam rubber boot is applied on the lateral surfaces of one or more extremities. The boot is held in place with elastic bandages. Weights are then attached to a spreader bar connecting the distal end of the boot.

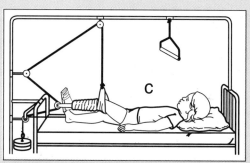

Russell's Traction

A modification of Buck's traction, with the addition of a sling under the affected leg. Allows more movement in bed and permits flexion of the knee joint.

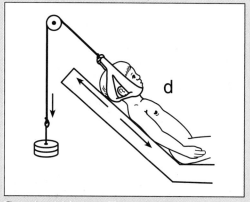

Cervical Halter Traction

Used to treat arthritic conditions of the cervical vertebrae and muscles.

A halter is fitted over the head and chin. Straps are attached to a spreader bar with ropes and weights attached to the spreader.

Figure 27–6   *Types of skin traction. (Illustrations from D. B. Broadwell Jackson and R. B. Saunders.* Child Health Nursing. *Philadelphia: J. B. Lippincott, 1993)*

Skeletal traction is applied directly to the bone by inserting a stainless steel pin or wire called a Steinmann pin or Kirschner wire (K-wire) through the end of the fractured long bone. The pin protrudes through the skin on both sides of the extremity, and weights are attached to a rope that is tied to a spreader bar for the purpose of traction. Examples of skeletal traction are 90-90 traction and Crutchfield tongs, Figure 27–7. Once initiated, traction must be maintained over long periods of time to be effective. Weights cannot be lifted or removed and must hang freely. Release of the weight could cause an increase in muscle spasms, displacing the fracture fragments (Morris et al. 1988b).

The site of the pin or wire insertion is prone to infection and must be cleansed to remove secretions and prevent infection (Jones-Walton 1991). The sites are monitored frequently for signs of infection and for loosening or slippage of the pins. The tips of the pins are covered with protective material to prevent puncture of other parts of the body.

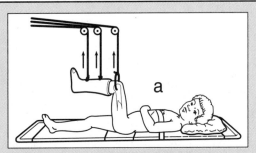

Ninety-Ninety Skeletal Traction

The most common type of skeletal traction. The lower leg is placed in a boot cast and a skeletal pin or wire is placed in the distal fragment of the femur. Traction is maintained so that the femur is positioned at a 90-degree angle to the bed.

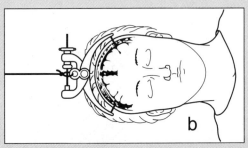

Cervical Traction

Usually accomplished with the use of Crutchfield tongs. The tongs are inserted through burr holes in the skull, and weights are attached to the hyperextended head. Immobilization of the fracture until healing takes place is essential.

Figure 27–7 *Types of skeletal traction (a adapted from D. B. Broadwell Jackson and R. B. Saunders.* Child Health Nursing. *Philadelphia: J. B. Lippincott, 1993.*

Nursing Care. Nursing interventions for children in traction include the following measures:

- Keep the child's body in proper alignment.
- Ensure that weights hang freely from the bed and are never removed without the physician's order.
- Check the pulse below the affected area and compare with the pulse in the opposite extremity.
- Report immediately any changes in color of the skin and nail bed and any alterations in sensation and motor ability.
- Observe for signs of pressure sores.

The child in traction may experience discomfort or pain because of muscle spasms. Pain relief is provided with muscle relaxants and analgesics. Limited mobility and forced confinement pose challenges to the child's care. Play, participation in self-care, encouragement with school work, and opportunities to socialize all stimulate the child and promote normal growth and development. Maintaining contact with peers is extremely important and is encouraged.

ADOLESCENT

SCOLIOSIS

Description.   **Scoliosis** is a lateral S-shaped curvature of the spine that occurs most often in adolescent girls. It is classified as structural or functional in origin. Structural scoliosis may be idiopathic, congenital, or secondary to other disorders such as muscular dystrophy. It results in loss of flexibility of the spine and deformity. Functional scoliosis results from poor posture, and treatment of the underlying problem usually corrects the misalignment.

Symptoms.   The lateral curvature of the spine results in uneven height of the shoulders and hips, which may be identified when the child bends forward at the waist, Figure 27–8. Pain is usually not present (Brosnon 1991).

Treatment.   Treatment involves straightening and realigning the spine through conservative measures, surgery, or a combination of both approaches. Conservative measures include exercises and bracing. The Milwaukee brace is one of the most successful types of braces for scoliosis. This brace is individually fitted from the neck to the hips and initially is worn continually except when bathing. The child wears the brace for six months to two years and should continue to perform normal activities of daily living while wearing the brace. In addition, exercises should be performed daily to maintain spinal and abdominal muscle tone. The brace is adjusted regularly as the child grows, and wearing time is gradually decreased as the bone matures.

Curvatures also may be corrected with casts or halofemoral traction. This form of traction consists of weights attached by a halo device to

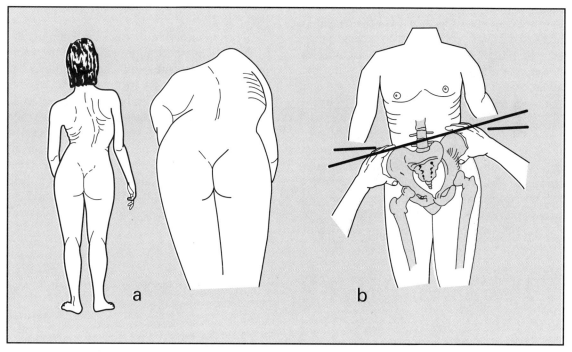

Figure 27–8   *Scoliosis (a) Lateral S-shaped curve with right rib hump on forward flexion and noticeable shoulder obliquity (b) Pelvic obliquity*

the skull with counterweights attached to the femur. Surgical treatment is used to realign and straighten the severely curved spine. During surgery, a Harrington rod or other device is inserted to correct the curve, and the spine is fused. The Harrington rod is a metal rod with clips that are attached to vertebrae to permanently fuse them. After surgery, the child is placed in a body cast or brace, which is worn for several months (Cotton 1991). More recently the Luque rod has been used. This rod is a flexible L-shaped metal rod attached with wires to the spinous process of the vertebrae. After surgery, the child does not have to be immobilized and may be up and walking within a few days (Cotton 1991).

Nursing Care. Scoliosis is a slowly progressive condition that may not be diagnosed until adolescence. Supportive care is needed to help the adolescent cope with concerns about body image and comply with the treatment program. Encourage the adolescent wearing a brace to maintain correct posture and perform exercises that strengthen the back muscles (Olsen et al. 1991). Teach both parents and the adolescent how to properly apply and wear the brace and to watch for signs of skin irritation from rubbing or chafing.

Adolescents who require surgical treatment need to be prepared with specific information about the surgical procedure and care after surgery. Postoperative nursing assessment focuses special attention on neurological and respiratory status. Assess the extremities for circulation, motion, and sensation frequently.

Encourage coughing and deep breathing at least every two hours. Surgery can be very painful and frequent administration of analgesics may be necessary. Physical therapy is begun as soon as possible after surgery, using range-of-motion exercises. Providing diversional activities and encouraging participation in decision making are important components of care of the adolescent patient (Mason 1991).

OSTEOSARCOMA

Osteosarcoma, also called osteogenic sarcoma, is a rapidly growing tumor of the bone that usually occurs in adolescent or young adult males. The primary tumor site is usually in an area of active bone growth, commonly the distal femur. The adolescent may complain of bone tenderness and increasing pain at the site that is not related to activity and may increase at night.

Treatment involves either limb amputation or removal of the tumor without amputation, called **limb salvage**, and chemotherapy. The prognosis depends on treatment, primary site, and whether metastasis has occurred. Overall, 50% of children with osteosarcoma survive long term. Nursing care centers on assisting the patient and family as they deal with a life-threatening condition and the potential for altered body image. Provide emotional support to help the family cope with the diagnosis and address concerns about surgery and treatment (Caswell and Ehland 1989).

REVIEW QUESTIONS

A. Multiple choice. Select the best answer.

1. Which of the following assessment data would indicate a cast properly applied to a lower extremity?
    a. pallor, cyanosis, or discoloration of the skin
    b. edema of the toes
    c. warm, dry toes
    d. loss of pedal pulse

2. An appropriate nursing intervention for a child in skeletal traction would be to
    a. reapply traction as needed
    b. observe pin sites for infection
    c. remove traction weights when repositioning the child
    d. rest weights on bed frame

3. Which of the following statements best describes Duchenne's muscular dystrophy?
    a. It is inherited as an autosomal dominant disorder.
    b. It is characterized by remissions and exacerbations.
    c. Symptoms include a waddling gait and lordosis.
    d. Onset is usually in late childhood.

4. Stress fractures are commonly caused by
    a. a rapid increase in a training activity over a short period
    b. excessive training activities over a long period of time
    c. jogging over rough terrain
    d. sudden change in weight distribution on impact with the ground

5. A muscular condition resulting from abnormal contraction or injury of the sterno-cleidomastoid muscle is
    a. brachial plexus palsy
    b. lordosis
    c. rickets
    d. torticollis

B. True or false. Write *T* for a true statement and *F* for a false statement.

1. ___ The purpose of the Harrington rod in scoliosis treatment is to straighten the spine.

2. ___ The Milwaukee brace is worn up to 16 hours a day until the spine stops growing.

3. Which of the following statements is (are) true about Legg-Calvé-Perthes disease?
    a. ___ It is more likely to occur in girls than in boys.
    b. ___ It requires long-term treatment.
    c. ___ It can result in permanent disability.
    d. ___ It is treated initially with rest.

4. ___ Osteomyelitis is an infection of the bone caused by bacterial infection.

5. ___ Musculoskeletal dysfunction can adversely affect the child's self-concept.

SUGGESTED ACTIVITIES

- Visit an orthopedic clinic to see how casts and braces are applied.

- Discuss ways to help parents provide care for children who are immobilized in casts or traction.

- Plan age-appropriate play activities for a child in a cast or traction.

- Invite a child with a musculoskeletal condition to the classroom to discuss his or her perception of the particular condition. Have students prepare their questions in advance and include a discussion of what nurses can do and say to make hospital stays easier for children with these conditions.

BIBLIOGRAPHY

Barrett, J. B., and B. H. Bryant. Fractures: Types, treatment, perioperative implications. *AORN Journal* 52 (1990): 755–771.

Brewer, K. Identifying and treating torticollis. *Clinical-Management* 10, no. 4 (1990): 19–21.

Broadwell Jackson, D., and R. B. Saunders. *Child Health Nursing*. Philadelphia: J. B. Lippincott, 1993.

Brosnon, H. Nursing management of the adolescent with idiopathic scoliosis. *Nursing Clinics of North America* 26, no. 1 (1991): 17–31.

Campbell, L. S., and J. D. Campbell. Musculoskeletal trauma in children. *Critical Care Nursing Clinics of North America* 3, no. 3 (1991): 445–456.

Caswell, L. J., and J. M. Ehland. Don't bump my bed, don't touch my feet. *Journal of Pediatric Oncology Nursing* 6, no. 4 (1989): 111–120.

Cotton, L. A. Unit rod segmental spinal instrumentation for the treatment of neuromuscular scoliosis. *Orthopaedic Nursing* 10, no. 5 (1991): 17–23.

Cunningham, N. Physical abuse in children: Recognition and management. *Emergency Pediatrics* 4, no. 1 (1991): 13–15.

Curry, L. C., and L. Y. Gibson. Congenital hip dislocation: The importance of early detection and comprehensive treatment. *Nurse Practitioner* 17, no. 5 (1992): 49–55.

Dunst, R. M. Legg-Calvé-Perthes disease. *Orthopaedic Nursing* 9, no. 2 (1990): 18–27.

Hensinger, R. N., and J. W. Fielding. The lower limb. Pp. 727–766 in R. T. Morrissy, ed. *Lovell and Winter's Pediatric Orthopaedics*, 3rd ed. Philadelphia: J. B. Lippincott, 1990.

Hiller, L. B., and C. K. Wade. Upper extremity functional assessment scales in children with Duchenne muscular dystrophy. *Archives of Physical Medicine and Rehabilitation* 73, no. 6 (1992): 523–534.

Jones-Walton, P. Clinical standards in skeletal traction pin site care. *Orthopaedic Nursing* 10, no. 2 (1991): 12–16.

Kyzer, S. Congenital idiopathic clubfoot. *Orthopaedic Nursing* 10, no. 4 (1991): 11–18.

Mason, K. J. Congenital orthopedic anomalies and their impact on the family. *Nursing Clinics of North America* 26, no. 1 (1991): 1–16.

Morris, L., S. Kraft, S. Tessem, and S. Reinisch. Nursing the patient in traction. *RN* 51, no. 1 (1988a): 26–31.

Morris, L., S. Kraft, S. Tessem, and S. Reinisch. Special care for skeletal traction. *RN* 51, no. 2 (1988b): 24–29.

Mosca, V. S., and D. D. Sherry. Juvenile rheumatoid arthritis. Pp. 298–324 in R. T. Morrissy, ed. *Lovell and Winter's Pediatric Orthopaedics*, 3rd ed. Philadelphia: J. B. Lippincott, 1990.

Mourad, L. A., and M. M. Droste. *The Nursing Process in the Care of Adults with Orthopaedic Conditions*, 3rd ed. Albany, NY: Delmar Publishers, 1993.

Olsen, B., L. Ustanko, and S. Warner. The patient in a halo brace: Striving for normalcy in body image and self-concept. *Orthopaedic Nursing* 10, no. 1 (1991): 44–50.

Page-Goertz, S. S. Even children have arthritis. *Pediatric Nursing* 15 (1989): 11–16.

Reilly, P. Juvenile rheumatoid arthritis. Pp. 336–354 in P. L. Jackson and J. Vessey, eds. *Primary Care of the Child with Chronic Conditions*. St. Louis, MO: C. V. Mosby, 1992.

Rudolph, A. M., J. I. E. Hoffman, and C. D. Rudolph. *Rudolph's Pediatrics*, 19th ed. Norwalk, CT: Appleton and Lange, 1991.

Schaming, D., et al. When babies are born with orthopedic problems. *RN* 53, no. 4 (1990): 62–66.

Scoles, P. V. *Pediatric Orthopedics in Clinical Practice*. Chicago: Year Book Medical Publishers, 1988.

Skale, N. *Manual of Pediatric Nursing Procedures.* Philadelphia: J. B. Lippincott, 1992.

Smrcina, C. M. Stress fractures in athletes. *Nursing Clinics of North America* 27, no. 1 (1992): 159–166.

Thompson, G. H., and R. B. Salter. Legg-Calvé-Perthes disease: Current concepts and controversies. *Orthopedic Clinics of North America* 18, no. 4 (1987): 617–635.

Wilkins, K. E. Changing patterns in the management of fractures in children. *Clinical Orthopaedics and Related Research* 232 (1991): 136.

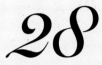

CHAPTER

28

Neurological Conditions

OBJECTIVES

AFTER STUDYING THIS CHAPTER, THE STUDENT SHOULD BE ABLE TO:

- IDENTIFY THREE TYPES OF NEURAL TUBE DEFECTS.

- COMPARE AND CONTRAST THE TYPES OF CEREBRAL PALSY AND DESCRIBE THEIR TREATMENT AND NURSING CARE.

- DESCRIBE THE TYPICAL BEHAVIORS ASSOCIATED WITH SEIZURES AND DISCUSS THEIR TREATMENT AND NURSING CARE.

- DESCRIBE THE CAUSE, SYMPTOMS, TREATMENT, AND NURSING CARE OF MENINGITIS.

- DISCUSS THE CAUSE, SYMPTOMS, TREATMENT, AND NURSING CARE OF NEUROBLASTOMA.

- DIFFERENTIATE BETWEEN THE TYPES OF HEAD INJURY AND DISCUSS THEIR TREATMENT AND NURSING CARE.

- DESCRIBE THE CAUSE, SYMPTOMS, TREATMENT, AND NURSING CARE OF ENCEPHALITIS.

- DISCUSS THE CAUSE, SYMPTOMS, TREATMENT, AND NURSING CARE OF REYE'S SYNDROME.

- DESCRIBE THE CAUSE, SYMPTOMS, TREATMENT, AND NURSING CARE OF BRAIN TUMORS.

- DESCRIBE THE TREATMENT AND NURSING CARE OF A CHILD IN A COMA.

*t*he neurological system is a complex system that is responsible for the control and coordination of body function. Changes in the neurological system may result from trauma, disease, or congenital anomalies. Early diagnosis of these potentially devastating conditions requires a complete history, good observation skills, and a thorough neurological assessment. By observing changes and recognizing differences, the nurse assists in early diagnosis and treatment of these conditions in infants and children.

OVERVIEW OF THE SYSTEM

The major structures of the nervous system are the spinal cord, spinal nerves, and brain, Figure 28–1. The spinal cord functions as a conductive pathway to and from the brain. Within the cord, connections are made between incoming and outgoing nerve fibers. Thirty-one pairs of nerves are connected to the cord.

The nervous system performs three general functions: (1) a sensory function (conveying information to the brain), (2) a conscious or integrative function (translating information into sensation, perception, thought, and memory), and (3) a motor function (stimulating muscle activity). Nervous system functioning thus enables us to see, hear, feel, respond, think, remember, and move.

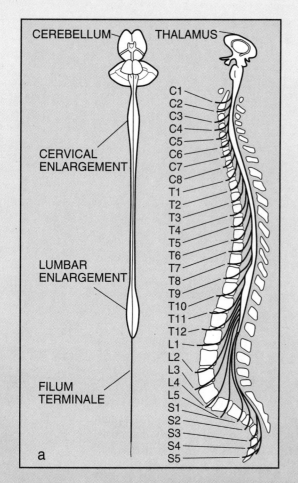
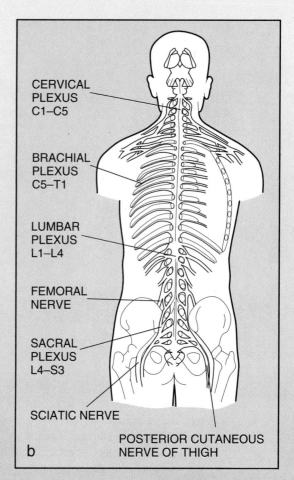

Figure 28–1 *(a) The spinal cord. (b) Spinal nerves. (c) Cross section of the brain.*

INFANT AND TODDLER

NEURAL TUBE DEFECTS

Neural tube defects are malformations that occur when the neural tube fails to close during fetal development. Another name for this malformation is spina bifida.

Neural tube defects may be further subdivided into spina bifida occulta, meningocele, and myelomeningocele. Spina bifida occulta involves a defect of the vertebrae, only. In a meningocele, a sac containing meninges and spinal fluid protrudes through an opening in the spinal column. In a myelomeningocele, the sac contains meninges, spinal fluid, and neural tissue.

A comprehensive, coordinated, interdisciplinary approach is necessary to provide care for children with neural tube defects. Infants

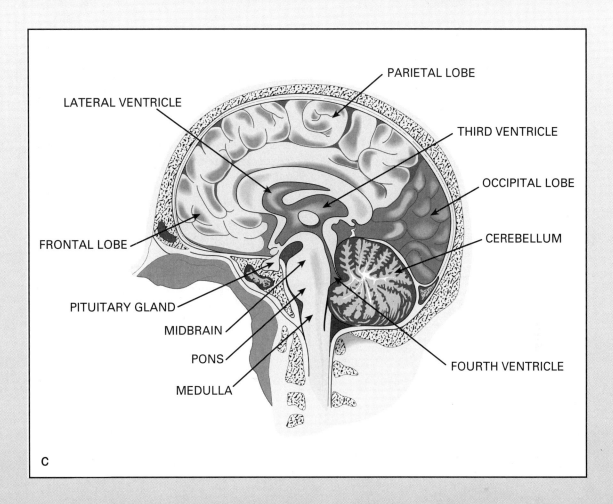

LATERAL VENTRICLE

PARIETAL LOBE

THIRD VENTRICLE

OCCIPITAL LOBE

CEREBELLUM

FRONTAL LOBE

PITUITARY GLAND

MIDBRAIN

PONS

MEDULLA

FOURTH VENTRICLE

C

Figure 28–1   continued

with myelomeningocele often are born with or develop hydrocephalus. Surgical placement of a shunt is necessary to drain the extra fluid from the brain. These children also require meticulous skin care because they lack or have limited feeling below the lesion. Bowel and bladder dysfunction is common. Management involves intermittent catheterization and a bowel stimulation program coupled with a nutritional program (Smith 1990). Depending on the type and location of the lesion, the child may be able to ambulate with assistive devices or may require a wheelchair.

Refer to Chapter 4 for additional discussion of spina bifida defects and their care.

CEREBRAL PALSY

Description. Cerebral palsy is a broad term for a nonprogressive neurological disorder that affects movement or posture. It is the most common childhood disability, occurring in 1.2 children per 1,000 live births (Nelson and Ellenberg 1978).

The disorder may be caused by developmental anomalies, cerebral trauma, or infections that occur before, during, or after birth. Failure of the brain to develop properly may result from chromosomal or genetic abnormalities or from a decrease in the blood supply to the brain of the developing fetus. Injuries to the brain are most often a result of ischemia and cerebral anoxia. Such injuries commonly occur in preterm or low-birth-weight infants, difficult deliveries, infections of the central nervous system, intraventricular hemorrhage, and as a result of toxins such as drugs and alcohol.

Children with cerebral palsy have damage to the brain that results in abnormal muscle tone. Muscle tone is required for balance, posture, and movement. Depending on the area of damage, the child may have increased muscle tone, decreased muscle tone, or a combination or fluctuation of increased and decreased muscle tone. There are four types of cerebral palsy: spastic, dyskinetic (or extrapyramidal), ataxic, and mixed.

Spastic Cerebral Palsy

This is the most common type of cerebral palsy, accounting for 50% to 60% of cases (Geralis 1991). Children with spastic cerebral palsy have sustained damage to the pyramidal tract (motor cortex) of the brain and the joints, resulting in increased resistance to passive movement. Movement is limited by the tight muscle groups. These children also display increased reflexes,

PATTERNS OF DISABILITY IN CEREBRAL PALSY

Hemiplegia
- One side of the body is involved
- Upper extremities are involved more than lower extremities
- Often associated with hemisensory deficit, a one-sided loss of sensation on the same side as the paralysis (paresis)
- Occurs in one-third of children with cerebral palsy

Diplegia
- Both sides of the body are involved
- Lower extremities are involved more than upper extremities
- Often associated with apraxia, inability to initiate voluntary movements

Quadriparesis
- All four limbs are involved

- Lower extremities are involved more than upper extremities
- Impairment of facial muscles results in feeding and speaking difficulties
- Often associated with significant mental retardation and seizures

Monoplegia
- Only one extremity is involved
- Usually mild and often goes away with time
- Rare

Paraplegia
- Only the legs are involved

Triplegia
- Three extremities are involved

Figure 28–2

persistent primitive reflexes, and a positive Babinski sign after 2 years of age. The signs and symptoms of spastic cerebral palsy are further defined by the pattern of disability, Figure 28–2.

Dyskinetic Cerebral Palsy

Dyskinetic, or extrapyramidal, cerebral palsy occurs when there is damage to the basal ganglia and cranial nerve VII (Whaley and Wong 1991). This damage causes abnormal involuntary and uncontrolled movements, especially in the face, tongue, neck, arms, and trunk, Figure 28–3. These abnormal movements often make speaking, eating, reaching, and holding objects very difficult. Muscle tone often is decreased, and thus maintaining posture for sitting and walking is difficult. The movements usually disappear in sleep and are worsened by stress.

Ataxic Cerebral Palsy

This is the least common form of cerebral palsy and is caused by a problem with coordination of voluntary movements. Children with ataxic cerebral palsy lose coordination in standing, walking, and balance and have a characteristic wide-based gait. The child has difficulty reaching for objects and performing rapid repetitive movements. There is delayed development during the first 3 to 5 years of life.

Mixed-Type Cerebral Palsy

Children with mixed-type cerebral palsy have spastic muscle tone and involuntary movements. Spasticity is often the first sign, followed by involuntary movements between 9 months and 3 years of age.

Treatment. Mild cases of cerebral palsy may not be diagnosed until a delay or absence of a gross motor skill such as standing or walking is seen. Diagnosis is made on the basis of the neurological examination and history. Physical assessment signs in neonates include decreased activity, poor suck and swallow reflexes, abnormal muscle tone (increased or decreased), periods of apnea, temperature instability, and seizures. Assessment signs in older infants and toddlers include leg extension and adduction when the child is lifted by the axillae, presence of the Moro reflex after 6 months of age, hand

MOVEMENTS ASSOCIATED WITH CEREBRAL PALSY		
Type	**Movement**	**Location**
Athetosis	Slow, writhing, wormlike	Wrists, fingers, face
Choreic	Abrupt, quick, jerky	Head, neck, arms, legs
Dystonia	Slow, rhythmic twisting or abnormal postures	Trunk or entire arm or leg
Hemiballismus	Flailing, circular movements	Arms, legs
Rigidity	Extremely high muscle tone in any position	Anywhere

Figure 28–3

dominance before 1 year of age, prolonged tonic neck reflex, toe walking, and hypotonia with brisk deep tendon reflexes.

The child is evaluated and treated by an interdisciplinary team consisting of the family, physician(s) (neurologist, pediatrician, rehabilitation physician), nurse, physical therapist, occupational therapist, psychologist, speech therapist, audiologist, nutritionist, social worker, teacher, and child life specialist.

The goal of treatment is to improve motor skills and minimize adverse effects. Independence is fostered by encouraging mobility, communication, education, and self-help skills to maximize the child's potential, Figure 28–4. Specific treatment approaches are listed in Figure 28–5.

Nursing Care. Nursing care focuses on observation, education of child and family, home care, psychosocial support, and referral of the family to support groups and community resources. Early recognition of developmental delays or failure to reach developmental milestones enables health care providers to begin therapy and teach the family how to care for the child. Encourage self care and participation in activities that promote developmental potential. Education of the family is essential as they will need to carry out a detailed home program involving feeding, exercises, positioning for play, dressing, and bathing. Encourage the family to express their frustrations and concerns.

SEIZURES

Description. A seizure is a sudden, uncontrolled episode of excess electrical activity in the brain. The excess electrical activity can produce a change in behavior, consciousness, movement, perception, or sensation. **Epilepsy** is the term given to recurrent seizures. Seizures may be idiopathic or a result of trauma, injury, or metabolic alterations such as hypoglycemia

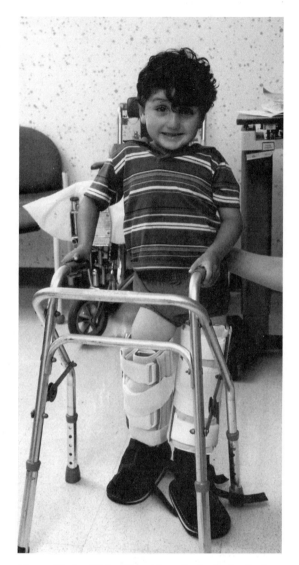

Figure 28–4 *This child with cerebral palsy has had surgery to improve muscle function. A walker assists with mobility.*

or hypocalcemia. A febrile seizure is transient and occurs with a rapid rise in fever over 101.8°F (38.8°C). Febrile seizures occur in children between 6 months and 5 years of age.

Symptoms. There are many types of seizures. Classification is based on the changes pro-

TREATMENT APPROACHES FOR CEREBRAL PALSY

Approach	Use
Casts and braces	Assist with positioning and mobility.
Mobility devices (scooter boards, wheelchairs)	Allow the child freedom of movement.
Orthopedic surgery	Improves function by lengthening tendons or releasing spastic muscles.
Medications (diazepam, dantrolene, baclofen) to modify and decrease spasticity	Of limited use. Diazepam frequently will relax muscle tone but has a tranquilizing effect. Dantrolene (Dantrium) and baclofen may also be used as skeletal muscle relaxants.

Figure 28–5

duced by the excess electrical activity and on the electroencephalogram (EEG), which shows the part of the brain involved. Seizures may be generalized (that is, the excess electrical activity affects the brain as a whole) or partial (confined to a certain area of the brain), Figure 28–6. **Status epilepticus** (a series of generalized tonic-clonic seizures in which the child does not regain consciousness between seizures) is an emergency situation that is life-threatening.

Treatment. The goal of treatment is to control recurrent seizures and reduce the frequency of occurrence. Complete control is possible in 50% to 75% of children. Medical management is based on using as few antiepileptic drugs as possible with the least amount of side effects (Santilli and Sierzant 1987). Medications are started slowly and increased gradually to desired levels that are measured by a blood test. Patient compliance is very important in treatment. Once a child is seizure-free for 2 to 3 years, the medication is tapered and discon-

tinued. If drugs are unsuccessful and the electrical discharge is limited to one place in the brain, surgical removal of the irritable brain tissue or lesion may be considered.

Nursing Care. Nursing care consists of observation skills, documentation of the seizures, and support and education of the child and family. Careful documentation of when and where the seizure began, what the child was doing, and how long the seizure lasted will help with diagnosis and treatment. Figure 28–7 outlines seizure first aid.

Educate the child and family about diagnostic tests and medications. It is essential that they understand the importance of the medication schedule and how to administer the medication. Parents also need to understand what happens during a seizure and how to help the child during a seizure. Encourage parents to allow the child to lead a regular life and not restrict activities. Teachers, babysitters, grandparents, and friends need the same information.

Types of Seizures

Type	Description
Generalized Seizures	Consciousness is impaired (may be brief and unnoticed).
Tonic-clonic seizure (Grand mal)	Characterized by a sudden fall to the ground with possibly a shrill cry. In the tonic phase, the body is rigid and the child is not breathing and may become cyanotic. This phase lasts about 10–20 seconds. In the clonic phase, the body begins to jerk and the child may lose control of bowel and bladder function and foam at the mouth. This phase lasts from 30 seconds to 30 minutes. After the seizure, the child is semiconscious and hard to arouse. The child may sleep for up to several hours, have a headache, or vomit, and has no memory of the seizure.
Absence seizure (petit mal)	A brief period when the normal activity of the brain stops with minimal or no changes in muscle tone; may be mistaken for daydreaming or inattention. The child has no memory of the seizure, but must catch up with the activity in which he or she was involved. These seizures may occur frequently during the day and interfere with school performance.
Myoclonic seizure	Sudden, brief jerks of a muscle or muscle group; may be mild or throw the child to the ground. These seizures are usually associated with worsening neurological conditions.
Atonic seizure	Drop attacks that involve a sudden loss of muscle tone, causing the child to slump and be unable to maintain an upright position. Injuries to the face and head are common, and children prone to these seizures often wear helmets for protection.
Partial Seizures	Confined to one hemisphere. Consciousness may or may not be impaired.
Simple partial seizure	The child remains conscious. If the discharge is located in the motor part of the brain, the leg may jerk.
Complex partial seizure	Like a simple partial seizure, except the child is not conscious. May be the result of a simple partial seizure that spreads to the part of the brain that determines consciousness. The child may manifest **automatisms** (involuntary movements that look purposeful), such as fumbling with clothes or chewing.

Figure 28–6

SEIZURE FIRST AID

Although a seizure cannot be stopped once it has begun, the following measures can be taken to protect the child from injury:

- Cushion the head and remove objects that could injure the child.

- *Do not* place anything in the child's mouth. (It is impossible to swallow your tongue.)

- Do not try to hold the child or stop the limbs from jerking.

- If possible, turn the child or the child's head to the side to let excess saliva drain from the mouth. This position helps to maintain a patent airway.

- After the seizure, stay with the child and offer reassurance. Tell other children who witnessed the seizures what happened to allay their fears.

Figure 28–7

There are many misconceptions about epilepsy, and the nurse can help encourage a healthy attitude toward the disorder. The Epilepsy Foundation of America (4351 Garden City Drive, Landover, MD 20785, 301-459-3700) is a resource for information and support. Many states have local chapters that provide educational programs and offer support groups.

Figure 28–8 summarizes nursing care for a child with seizures.

MENINGITIS

Description. Meningitis is an acute inflammation of the meninges (the surrounding membranes of the brain and spinal cord) that usually occurs in infants between 6 and 12 months of age. There are three main types: bacterial, tuberculous, and viral, Figure 28–9.

The central nervous system is at risk for infection by the same organisms that affect the other organs of the body. In 95% of children over 2 months, meningitis is caused by one of three bacterial organisms. Beta-streptococci and *Escherichia coli* are the prevalent organisms in neonates. *Hemophilus influenzae* is the predomi-

nant organism in children from 3 months to 3 years of age.

The most common route of infection is vascular spread from an infection located elsewhere (most often the nasopharynx). Bacteria can also enter the body through skull fractures, penetrating head wounds, lumbar puncture, or surgical procedures (Wong 1993).

Symptoms. Symptoms vary depending on the age of the child. In neonates the symptoms are vague. The neonate usually appears healthy for a few days and then develops symptoms of poor suck, weak cry, vomiting, diarrhea, jaundice, irritability, and lack of movement. In infants and young children, symptoms include seizures, irritability, fever, poor feeding patterns or loss of appetite, and vomiting. In infants under the age of 18 months, bulging fontanel is the most significant sign. Parents may report a resistance to diaper changes and to being held or cuddled.

In older children and adolescents, the illness is usually abrupt and the child appears very ill. Fever, chills, headache, vomiting, and sensory changes are usually present.

NURSING CARE PLAN: Seizures

NURSING DIAGNOSIS	GOAL(S)
Risk for injury resulting from seizure	The child will not experience injury during a seizure.
Anxiety (child's and parents') related to home management of seizures	The child (at appropriate age) and family will be able to state information about seizure disorder. Anxiety will lessen as knowledge about the disorder increases. The parents will be able to list prescribed medication(s), dosages, frequency of administration, and side effects. The parents will be able to state first aid for seizures (see Figure 28–7). The child and parents will contact appropriate support groups.

Figure 28–8

NURSING INTERVENTION	RATIONALE
Initiate seizure first aid (see Figure 28–7).	Seizure first aid helps to prevent injury and maintain a patent airway.
Avoid placing anything in the child's mouth.	Injury can occur when objects are placed in the mouth. Teeth may be knocked out, the object may be bitten, or it may injure the child's mouth.
Do not try to restrain or stop movement.	A seizure cannot be stopped and must be allowed to run its course.
Explain to child and family (in terms they can understand) the cause of seizures. Provide written information and brochures about the disorder.	Knowledge of the disorder and its management will enable child and family to return to normal routine and patterns of activity.
Explain medications and provide a list including purpose, dose, frequency, and side effects. Help parents develop a system or chart for administering medication.	Medications must be given as ordered to obtain a therapeutic blood level of drug(s).
Explain first aid for seizures and provide written instructions or brochures.	Knowledge of how to manage a seizure makes the family more comfortable and able to encourage the child to lead an unrestricted life.
Provide name and telephone number of local support group. If one does not exist, arrange for parents to talk to parents of another child with epilepsy.	Support group and other parents of epileptic children provide ongoing support to parents once the child has been discharged.

Figure 28–8   continued

COMMON TYPES OF MENINGITIS

Bacterial: Caused by pus-forming bacteria:

Hemophilus influenzae (*H. influenzae* meningitis)

Neisseria meningitidis (meningococcal meningitis)

Streptococcus pneumoniae (pneumo-coccal meningitis)

H. influenzae occurs from autumn to early winter; *N. meningitidis* and *S. pneumoniae* occur from late winter to early spring.

Tuberculous: Caused by the tubercle bacillus (*Mycobacterium tuberculosis*)

Viral or aseptic: Caused by a wide variety of viruses.

Figure 28–9

Treatment. A lumbar puncture to examine cerebrospinal fluid is required for diagnosis of meningitis. A culture and gram stain are used to identify the causative organism. A blood culture, computerized axial tomographic (CAT) scan, and EEG may also be obtained.

Treatment depends on the causative organism. Intravenous antibiotics are administered for 10 to 14 days. In addition, the child is usually placed in respiratory isolation for 24 to 48 hours after initiation of antibiotic therapy.

Nursing Care. Specific nursing care depends on the neurological status of the child. For the child who is placed in respiratory isolation, nursing care should be organized in order to provide minimum stimulation to the child. Keep the room darkened and quiet. The child will be most comfortable without a pillow, with the head of the bed slightly raised, and in a side-lying position. Care should be taken not to move the child's head and neck because moving them is very painful.

Mild analgesics such as acetaminophen are used to decrease pain and irritability. Stronger medications are not used because they can change the neurological status of the child. Fluids are restricted initially to reduce central blood volume and intracranial pressure. It is important to maintain a strict record of intake and output. Maintain the IV line at all times. In the infant, head circumferences should be measured every 8 hours to identify the early signs of developing hydrocephalus. Because of the decreased level of consciousness, all children with meningitis are at increased risk for injury. Children must also be observed for seizures. Assess neurologic status.

The child's disease and symptoms should be explained to the parents. Parents also require emotional support during the initial phase of the illness. The child may be irritable and in pain, and parents may have difficulty comforting the child. Encourage them to bring the child's "security items," such as a blanket or teddy bear, from home.

Visitors should be kept to a minimum during the initial phase of the illness. Advise parents that the risk of an adult contracting meningitis is slight. There is some risk, however, to children and siblings exposed to the infected child, and prophylactic treatment may be suggested.

During recovery, encourage diversional activities and visits by parents and siblings to help prevent the effects of long-term hospitalization, such as regression, dependence, and boredom.

Parents often have many questions and fears related to the prognosis. The age of the child and the speed with which the diagnosis is made affect outcome. Complications that can occur as a result of meningitis include mental retardation, learning disabilities, physical or motor disabilities, and alterations in vision and hearing.

Figure 28–10 summarizes nursing care for the child with meningitis.

NEUROBLASTOMA

Description. Neuroblastoma, the most common malignant tumor of infancy, occurs in 1 child per 1,000 and slightly more often in boys than in girls. Half of all cases occur in children under 2 years of age, and one-quarter in children under 4 (Whaley and Wong 1991). Because these tumors arise from cells that, in the embryo, make up the adrenal glands and part of the sympathetic nervous system, they are usually located in the abdominal cavity. Other sites include the pelvis, chest, and neck.

Symptoms. Symptoms depend on the primary tumor site. A tumor in the abdomen causes a mass, pain, decrease in appetite, and bladder and bowel changes. A tumor in the chest may cause pain, cough, and shortness of breath. A tumor in the neck may cause pain and difficulty in swallowing. Metastases are often present at diagnosis and account for joint and bone pain. In infants, the presenting symptoms are hepatomegaly, anemia, poor feeding patterns, and dyspnea. Children may have weight loss, fever, and anemia.

A clinical staging classification system has been developed to establish an appropriate treatment plan for the child with a neuroblastoma. Tumors are classified into four stages, ranging from stage I (no metastasis) to stages IV and IV-S (metastases to other body sites).

Treatment. Prognosis and treatment are based on the stage of the tumor. Children younger than 2 years and those with localized disease (stage I or II) have the best prognosis. The goal of treatment is to remove the tumor. In half of the cases, however, metastasis is present and total surgical removal is impossible. Radiation and chemotherapy may also be used.

Nursing Care. Nursing care includes supportive care, preparing the child and family for diagnostic tests and treatment, and planning for a return to normal activities upon discharge. Analgesics are used judiciously with the realization that they may alter neurological functioning. Provide a quiet room with dim lights, limit visitors, and avoid sudden movements. Ice compresses may provide comfort and relieve pain, especially if edema is present.

If possible, the nurse should be present during physician visits to reinforce and clarify information presented. Encourage the family to verbalize fears and questions. Parents and siblings will need emotional support. The nurse and other interdisciplinary team members (social worker, psychologist, child life specialist, and clergy) can help the family discuss the illness with the child and siblings.

HEAD INJURY

Head injury — an injury of the scalp, skull, or brain — is one of the most common causes of disability and death of children (Patterson et al. 1992). Each year, 200,000 children sustain head injuries, 4,000 of which are fatal (Patterson et al. 1992).

Common head injuries include concussions, contusions and lacerations, vascular injuries, skull fractures, and coma. Falls and motor vehicle crashes are the primary causes of head injuries. Other causes are child abuse, unhelmeted biking accidents, diving accidents, and sports injuries.

Hitting the head is a common occurrence in childhood. In infants and very young children, the head is large in proportion to the rest of the body. Infants often fall from beds and high chairs, landing on their heads. Toddlers, who are unsteady on their feet, often bump their heads.

NURSING CARE PLAN: Meningitis

NURSING DIAGNOSIS	GOAL(S)
Irritability, altered consciousness, and disorientation	The child's neurological status will remain stable and/or improve each day.
Pain and discomfort	The child will state or demonstrate comfort.

Figure 28–10

Nursing Intervention	Rationale
Assess neurological status and vital signs as ordered. Maintain a quiet environment in room and hallway. Keep the lights low. Avoid jarring the bed, and group nursing care activities to avoid unnecessary disturbances.	A quiet environment with minimal disturbances facilitates recovery.
Approach the child in a calm manner and limit the number of caregivers. Tell the child who you are and what you are going to do. Have parents bring the child's favorite toys and objects from home.	Reorientation helps the child adjust to the new environment.
Encourage parents to limit visitors until the child's neurological status improves.	Limiting visitors helps maintain a quiet environment.
Administer analgesics or antipyretics as ordered and assess effectiveness and side effects.	Medications should be given on schedule and monitored for effectiveness and side effects.
Avoid moving the child, and minimize movements of the head and neck. Do not use pillows, and keep the head of the bed elevated 30 degrees. Assist the child to avoid straining, coughing, or nose blowing.	Sudden movements cause pain and discomfort.
Provide age-appropriate diversional activities.	If distracted, the child may relax and feel more comfortable.

Figure 28–10 continued

The skull serves as protection to the brain. When the head is hit, the skull accelerates, causing the brain to move. When the head stops, the skull decelerates, and the brain strikes sharp edges of the skull, causing damage. The technical term for this type of injury is coup-contrecoup injury, Figure 28–11. Rotational injury is also possible from twisting of the brain within the skull.

Concussion. In a concussion (the most common head injury), acceleration-deceleration produces a loss of consciousness that lasts for seconds to hours. There is no structural damage to the brain, Figure 28–12. Amnesia is common but normally disappears by 24 hours after the injury. Postconcussion syndrome occurs when the amnesia lasts longer than 24 hours or the loss of consciousness is prolonged. Symptoms of postconcussion syndrome include vertigo,

visual disturbances, light-headedness, memory and concentration problems, mood alterations, and fatigue. These symptoms may last for days to months, but usually resolve.

Contusion and Laceration. A contusion is a bruising or hemorrhage of the brain, Figure 28–12. In a serious injury, there may be many sites of hemorrhage, causing changes in motor, sensory, or visual functioning. A laceration is a traumatic tearing of the brain that causes bleeding that leads to a more severe injury and often permanent disability. Contusions and lacerations are usually caused by blunt trauma and penetrating injuries to the head.

Vascular Injuries. Hemorrhage occurs in about 7% of all head injuries (Whaley and Wong 1991). Bleeding may result in an intracranial, epidural, or subdural hemorrhage.

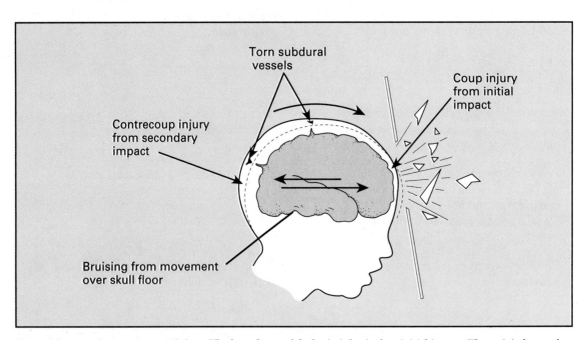

Figure 28–11   *Coup-contrecoup injury. The frontal area of the brain is bruised on initial impact. The occipital area of the brain is bruised as the brain bounces back and strikes the back of the skull. (From M. R. Eichelberger, J. W. Ball, G. S. Pratsch, and E. Runion. Pediatric Emergencies: A Manual for Prehospital Care Providers. Reprinted by permission of Prentice-Hall. Englewood Cliffs, NJ: Brady/Prentice-Hall, 1992.)*

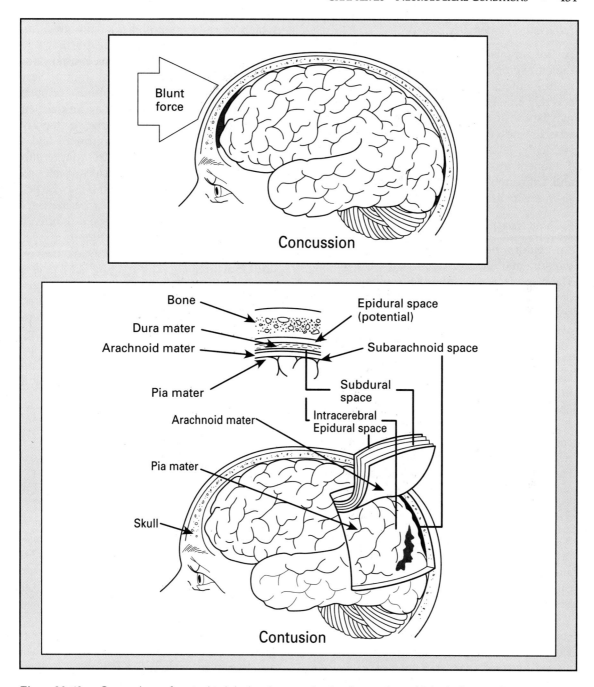

Figure 28–12   *Concussion and contusion injuries. A concussion involves no detectable brain damage. A contusion involves bruising or rupturing of the brain tissue and vessels at any of the identified levels. (From M. R. Eichelberger, J. W. Ball, G. S. Pratsch, and E. Runion.* Pediatric Emergencies: A Manual for Prehospital Care Providers. *Reprinted by permission of Prentice-Hall. Englewood Cliffs, NJ: Brady/Prentice-Hall, 1992.)*

Intracranial Hemorrhage

An intracranial hemorrhage is bleeding into the intraventricular space. It may occur in premature infants as a result of trauma or in severely injured children. The child initially may be able to respond to commands, but then consciousness deteriorates. Seizures may begin suddenly, followed by respiratory difficulties. Treatment involves cardiorespiratory support and anticonvulsive medications. The prognosis in severe hemorrhage is poor.

Epidural Hemorrhage

An epidural hemorrhage is bleeding between the dura and the skull that forms a hematoma. The blood is usually from the meningeal artery or vein. As the blood expands, the brain is compressed. The child usually has a momentary loss of consciousness, followed by a return to normal consciousness for a few hours or several days. How long the period of normal consciousness lasts depends on the rapidity of bleeding. Impaired consciousness follows, beginning with drowsiness that progresses to confusion and coma. There may also be headache, vomiting, and seizures. Treatment involves surgery to remove the clot and to stop the bleeding. Early diagnosis and treatment lead to a positive outcome.

Subdural Hemorrhage

A subdural hemorrhage is venous bleeding between the dura and the cerebrum that creates pressure on the brain. The hemorrhage causes a subdural hematoma, which can be acute or chronic.

In an acute hemorrhage, an underlying contusion or laceration usually is present. Hemorrhage also may occur from damage caused by rapid shaking of the head, which is common in child abuse. Symptoms include headache, drowsiness, agitation, confusion, and fixation and dilation of the ipsilateral pupil (the pupil on the same side as the hematoma).

A high mortality rate and poor prognosis are associated with acute subdural hemorrhage.

Chronic subdural hematoma is more common and may develop from minor head injuries. If the fontanels and sutures are open, the occurrence of symptoms may be delayed. The child may exhibit headache, irritability, full fontanel, increased head growth, and a low hematocrit. In older children, large subdural hematomas are surgically removed, whereas in infants, a subdural tap may be performed. A small hematoma may be managed without surgery because the bleeding often is reabsorbed by the surrounding tissue.

Skull Fracture. A skull fracture is a break in the cranial bones. Skull fractures may be minor or life-threatening. A child with a skull fracture may have an accompanying scalp laceration, which can be a major source of bleeding. In fact, a skull fracture with a major scalp laceration can cause a child to bleed to death. Figure 28–13 describes four common skull fractures and their management.

PRESCHOOL AND SCHOOL-AGE CHILD

ENCEPHALITIS

Encephalitis, an inflammation of the brain, is most often caused by viruses but may also be caused by bacteria, fungi, or parasites. Ingestion of lead, inhalation of carbon monoxide, certain vaccines, and complications from measles, mumps, rubella, and rabies may also produce encephalitis.

Signs and symptoms of encephalitis are similar regardless of the causative agent. The causative agent enters the lymphatic system, infects the blood, and produces an inflammatory response that results in cellular damage, cerebral edema, and temporary neurological dysfunction. The child presents with a headache, fever,

COMMON SKULL FRACTURES

Type	Description	Treatment
Linear (or simple) skull fracture	A line or crack in the skull.	Usually heals on its own in 3–4 months.
Depressed skull fracture	Involves a broken bone with fragments that are pushed in and toward the brain. The skull is indented, and brain tissue below the indentation is injured. The bone may be broken in several places or comminuted.	If the depression is very deep, surgery is necessary.
Compound skull fracture	A laceration of the scalp with a depressed skull fracture that allows access to the cranium. Debris may enter the cranium.	Requires surgery and antibiotics.
Basilar skull fracture	The most serious type of skull fracture. Occurs at the base of the skull and may be linear, depressed, or comminuted. Cerebrospinal fluid is often noted leaking from the child's nose or ear. "Raccoon eyes," caused by blood leaking into the frontal sinuses, often are present. Bruising behind the ear may also be present because of blood leaking into the mastoid sinus. This bruising is called the battle sign.	Children with a basilar skull fracture are at risk for meningitis. Frequent neurological assessment is required. Safety must also be considered because the child may be disoriented and restless. The room should be kept dim and quiet, and visitors should be limited.

Figure 28–13

irritability, gastrointestinal distress, and often mild respiratory symptoms. The onset of symptoms may be sudden or gradual. In severe cases, the child has a high fever, seizures, disorientation, and possibly lapses into a coma. Other symptoms include alterations in motor function, such as inability to walk or changes in balance and coordination.

Diagnosis is made on the basis of the history, physical examination, lumbar puncture, and laboratory tests, including cultures of cerebrospinal fluid (CSF) and blood. The child is hospitalized for neurological assessment and supportive care. Cerebral symptoms are managed as for a child with meningitis. Nursing care is also similar.

REYE'S SYNDROME

Reye's syndrome is a multisystem disease that is damaging to the liver and brain. The liver fails to convert ammonia to urea, resulting in toxic uremia. Diagnosis is made by liver biopsy, which shows hepatic fatty degeneration. Children between the ages of 5 and 10 years are at greatest risk. Public education about the disorder and its symptoms has resulted in a decline in the number of reported cases.

Most cases of Reye's syndrome occur during the winter flu season. The disease usually follows a viral illness (most often influenza or varicella). The child is usually ill with flu-like symptoms for a week, is healthy for several days, and then experiences prolonged vomiting for 2 to 3 days. The child's level of consciousness decreases each day. Symptoms progress to include persistent or continuous vomiting, listlessness, personality change, disorientation, delirium, convulsions, and coma. Infants with Reye's syndrome may have diarrhea or respiratory distress but no vomiting. Because of the possible link between aspirin use and Reye's syndrome, aspirin should not be given to children less than 18 years of age to relieve symptoms of cold, flu, or varicella.

At the onset of symptoms, the child should be evaluated by a health care provider. Medications to reduce fever or pain should not be given, because they may mask the symptoms of the disease. Recovery depends on early diagnosis and treatment to control cerebral edema, reverse metabolic injury, and prevent respiratory compromise. Symptoms may progress rapidly without intervention and treatment.

Treatment for mild symptoms is supportive, involving return to normal acid-base balance, control cerebral edema, and decreasing the risk of intracranial pressure. More severe symptoms require aggressive management in a pediatric intensive care unit. Measures to maintain a patent airway and control cerebral edema are necessary to prevent irreversible brain damage.

Prognosis and sequelae are based on the amount of cerebral edema. The child may recover completely or have slight to severe brain damage. If the child has a rapid progression of symptoms or becomes comatose, the prognosis is worse. Neurological sequelae include speech and language disorders, fine and gross motor skill problems, and problems with memory, concentration, and attention.

Brain Tumor

Brain tumors originate in the neural tissue and are the most common type of solid tumors in children (Shiminski-Maher 1990). They account for 20% of childhood cancers and occur in 1,000 to 1,500 children each year (Shiminski-Maher 1990). Most brain tumors occur in children between 5 and 10 years of age. The prognosis depends on the age of the child, and the type, anatomical location, and size of the tumor. Figure 28–14 lists common pediatric brain tumors.

Accurate diagnosis of a brain tumor can be difficult because symptoms often are vague. In infants, the sutures and fontanels are open, and early signs of increased intracranial pressure are not noticeable. In older children, the symptoms may resemble those of other common illnesses.

Classic symptoms are a recurrent and progressive headache that is present in the morning and projectile vomiting. Other symptoms include muscular disturbances such as clumsiness, unsteady gait, and a decrease in fine motor coordination. The child's personality may also change, and vision and speech changes and seizures may occur.

Diagnosis is based on a detailed history combined with CAT scan or magnetic resonance imaging (MRI). Nursing care for children undergoing these tests includes patient and family education as well as administration of any medication that may be needed for sedation.

Treatment options include surgery, radiation therapy, and chemotherapy, all of which have risks.

COMMON PEDIATRIC BRAIN TUMORS	
Type	**Description**
Medulloblastoma	Fastest-growing, malignant brain tumor. Located in the cerebellum.
Cerebellar astrocytoma	Cystic or benign and slow-growing tumor.
Brain-stem glioma	Often grows very large before resulting in symptoms. Hard to resect surgically because of location.
Ependymoma	Grows at varying rates. Located in the ventricles.
Craniopharyngioma	Located near the pituitary. Removal may necessitate hormone replacement.

Figure 28–14

- *Surgery*: The tumor needs to be removed as completely as possible without causing residual neurological damage.
- *Radiation*: Children undergoing radiation treatment receive treatment twice a day for eight weeks. It is important to orient children to the procedure so they will not be frightened during the treatment. Side effects include nausea and vomiting, decreased oral intake, fatigue, hair loss, skin sensitivity, and possible loss of cognition.
- *Chemotherapy*: The goal of chemotherapy is to destroy tumor cells and spare healthy cells. The types, amounts, and frequency of chemotherapy vary with the particular hospital and pediatric oncologist, but the side effects of nausea, vomiting, and immunosuppression remain the same.

Regardless of the treatment, nurses play a major role in the support, education, and discharge planning of children with brain tumors. The goal is for the child to return to a normal routine, activities, and school as soon as possible.

COMA

Coma is a state of unconsciousness in which the child cannot open the eyes, speak, obey commands, or be aroused by any measure. The Glasgow Coma Scale (GCS) is a well-known scale used to assess the neurological responses of patients with head injuries. The scale relies on the best response to eye opening, motor, and verbalization requests, and the score can range from 3 points to 15 points. Because the original GCS does not take into consideration the developmental levels of children, many hospitals use a modified GCS for pediatric patients, Figure 28–15. Neurological assessments are performed frequently. Nurses who care for a child in a coma must work closely with parents to identify the child's normal behaviors. These behaviors provide a measure for assessing return to normal functioning.

Family support is essential to the nursing care of the child in a coma. Parents exhibit a wide range of feelings and emotions intensified by the uncertain prognosis for the child.

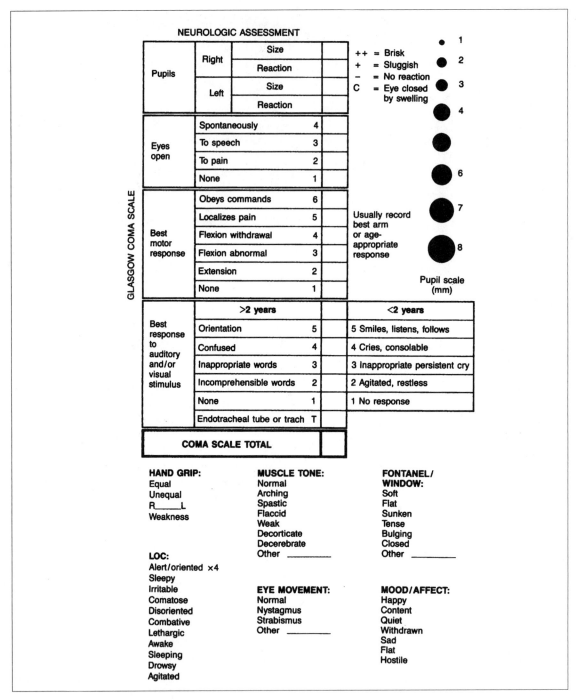

Figure 28–15 *Pediatric coma scale (From D. Wong,* Whaley & Wong's Essentials of Pediatric Nursing, *4th ed. St. Louis, MO: Mosby-Year Book, 1993.)*

Fear of death, and physical and mental disability are foremost. If the child dies, the family needs support to cope with the loss. If the child remains comatose, parents must decide whether to place the child in a long-term care facility or care for the child at home.

Parents of a child in a coma face many difficult decisions. The brain may be damaged so severely that life is maintained only through life-support systems. On the other hand, the coma may resolve, but the child may be physically or mentally disabled and require long-term care and rehabilitation.

Nurses can help parents during this decision-making process by listening and providing information. Regardless of the outcome, parents should be encouraged and taught to provide physical care for the child through bathing, skin care, and range-of-motion exercises. Parents should also be encouraged to bring items from home (such as toys and blankets) and to talk with, read to, and touch the child. When parents or siblings cannot visit, they should be encouraged to send tapes to be played for the child.

REVIEW QUESTIONS

A. Multiple choice. Select the best answer.

1. Children with cerebral palsy usually
    a. die before the age of 2
    b. have progressive worsening of symptoms
    c. have developmental problems
    d. get better over time with therapy

2. A child with cerebral palsy who has quadriparesis will not have
    a. limited function in all four extremities
    b. impairment of facial muscles
    c. mental deficits or delays
    d. disappearance of symptoms over time

3. Which of the following best describes the appearance of a child experiencing a tonic-clonic seizure?
    a. is confused and sleepy after the seizure
    b. is initially flaccid followed by jerking motions
    c. stares blankly into space
    d. has unimpaired consciousness

4. First aid for a seizure involves which of the following actions?
    a. placing an object in the mouth to protect the tongue
    b. attempting to stop the seizure
    c. loosening tight clothing and turning the head to the side
    d. putting your fingers in the mouth to keep the child from biting the tongue

5. Nursing care for the child with meningitis includes
    a. elevating the head with two pillows
    b. restricting fluids
    c. encouraging visitors
    d. administering strong sedatives to alleviate pain

6. Children who are at risk of developing Reye's syndrome have usually
   a. taken acetaminophen to treat cold, flu, or varicella
   b. been healthy before developing Reye's syndrome symptoms
   c. taken aspirin to treat cold, flu, or varicella
   d. been exposed to bacteria

7. A child with a brain tumor may have which of the following symptoms?
   a. projectile vomiting
   b. a recurrent and progressive pain behind the ears
   c. increasing difficulty in being awakened in the morning
   d. constipation

8. Treatment for brain tumors may include all of the following except
   a. chemotherapy
   b. antibiotic therapy
   c. radiation therapy
   d. surgery

9. Which of the following is true of neuroblastoma?
   a. usually involves metastases
   b. cannot be treated with surgery
   c. commonly presents in the brain
   d. is always fatal

10. Damage from a head injury may result from
    a. rapid acceleration followed by rapid deceleration
    b. seizures
    c. being in a coma
    d. lack of nutrition

Suggested Activities

- Contact a local outpatient facility or infant intervention program and arrange to observe a child with cerebral palsy during physical therapy, occupational therapy, and speech therapy.

- Call the Epilepsy Foundation of America (1-800-EFA-1000) and request brochures about children with epilepsy. Investigate an area such as school issues, psychosocial issues, or first aid.

- Call a local school system and make arrangements to observe in a classroom with disabled students.

- Arrange a tour of a pediatric intensive care unit. Talk with the nursing staff about management issues for children with meningitis or brain tumors.

BIBLIOGRAPHY

American Association of Neuroscience Nursing. *Core Curriculum for Neuroscience Nursing*, 3rd ed. Chicago: Chicago University Press, 1990.

Avery, M., and L. First, eds. *Pediatric Medicine*. Baltimore: Williams and Wilkins, 1989.

David, R. *Pediatric Neurology for the Clinician*. Norwalk, CT: Appleton and Lange, 1992.

Foster, R. L., M. M. Hunsberger, and J. J. Anderson. *Family-Centered Nursing Care of Children*. Philadelphia: W. B. Saunders, 1989.

Geralis, E., ed. *Children with Cerebral Palsy: A Parent's Guide*. Kensington, MD: Woodbine House, 1991.

Hazinski, M. *Nursing Care of the Critically Ill Child*. St. Louis, MO: C. V. Mosby, 1987.

Hockenberry, M., D. Coody, and B. Bennett. Childhood cancers: Incidence, etiology, diagnosis, and treatment. *Pediatric Nursing* 16, no 3 (1990): 239–246.

Lovejoy, F., A. L. Smith, M. J. Bresnan, J. M. Wood, D. I. Victor, and P. C. Adams. Clinical stages in Reye's syndrome. *American Journal of Diseases of Childhood* 128, no. 2 (1974): 36–41.

Maheady, D. Reye's syndrome: Review and update. *Journal of Pediatric Health Care* 3, no. 5 (1985): 246–250.

National Reye's Syndrome Foundation. *Be Wise about Reye's*, Awareness Bulletin. Bryan, OH: National Reye's Syndrome Foundation, 1983.

Nelson, K., and J. Ellenberg. Epidemiology of cerebral palsy. *Advances in Neurology* 19, no. 3 (1978): 421–435.

Patterson, R., G. Brown, M. Salassi-Scotter, and D. Middaugh. Head injury in the conscious child. *American Journal of Nursing* 92, no. 8 (1992): 22–27.

Peacock, W., L. Arens, and B. Berman. Cerebral palsy, spasticity and selective posterior rhizotomy. *Pediatric Neuroscience* 13, no. 2 (1987): 61–66.

Reisner, H., ed. *Children with Epilepsy: A Parent's Guide*. Kensington, MD: Woodbine House, 1988.

Santilli, N., and T. Sierzant. Advances in the treatment of epilepsy. *Journal of Neuroscience Nursing* 19, no. 3 (1987): 141–157.

Shiminski-Maher, T. Brain tumors in childhood: Implications for nursing practice. *Journal of Pediatric Health Care* 14, no. 3 (1990): 122–130.

Smith, K. A. Bowel and bladder management of the child with myelomeningocele in the school setting. *Journal of Pediatric Health Care* 4, no. 4 (1990): 175–180.

United Cerebral Palsy. *What Everyone Should Know about Cerebral Palsy*. Boston: Channing L. Bete, 1992.

Whaley, L., and D. Wong, eds. *Nursing Care of Infants and Children*, 4th ed. St. Louis, MO: Mosby-Year Book, 1991.

Wong, D. L. *Whaley & Wong's Essentials of Pediatric Nursing*, 4th ed. St. Louis, MO: Mosby-Year Book, 1993.

CHAPTER

Conditions of the Blood and Blood-Forming Organs

OBJECTIVES

AFTER STUDYING THIS CHAPTER, THE STUDENT SHOULD BE ABLE TO:

- DESCRIBE THE COMPONENTS OF BLOOD AND THEIR FUNCTIONS.
- IDENTIFY THE CAUSE, SYMPTOMS, TREATMENT, AND NURSING CARE OF IRON DEFICIENCY ANEMIA.
- IDENTIFY THE CAUSE, SYMPTOMS, TREATMENT, AND NURSING CARE OF SICKLE CELL ANEMIA.
- DEFINE HEMOPHILIA AND DISCUSS ITS TREATMENT AND NURSING CARE.
- IDENTIFY THE CAUSE, SYMPTOMS, TREATMENT, AND NURSING CARE OF LEUKEMIA.
- DEFINE IDIOPATHIC THROMBOCYTOPENIA PURPURA AND DISCUSS ITS TREATMENT AND NURSING CARE.
- IDENTIFY THE CAUSE, SYMPTOMS, TREATMENT, AND NURSING CARE OF HODGKIN'S DISEASE.

KEY TERMS

PLASMA

ERYTHROCYTES

LEUKOCYTES

THROMBOCYTES

GRANULOCYTES

LEUKOPENIA

AGRANULOCYTES

PETECHIAE

ECCHYMOSIS

*t*he blood and blood-forming organs (hematologic system) help to regulate, directly or indirectly, all other body functions. Thus, changes in this system may compromise the functioning of many other body systems and organs. Because signs of altered hematologic functioning are often subtle, a careful history and thorough physical assessment are essential for accurate diagnosis. Nurses can play an important role in ensuring prompt diagnosis and treatment of these conditions, and in providing necessary teaching and emotional support to children with these conditions and their parents.

OVERVIEW OF THE SYSTEM

Blood is composed of two parts, a liquid and a solid portion. The liquid portion, called **plasma**, contains protein, clotting factors, and electrolytes. The solid portion is made up of red blood cells **(erythrocytes)**, white blood cells **(leukocytes)**, and platelets **(thrombocytes)**. The plasma transports the solid elements of the blood throughout the body. Plasma also aids in distributing heat throughout the body.

Red blood cells (RBCs) are responsible for transporting oxygen to the tissues of the body. They do this by synthesizing hemoglobin, which then binds with oxygen and carbon dioxide to carry gases to and from the tissues. Mature RBCs live approximately 120 days. Because they are destroyed at approximately the same rate at which they are produced, the number of circulating RBCs remains relatively constant. This number, however, varies according to the age of the child.

White blood cells (WBCs) are responsible for fighting infection. There are two major classifications of WBCs: granulocytes and agranulocytes. The **granulocytes** consist of neutrophils, which are responsible for fighting bacterial and fungal infections, and eosinophils. The exact function of eosinophils is unknown, although they are elevated in parasitic infections as well as in allergic conditions. **Leukopenia**, a reduction in WBCs, decreases the ability of the body to fight infection.

The **agranulocytes** consist of lymphocytes and monocytes. Lymphocytes, which are divided into B-cells and T-cells, are necessary for the maintenance of the immune system. Monocytes serve as "back-up" to the neutrophils when the body is faced with an infection.

Platelets are necessary for clotting. When the body is injured, platelets form a "plug" at the site of the injury. Platelets alone, however, cannot stop bleeding; blood coagulation factors also are necessary. (Deficiencies of factors VIII and IX are discussed later in the section on hemophilia.) Children with low platelet counts may develop **petechiae** (pinpoint hemorrhages) and **ecchymoses** (bruises).

INFANT AND TODDLER

IRON DEFICIENCY ANEMIA

Description. Iron deficiency anemia is a reduction in RBCs that occurs as a result of inadequate dietary intake of iron. It is the most common type of anemia in children and usually occurs between 6 months and 3 years of age. Young children are at higher risk for this disorder because of their proportionately higher need for iron compared with adults as well as their high consumption of milk (which decreases absorption of iron). The incidence of iron deficiency anemia is also higher in adolescent girls. This higher incidence is due to the combination of the increased need for iron once menstruation begins, rapid growth, and the often poor dietary habits of teenagers.

Symptoms. Children with iron deficiency anemia may have few or no symptoms until their anemia is quite profound. On physical examination, the conjunctiva appear pale. Parents may also comment on the child's decreased activity level. Children with mild anemia usually compensate so effectively that few other symptoms are seen (Stockman 1992). If the anemia has been present for some time, cardiomegaly, splenomegaly, and tachycardia may be present. The definitive diagnosis is made using laboratory data. A complete blood count, serum iron, and iron-binding capacity will probably be ordered.

Treatment. The best treatment is prevention. All breast-fed infants should receive iron supplementation. Formula-fed infants should receive iron-rich formula. When the child is started on solids, iron-enriched cereals and other foods high in iron should be encouraged. Parents should be advised to decrease the amount of formula or breast milk ingested as the child moves into the second year. Children with iron deficiency anemia are given iron supplements such as ferrous sulfate. Occasionally intramuscular iron is prescribed. There is no indication, however, that response is any more complete with parenteral iron than with oral iron (Stockman 1992).

Nursing Care. The primary focus of nursing care is education. Teach parents about good dietary sources of iron (see Figure 29–1) and about side effects of the iron medication. In particular, parents should be told that iron can turn the child's stools green or black and that this color is not a sign that something is wrong with the child. Other side effects include nausea and diarrhea or constipation.

Teach parents to give iron between meals with a source of vitamin C (such as orange juice) to enhance absorption. Liquid iron should be given with a straw or dropper to avoid staining the teeth.

Treatment and nursing care for adolescents with iron deficiency anemia are similar to treatment and care for young children: iron supplementation or improved dietary intake of iron, or both.

IRON-RICH FOODS

Apricots	Poultry
Eggs	Prunes
Fish	Raisins
Iron-fortified cereal	Red meat
Liver	Spinach
Oysters	

Figure 29–1

SICKLE CELL ANEMIA

Description. Sickle cell anemia is an autosomal recessive disease that occurs primarily in black children. Both parents must be carriers for the disease to be present in the child. There is a one in four chance with each pregnancy that the child will have the disease, a one in two chance of being a carrier, and a one in four chance of being neither a carrier nor an affected individual.

In sickle cell anemia, the red blood cell is elongated and sickle-shaped. This configuration decreases its oxygen-carrying capacity. From 80% to 95% of the hemoglobin may be sickled. This percentage increases when the cells are hypoxic (Stockman 1992). Once sickled, the cells are more fragile and more easily destroyed. The life span of the sickled cell averages only 10 to 20 days, as compared with a normal cell life span of 120 days. The altered shape also

SICKLE CELL CRISES

Crisis	Symptoms	Treatment
Vasoocclusive crisis Clumped RBCs occlude (or block) the vessels, resulting in tissue death. May be caused by infection, dehydration, acidosis, stress, or exertion.	Severe pain (due to hypoxia distal to the occlusion); fever; swelling; respiratory distress; priapism (prolonged painful erection of the penis)	Alleviate underlying cause of the occlusion. Relieve pain. Antibiotics. Blood transfusion may be necessary to correct anemia. Supplemental oxygen is given to severely hypoxic children.
Splenic sequestration crisis Occurs when large volumes of blood are sequestered (trapped) in the spleen. May result in death.	Splenomegaly (enlarged spleen); shock; decreased hemoglobin	Blood transfusion. Splenectomy (removal of the spleen), if indicated. Supportive care.
Aplastic crisis Occurs rarely, but may be life-threatening. Bone marrow shuts down despite increased destruction of RBCs.	Anemia; rapid heart rate; weakness	Blood transfusions are given until the marrow begins to function.

Figure 29–2

increases the chances of the cells' becoming caught in the capillaries, causing decreased circulation distal to the site of the occlusion.

Sickle cell anemia can be diagnosed in utero or during the newborn period. An infant will not, however, be symptomatic until 4 to 6 months of age (when fetal hemoglobin is replaced by adult hemoglobin).

Symptoms. Symptoms vary depending on the severity of the disease and the age at which the diagnosis is made. In infants, symptoms may include pallor, irritability, and jaundice. In older children splenomegaly, hepatomegaly, and cardiomegaly may occur. Children may also present with anemia or bacterial infections. Leg ulcers are a characteristic finding in adolescents. During a sickle cell crisis, symptoms commonly include abdominal pain, fever, and leg pain.

Treatment. Treatment will vary according to the symptoms that are present. Sickle cell disease is a chronic disease, and children usually require hospitalization only for acute crises. Three different types of sickle cell crises may occur: splenic sequestration crisis, aplastic crisis, and vasoocclusive crisis, Figure 29–2. The most common is vasoocclusive crisis; however, aplastic crisis may be life-threatening. Infection, dehydration, and acidosis are the most common factors precipitating vasoocclusive crises.

Nursing Care. Nursing care focuses on the immediate problems of relieving pain and replacing lost fluids. An intravenous line is started for rehydration and to administer pain medication. Replacement of fluids helps decrease viscosity of blood, decreasing occlusion of the blood vessels by the sickled cells. Morphine is usually the drug of choice for pain management. Older children may be able to use patient-controlled analgesia pumps; whereas younger children may receive a continuous morphine drip or IV push morphine at regularly scheduled intervals. Guided imagery (the use of mental images and imagination to reduce pain) and heat may also be helpful in managing pain.

The nurse should monitor intravenous fluids, intake and output, and urine specific gravity, and should weigh the child daily. Remember that the baseline urine specific gravity in these children will be lower than normal because of their inability to concentrate urine.

After the child is stabilized, attention should be paid to educating the child and family about the disease as well as establishing a home health maintenance program. Long-term management includes nutritional counseling and education about the need for increased fluid intake and preventing infection. Maintaining adequate hydration is of prime importance in preventing further complications. Figure 29–3 presents several topics to be addressed in teaching parents of children with sickle cell anemia.

HEMOPHILIA

Hemophilia is inherited as an X-linked recessive trait. Women are carriers who generally transmit the disease only to sons. A man who has the disease and a woman who is a carrier could produce a daughter who has the disease.

The two most common types of hemophilia are hemophilia A (or classic hemophilia), which results from a deficiency of factor VIII, and hemophilia B, which is a deficiency of factor IX. Although diagnostic criteria and replacement therapy differ depending on the type of hemophilia, the nursing care for the two types is virtually the same.

The diagnosis is usually made when the child has prolonged bleeding from a minor injury. Bleeding may occur when the infant is circumcised or when the child becomes more mobile and sustains one of the many injuries that occur in toddlerhood. Typically, these children bleed into the joints. The joint appears

PARENT TEACHING: SICKLE CELL ANEMIA

- Encourage parents to offer children fruit juice, flavored ices, frozen slushes, gelatin desserts, broth, soup, and fruits with a high fluid content, such as oranges and grapefruit, to increase fluid intake.

- Caution parents to keep the child away from persons with known infections and from large crowds, and to keep the child's immunizations up to date.

- Children with asplenia (a nonfunctioning spleen) or who have had their spleen surgically removed should receive the pneumococcal vaccine. These children are often placed on prophylactic antibiotics. Emphasize the importance of taking antibiotics at the designated times to child and parents.

- Teach parents to monitor the child for signs of infection, such as temperature elevation, cough, or change in behavior. If any of these occur, parents should take the child to a health care provider promptly.

- Counsel parents that the child should avoid high altitudes and unpressurized aircraft; these can cause increased sickling. Activities that result in hypoxia — for example, strenuous exercise or surgery — should be monitored carefully. Caution is needed in the summer months, in particular, because high temperatures combined with increased activity heighten chances of dehydration.

Figure 29–3

swollen, and the child keeps the joint flexed. The definitive diagnosis is made when the child's activated partial thromboplastin time is prolonged and specific clotting factors are found to be deficient.

Nursing care focuses on educating parents to care for the child at home. Parents must learn many skills, including home infusion of replacement factors and manipulation of the environment to prevent additional injuries to the child. Parents must also learn appropriate first-aid techniques, including the application of ice and elastic bandages to an affected joint, and they must know when to seek help from the health care team. As children become older, they can be taught to perform self-infusion.

Genetic counseling should be offered so parents can make informed decisions about future pregnancies.

PRESCHOOL AND SCHOOL-AGE CHILD

LEUKEMIA

Description. Leukemia is marked by the rapid growth of immature white blood cells, called blasts. Because the blast cells are unable to carry out the usual functions of the mature white blood cells, children with leukemia are prone to repeated infections. The immature white blood cells also crowd out the other elements of the bone marrow, causing the child to exhibit symptoms of anemia and thrombocytopenia (for example, fatigue and easy bruising). The peak incidence of leukemia is in children between 3 and 5 years of age.

Leukemia may occur as an acute or chronic disease. Chronic leukemia is rare in children, accounting for only 1% to 5% of all leukemias. Acute leukemia has a more rapid onset and is, without treatment, fatal. There are two main types of acute leukemia: acute lymphocytic leukemia (ALL) and acute nonlymphocytic leukemia (ANLL). ALL is the most common type, but ANLL is more deadly.

The cause of leukemia is unknown. Children with chromosomal defects or immunologic deficiencies, however, are at increased risk for ALL.

Symptoms. Children with leukemia often present with very subtle symptoms. Parents may report repeated infections or bruising, but because these signs also occur in well children, they may be ignored. When leukemia is suspected, a complete blood count is ordered. The WBC count may be low or elevated. The child is anemic and thrombocytopenic, and may have enlarged lymph nodes, spleen, and liver. Bone marrow aspiration and lumbar puncture confirm the diagnosis.

Treatment. Treatment includes chemotherapy and, occasionally, radiation. Bone marrow transplantation may also be performed. The long-term prognosis for children with ALL has improved dramatically with the advent of aggressive chemotherapy. Chemo-therapy is administered to induce remission. There are three phases of chemotherapy: remission induction, sanctuary therapy (or central nervous system prophylaxis), and maintenance.

Remission Induction

The actual drugs used will vary according to the type of leukemia and chemotherapy protocol (treatment plan), but almost all protocols include prednisone. Parents should be educated about the possible side effects

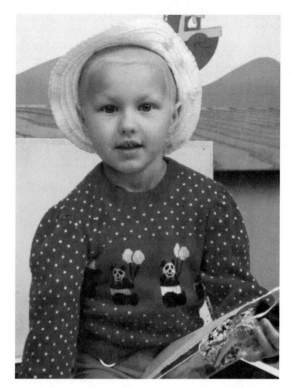

Figure 29–4   *This child has alopecia resulting from chemotherapy.*

of chemotherapy, including the cushingoid features (moon face) and alopecia, Figure 29–4, increased appetite, and growth retardation.

Sanctuary Therapy (CNS Prophylaxis)

The goal of sanctuary therapy is to prevent leukemic cells from seeking sanctuary in the central nervous system (CNS). At one time both intrathecal (into the spinal canal) methotrexate and CNS irradiation were used to prevent this occurrence. Because of the link between learning disabilities and CNS irradiation, however, most facilities now give only intrathecal drugs except for high-risk patients (Leventhol 1992).

Maintenance

During the maintenance phase, the child continues to receive chemotherapy as well as periodic bone marrow examinations to monitor for recurrence of the disease.

Nursing Care. Nursing care varies depending on the specific drugs used and the family's response to the disease. All families need emotional support as they learn more about the disease and its treatment. Families need to be made aware of other problems that could occur in response to chemotherapy and its side effects, which may include increased bleeding tendencies, infection, and anemia. Changes in body image resulting from alopecia and cushingoid features present problems, particularly for older children. Figure 29–5 summarizes nursing care for the child with leukemia.

IDIOPATHIC THROMBOCYTOPENIA PURPURA

Idiopathic thrombocytopenia purpura is a commonly occurring blood disorder characterized by a decrease in thrombocytes. In approximately 30% of cases, the onset can be traced to medications or a viral infection. In most cases, however, the cause is unknown.

Idiopathic thrombocytopenia purpura may be acute or chronic. In children with the disorder, the platelet count is reduced. Ecchymoses and petechiae are common. Bleeding from the mucous membranes of the mouth, such as the gums, or the nose (epistaxis) and internal hemorrhage may also occur.

Many cases resolve spontaneously, but some are treated with prednisone or intravenous gamma globulin. Splenectomy is performed in chronic cases that do not respond to therapy.

Nursing care focuses on protecting the child from injury and on education. Children should be cautioned to avoid contact sports, to brush their teeth with a soft-bristled toothbrush, and to avoid drugs such as aspirin, which can damage platelets.

ADOLESCENT

HODGKIN'S DISEASE

Description. Hodgkin's disease, or cancer of the lymphatic system, occurs most often in late adolescence or young adulthood and is twice as common in boys as in girls.

Symptoms. Symptoms initially include painless lymphadenopathy, followed by shortness of breath, cough, and splenomegaly. The diagnosis is made by lymph node biopsy. Exploratory laparotomy is often performed to assess the extent of the disease.

Treatment. Once the diagnosis has been made and the extent of disease (staging) determined, the child is treated with either short-term radiation or, for more advanced disease, with a combination of chemotherapy (such as MOPP — mustargen, Oncovin, procarbazine, and prednisone) and radiation. Children with less-advanced disease (stage I or II) have an excellent prognosis.

Nursing Care. Nursing care for the child with Hodgkin's disease is similar to that for the child with leukemia. Because children with Hodgkin's disease are older, they may have more difficulty with problems of body image as well as difficulty facing their own death. The adolescent who is diagnosed with advanced (stage III or IV) disease may benefit from counseling resources. Oncology nurses, clinical nurse specialists, social workers, members of the clergy, or the hospital chaplain may provide support to the child and family. It is important that the adolescent and family be kept informed of the child's progress and prognosis at all times.

NURSING CARE PLAN: Leukemia

NURSING DIAGNOSIS	GOAL(S)
Anxiety (child) related to invasive diagnostic procedure (bone marrow aspiration)	Before bone marrow procedure, the child will understand the need for diagnostic tests.
Anxiety (parent) related to potentially life-threatening condition of child	The parents will be able to explain treatment for leukemia and hoped-for response.
Immunosuppression related to chemotherapy and disease process	The child will remain infection-free. The parents will be able to identify signs of infection.

Figure 29–5

NURSING INTERVENTION	RATIONALE
Before each procedure, explain exactly what is happening and what the child's role will be.	Knowledge decreases anxiety, which in turn decreases pain.
Discuss use of Lidocaine patch. Let child put Lidocaine cream on arm and feel the effect. Teach guided imagery techniques and breathing exercises.	Lidocaine decreases pain perception. Control over what is happening increases child's ability to manage pain.
Explain cause and common symptoms of leukemia. Give parents written information on leukemia and its treatment. Identify usual side effects of treatment.	Knowledge decreases anxiety. Written information gives parents something to refer to.
Introduce parents to parents of other children with leukemia and to resources such as chaplain and social worker.	Provides support and comfort.
Instruct child and parents on the need to wash hands frequently and the need to limit visitors, particularly those with infections.	Handwashing and limitation of visitors decrease child's contact with organisms, which decreases chance of developing an infection.
Teach parents to monitor child for signs of infection, such as cough, fever, or earache.	Early identification of infection allows for prompt treatment.

Figure 29–5 continued

NURSING DIAGNOSIS	GOAL(S)
Side effects of chemotherapy (e.g., constipation and oral ulcers)	The child will maintain a normal stool pattern. The child's mouth will be kept clean, and child will experience minimal oral ulcers.
Body image disturbance related to hair loss and cushingoid appearance	The child will cope with changed appearance.
Weight loss related to nausea and vomiting associated with chemotherapy	The child will: maintain current weight during hospitalization; gain 1 lb per month when home; eat a nutritious diet high in protein and complex carbohydrates.
Risk for hemorrhage related to decreased platelets as a result of chemotherapy	The child will not sustain injury or hemorrhage.

Figure 29–5 *continued*

NURSING INTERVENTION	RATIONALE
Keep a record of daily stool pattern. Encourage 8 glasses of preferred beverage daily. Encourage fruits and vegetables.	Increasing fluid and fiber intake will increase bowel motility.
Instruct child to brush teeth with soft-bristled toothbrush after eating, before bed, and on awakening.	A clean mouth decreases the chance of oral ulcers developing.
Teach parents to inspect child's mouth daily for oral ulcers.	Early identification allows for prompt treatment.
Reassure child that hair loss is temporary. Suggest use of hats or scarves if child wants to cover head. If child wants to wear a wig, advise parents to purchase it before hair loss occurs.	Knowing that hair loss is temporary decreases child's concern. Hats and scarves are colorful and cheaper than wigs. If a wig is worn, child should start wearing it before loosing all hair so that the contrast is not so apparent.
Premedicate child with antiemetic before chemotherapy.	Prevention is the best treatment for nausea and vomiting related to therapy.
Keep room odor-free.	Noxious stimuli can cause nausea.
Offer preferred foods. Encourage parents to bring favorite foods from home.	Child is more apt to eat favorite foods than hospital food.
Provide parents with handouts identifying foods high in protein and complex carbo-hydrates. Encourage high-calorie foods such as milk shakes, cheese cake, ice cream, and eggnog.	Gives parents information they can refer to. Milk-based foods are packed with calories and protein.
Discourage rough play or contact sports.	Unintentional injury causes bleeding.
Teach first aid for bleeding (ice, pressure, elevation).	Minor bleeding may be managed at home.
Administer platelets per physician's order.	When platelets fall to predetermined level, replacement must be given.

Figure 29–5   *continued*

Review Questions

A. Multiple choice. Select the best answer.

1. Johnny is a 2-year-old diagnosed with iron deficiency anemia. His mother states that he loves milk, and since "milk is nature's most nearly perfect food" she sometimes allows him to drink milk in place of meals. What will you tell Johnny's mother?
   a. "Milk is an excellent food for children Johnny's age. I cannot understand why Johnny is anemic."
   b. "Milk is an excellent source of calcium, but not iron. Let's review some iron-rich foods."
   c. "Whatever made you think that milk could be used in place of meals? Johnny needs to eat from the basic food groups every day."
   d. "The amount of milk Johnny drinks each day should be limited to no more than 12 ounces."

2. Shamiqua is admitted to the hospital in sickle cell crisis. She is 4 years old and was diagnosed with sickle cell anemia at age 2. This is Shamiqua's third hospitalization in 6 months. Her mother asks what she can do to decrease the chance that Shamiqua will be hospitalized again in the near future. What will you tell her?
   a. "There really isn't much you can do about sickle cell crisis. It just happens."
   b. "You must feel bad about Shamiqua's hospitalizations. Do you attend a support group?"
   c. "The two most common reasons for hospitalization are dehydration and infection. If you can see to it that Shamiqua avoids crowds and drinks plenty of fluids you may see a decrease in her hospitalizations."
   d. "Is Shamiqua up-to-date on all of her immunizations? If you can prevent some of these infections, she should be able to stay out of the hospital."

3. The child with idiopathic thrombocytopenic purpura usually does not receive intramuscular injections or venipunctures unless absolutely necessary. Why?
   a. The child's blood does not clot properly. Intrusive procedures are avoided because of the danger that blood will ooze from the puncture site and the increased risk of bruising.
   b. The child already has bruising and it is difficult to identify anatomical landmarks, so it is difficult to find an appropriate site.
   c. The child has already had so many injections that an attempt is made to avoid any more.
   d. The child is at risk for bleeding. Therefore, injections are avoided to decrease the danger of a fatal hemorrhage.

4. Jonathan is a 10-year-old with hemophilia A. His mother states, "I don't understand how this happened. Neither his father nor I have hemophilia." What will you tell them about the disease?
   a. "Hemophilia occurs randomly, and there is no way to predict who will have it."
   b. "Hemophilia is usually transmitted genetically from father to son."
   c. "This must be confusing for you. I'll tell the doctor you have some questions."
   d. "The most common method of transmission is from a carrier mother to her son. The mother may be unaware that she is a carrier."

5. The child with an infection normally has an increase in
   a. RBCs
   b. WBCs
   c. platelets
   d. hemoglobin

6. The white blood cells that are responsible for fighting infection are the
   a. neutrophils
   b. erythrocytes
   c. thrombocytes
   d. electrolytes

7. Which of the following orders should you question when your patient has a diagnosis of idiopathic thrombocytopenia purpura?
   a. oral acetaminophen
   b. platelet count
   c. oral aspirin
   d. oral prednisone

B. True or false. Write *T* for a true statement and *F* for a false statement.

1. ___ Iron deficiency anemia is common in preschoolers.

2. ___ Sickle cell anemia is a chronic disease.

3. ___ Hemophilia is equally common in boys and girls.

4. ___ Children with acute lymphocytic leukemia have an invariably poor prognosis.

5. ___ Hodgkin's disease is cancer of the lymphatic system.

SUGGESTED ACTIVITIES

• Arrange to observe a pediatric hematology clinic. Note how the children cope with painful procedures.

• Plan to spend a day with a pediatric oncology clinical nurse specialist or clinician. Make careful note of his or her role on the pediatric oncology team.

• Role play the necessary explanation and teaching to a parent of a child with a disorder of the blood or blood-forming organs.

BIBLIOGRAPHY

Diamond, C. A., and K. K. Matthay. Childhood acute lymphoblastic leukemia. *Pediatric Annals* 17 (1988): 156.

Dudek, S. *Nutrition Handbook for Nursing Practice.* Philadelphia: J. B. Lippincott, 1993.

Fochtman, D., G. V. Foley, and K. Mooney, eds. *Nursing Care of the Child with Cancer.* Boston: Little, Brown, 1993.

Foster, R. L., M. M. Hunsberger, and J. J. Anderson. *Family-Centered Nursing Care of Children.* Philadelphia: W. B. Saunders, 1989.

James, S. R., and S. R. Mott. *Child Health Nursing.* San Francisco: Addison-Wesley, 1988.

Leventhol, B. Neoplasms and neoplasm-like structures. In R. E. Behrman and V. C. Vaughan, eds. *Nelson's Textbook of Pediatrics*, 14th ed. Philadelphia: W. B. Saunders, 1992.

Morrison, R. A., and D. A. Vedro. Pain management in the child with sickle cell disease. *Pediatric Nursing* 15, no. 5 (1989): 595–599, 613.

Shapiro, B. S. The management of pain in sickle cell disease. *Pediatric Clinics of North America* 36, no. 4 (1989): 1029–1043.

Stockman, J. Diseases of the blood. In R. E. Behrman and V. C. Vaughan, eds. *Nelson's Textbook of Pediatrics*, 14th ed. Philadelphia: W. B. Saunders, 1992.

*E*motional and Behavioral Conditions

OBJECTIVES

AFTER STUDYING THIS CHAPTER, THE STUDENT SHOULD BE ABLE TO:

- DESCRIBE BEHAVIORS AND RESPONSES OF AN INFANT OR TODDLER WITH FAILURE TO THRIVE.

- FORMULATE A BASIC PLAN OF CARE FOR THE INFANT WITH FAILURE TO THRIVE THAT WILL NURTURE THE INFANT AND PROMOTE ATTACHMENT.

- BRIEFLY DESCRIBE ATTENTION DEFICIT HYPERACTIVITY DISORDER AND DISCUSS ITS SYMPTOMS, TREATMENT, AND NURSING CARE.

- DISCUSS THE CAUSE, SYMPTOMS, AND TREATMENT OF SCHOOL PHOBIA.

- NAME THREE EATING CONDITIONS THAT AFFECT SCHOOL-AGE CHILDREN AND ADOLESCENTS AND DESCRIBE THEIR CAUSES, SYMPTOMS, AND TREATMENT.

- DESCRIBE SYMPTOMS OF DEPRESSION AND SUICIDAL BEHAVIOR IN ADOLESCENTS AND DISCUSS TREATMENT AND NURSING CARE FOR THESE PATIENTS.

- IDENTIFY CAUSES AND SYMPTOMS OF SUBSTANCE ABUSE AND DESCRIBE TREATMENT AND NURSING CARE FOR THE SUBSTANCE-ABUSING ADOLESCENT.

Key Terms

FAILURE TO THRIVE

ATTACHMENT

PHOBIA

SEPARATION ANXIETY

BINGING

PURGING

DYSPHORIA

ANHEDONIA

PSYCHOACTIVE

*a*s the health care provider who first establishes rapport with a child and family in the health care system, the nurse needs to be able to use basic communication skills as a tool to gather assessment data. The nurse must also be knowledgeable about general norms of behavior, stages of growth and development, and signs and symptoms of disease. Finally the nurse needs to know when and where to refer a patient for further assessment and treatment.

It is not always clear whether an individual's responses or symptoms have a physiological (organic) cause or are related to emotional and psychological factors. It is not unusual for symptoms of the infant, child, and adolescent to present as a physical problem, at least initially.

The conditions discussed in this chapter are considered to be primarily behavioral and emotional problems. For some conditions, however, there is a strong physiological component. The nurse must be constantly aware of this component and address physiological needs while responding to and being supportive of emotional and psychological needs and behavioral responses.

Overview of Emotional and Behavioral Conditions

For a newborn infant to become an integrated and emotionally healthy person, the infant must be perceived as an individual, with separate needs who, through his or her behavior, tells the parents what those needs are. Parents must, in turn, observe and interpret the infant's cues to find out what the infant is "telling" them through these sounds and behaviors.

Before an infant is born, parents may plan for the infant's characteristics — gender, personality, talent — sometimes going so far as planning a role the infant will play in life. This role may be one that parents believe will correct for disappointments in their own lives. Each child, of course, has his or her own way of responding to life. Some children may accept and respond more or less comfortably to the role given by their parents; others may be unsuited for the chosen role. These children may be at risk for behavioral or emotional problems.

When parents are unable to relate to the infant as a separate person, they may respond in ways that interfere with the infant's emotional well-being. Such a response may create difficulties as the child matures, ranging from emotional "hang-ups" to pervasive childhood behavioral conditions.

Figure 30–1 presents general principles that may assist the nurse in relating to and gathering information about a child with an emotional or behavioral condition.

GENERAL ASSESSMENT PRINCIPLES

- Be knowledgeable about the norms for each stage of growth and development.

- Remember that each child and each situation is unique.

- Show willingness and patience to listen to the child's story. Often stories are "told" through emotions and behavior. Many important messages are transmitted by the way we sit, stand, walk, and respond, as well as by how we say things (tone, affect) and what we say (words). Because the child's vocabulary is not well developed, it is essential to pay attention to other cues.

- Be willing to see the problem through the child's eyes.

- Demonstrate a belief that the child has the ability to solve his or her own problem.

- Show willingness and patience to help parents make the changes needed to lessen the difficulty the child is experiencing. (Helping the parents to change may be particularly difficult if they are embarrassed, angry, protective, or refuse to or cannot separate themselves from the child and the child's needs.)

- Be aware of cultural differences that can cause misinterpretations of cues (e.g., stoicism, hysteria).

Figure 30–1 *General principles in assessment of children with emotional and behavioral conditions*

INFANT AND TODDLER

FAILURE TO THRIVE

Description. **Failure to thrive** (FTT) is a condition of infants and children under 2 years of age characterized by a weight for age that is below the third percentile. (Because National Center for Health Statistic growth charts do not give values below the fifth percentile, some authorities use weight below the fifth percentile as the criterion for FTT.) Failure to thrive may have an organic (physical) or nonorganic basis. This discussion focuses on children with nonorganic FTT. In these cases, the infant, parents, and environment interact in a way that results in emotional deprivation and, often, an accompanying lack of food. Sometimes an infant is offered sufficient food, but the emotional interaction and environment are not conducive to well-being. Sometimes the infant is too lethargic to eat. At other times, parents do not feed the infant properly because they lack knowledge about nutritional needs or feeding techniques, are unconcerned, or are neglectful.

The period immediately following birth has been described as the maternal sensitive period (Olds et al. 1992, Wong 1993). Predictable behaviors occur when mothers (and fathers) are with their infants soon after birth. These include touching the infant, examining the infant with the fingers, observing, and having direct eye contact while holding the infant in front of them, Figure 30–2. The infant responds to these behaviors, creating a reciprocal interaction. This interaction results in **attachment** (the emotional ties from infant to parent) and bonding (the ties from parent to infant).

Neglect of the infant and a lack of attachment and bonding can result in poor future parent-child relationships. When care is irregular, inconsistent, or mostly absent, attachment and bonding do not occur. The infant does not learn to trust or may perceive the world as confusing and unstable. As the child matures, this

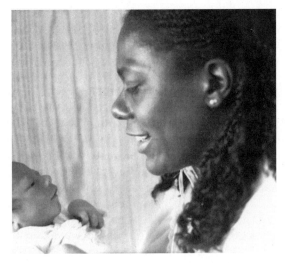

Figure 30–2 *Attachment and bonding behaviors occur in the period immediately after birth. (Courtesy Carol Toussie Weingarten)*

perception may lead to difficulties in trusting himself or herself and problems with self-esteem. The child may demonstrate social and behavioral delays and cognitive difficulties.

Symptoms. The weight of a child with FTT is below the third percentile. Infants with long-standing FTT are also below average in height. Infants with FTT may be listless, apathetic, and passive, or hyperalert to the environment. They may avoid (or have minimal) eye contact and demonstrate a lack of stranger anxiety (do not cry when they see a stranger). Sucking responses, cooing, and crying may be minimal or absent. Older infants may demonstrate reluctance to reach, crawl, or pull themselves to standing. A lack of interest in toys or play is common. Toddlers or preschool children may demonstrate delayed speech.

Treatment. The goals of treatment are to ensure adequate nutrition, provide support to parents, encourage parental involvement in care of the child, and teach the parents about developmental patterns and nutritional needs of infants and children. Continued support by health care providers and family counseling may be necessary.

Nursing Care. Assess the infant's behavior for cues to determine whether attachment and bonding have occurred, Figure 30–3. Assessment of the infant or toddler can be performed by observing the mother and child at feeding and visiting times to determine interaction patterns. Assessment should include several observations to avoid basing conclusions on random and isolated behavior. Observe the infant for approach and responses to the parent and others. Abnormal attachment behaviors include listlessness, lack of interest in the environment and parent, lack of cooing and eye contact, and lack of crying. The assessment must also include data on the weight and height of the infant and a comparison with norms and the infant's own growth rate.

Observe the parent(s) for affect (feeling state), ability to give care, concerns (voiced or not), and ways of relating and responding to the infant. Negative comments — including disappointments about the infant, not looking at the infant, not wanting to hold the infant, not asking questions about the infant, and general lack of interest and withdrawal — are all possible signs of impaired bonding to the infant.

Many factors have an effect on the bonding process. Cultural and ethnic differences may influence the ways in which mothers relate to their infants. Determine whether the behavior of the mother is related to a lack of knowledge about care of the infant, fear of hurting the infant, or anxiety over being a parent. Other barriers to the bonding process are physical illness of either the mother or infant, drug abuse (of parents or withdrawal in the infant), AIDS, premature birth, and the parent's feelings of guilt and failure (Olds et al. 1992, Pillitteri 1992, Wong 1993).

Nursing care includes giving parents information about the infant, telling them what is normal, helping them to interpret the infant's cues, listening to expressions of concern and feelings, and teaching parents how to care for the infant.

The infant is placed on a diet specific for his or her needs. Parents are incorporated into the plan of care and encouraged and assisted as necessary to care for their infant. Some parents may need continuing support or counseling to become effective parents. Figure 30–4 summarizes nursing care for an infant with failure to thrive.

ATTACHMENT BEHAVIORS

Newborns	Infants (1–12 months)	Toddlers (2–3 years)
• Visually follow the caregiver	• Imitate (imprint)	• Curious
• Smile	• Need visual or tactile contact with the parent while exploring an unfamiliar environment	• Cooperative
• Reach	• Fear of strangers (cry when looking at strangers)	• Responses indicate separation anxiety (cry when parent leaves)
• Grasp		• Adapt to changes, even when the parent is out of sight

Figure 30–3

NURSING CARE PLAN: Failure to Thrive

NURSING DIAGNOSIS	GOAL(S)
Body weight below third percentile for age, height, and gender	Infant receives adequate oral intake and experiences weight gain of 1 to 2 oz. daily.
Altered growth and development (listless, absence of cooing, diminished sucking response)	Infant's responses are within normal range for chronological age.

Figure 30–4

Nursing Intervention	Rationale
Select one caregiver to care for child.	Encourages development of trust and attachment.
Model positive parenting techniques: cuddle, talk with, and have eye contact with infant during feeding.	These techniques stimulate interaction and relating, promote bonding, and stimulate development.
Establish consistent caregiving routine.	Consistency provides structure, lessens anxiety, and promotes trust (infant knows what to expect).
Avoid interruptions and minimize environmental stimulation during care and feeding.	Minimizes unwanted stimuli that might distract from the feeding process.
Give prescribed formula. Record schedule, intake, daily weight, and responses to staff, parent, and environment.	This information provides a baseline for evaluating progress and determining whether to continue or change approach and management of care.
Have the same caregiver provide care to the infant.	Frequent contacts with the same caregiver help establish a relationship of trust and promote attachment.
Encourage play times and use of developmentally appropriate stimuli.	Play and stimulation encourage development and growth.
Handle the infant gently, lovingly, with confidence, and with consistency: cuddle, soothe, coo, talk with, and make eye contact with infant.	These types of contacts will promote a sense of safety, comfort, and belonging in the infant.

Figure 30–4 *continued*

Nursing Diagnosis	Goal(s)
Inappropriate parenting practices	Parents are able to state feelings and concerns related to care of the infant.
	Parents request information about proper care of the infant.
	Parents participate in care of the infant.

Figure 30–4   continued

NURSING INTERVENTION	RATIONALE
Set aside time during each visit to listen to parents' concerns.	A consistent and designated time period allows parents to express feelings and concerns and promotes interaction and formation of a trusting relationship with the caregiver.
Encourage parents to discuss concerns, frustrations, and fears; acknowledge parental difficulties and frustrations.	Expressing feelings (especially negative) and receiving acknowledgment of feelings lessens anxiety and resentment and promotes the expression of positive feelings.
Nurture and give emotional support to parents.	Providing emotional support will enhance parents' self-esteem and confidence.
Identify needs and determine readiness to receive information.	Before any health teaching takes place, it is necessary to identify what information is needed and determine learner readiness.
Encourage questions by parents about infant.	Parents may be reluctant to admit they don't know how to care for the infant; encouraging parents' questions helps to provide this information.
Provide information and guidance about normal infant development and growth; teach parenting skills (for example, holding, touching, talking, physical care techniques, feeding, etc.).	Be clear with information given. Provide information at a level geared to parents' level of understanding; do not overload parents with too much information at one time (more sessions are better than too much information at one time). Provide diagrams and written information that parents can refer to at a later time. Follow up the next day to assess understanding and retention by having parents repeat information.
Model appropriate parenting behaviors; encourage parental caregiving; assist parents to recognize infant cues and interpret these cues when necessary.	Giving encouragement, feedback, positive comments, and helpful hints promotes confidence in parents and reinforces their efforts.

Figure 30–4   continued

NURSING DIAGNOSIS	GOAL(S)
Inappropriate parenting practices *(continued)*	Parents participate in care of the infant.

Identify and contact appropriate referral resources for follow-up support, as appropriate. |

Figure 30–4 *continued*

SCHOOL-AGE CHILD

ATTENTION DEFICIT HYPERACTIVITY DISORDER

Description. Attention deficit hyperactivity disorder (ADHD) is characterized by excessive and constant motor activity with little or no ability to concentrate. The condition occurs in boys more often than girls and affects approximately 3% of the school-age population (Townsend 1993). The cause is unknown but may be linked to biochemical or genetic factors.

Symptoms. Although symptoms usually appear before the child is 7 years of age (Rudolph et al. 1991), hyperactivity is often first observed by the child's teacher and reported to the school nurse, counselor, or parent because of difficulties in the classroom. The following behaviors may be seen:

exaggerated muscle activity
unfocused or aimless motion
interruption of and intrusion on others

- impulsive and unpredictable behavior
- fidgeting
- squirming
- difficulty finishing a task or remaining seated when asked to do so

Symptoms can result in impaired emotional and psychological development, as parents often become frustrated with the child, which in turn can affect the child's self-esteem and ability to cope.

Cognitively, children with ADHD have difficulty concentrating, do not seem to listen when spoken to, blurt out information, and often have difficulty with space perception (right-left and front-back), which may be revealed by difficulty in turning faucets on or off, turning doorknobs to open or close, or by reaching beyond an object and tipping the object over. Written work may be messy, with poorly formed and reversed letters (b/d, g/p/q). These children may have difficulty putting words in sequence and using conjunctions and prepositions. They have difficulty learning to read and learning rules of math

NURSING INTERVENTION	RATIONALE
Assess parental and infant responses and behaviors to determine whether attachment and bonding are occurring.	Continual assessment by the nurse assists in evaluating progress and determining whether any changes in the management plan are needed.
Assess (discuss) home environment (situation, stressors) and support system. Identify resources available to parents for support after discharge.	Knowledge about the home environment and resources for support when infant is discharged and parents are on their own will often help parents continue to give the care learned in the hospital or other structured setting.

Figure 30–4   continued

and language because they cannot remember the information (for example, a child will be unable to remember two numbers in order to add them to a third number and find the total). Environmental stimuli seem to compound these difficulties. Children with ADHD seem to be less able than "normal" children to filter out irrelevant stimuli to concentrate on a task.

Treatment. Diagnosis includes a medical workup (neurological examination, electro-encephalogram) to rule out a physical problem, psychological testing, and testing for learning disabilities. A safe, nonstimulating, structured though relaxed, and consistent environment is essential.

Management is directed toward enhancing self-esteem and self-control and decreasing anxiety. Medication may be used to control symptoms. Care of the child with ADHD requires patience, warmth, and discipline mixed with love. Parents need support in managing their feelings (often anger and frustration, sometimes a sense of failure) and in maintaining consistency.

Nursing Care. In order to best support and meet the child's needs, all the people who have responsibility for the child's development should be involved in the treatment plan. Frequent meetings allow for verbalization of feelings and concerns, communication of changes, and maintenance of consistency. Limits for the child will need to be set and adhered to. Instructions should be given clearly and concisely. Choices need to be limited and distractions minimized. Reminders, preparation for changes in routines, and planned periods of exercise enhance the child's well-being, as do praise, promotion of self-control, and immediate discipline when warranted (e.g., when the child deliberately does something wrong).

SCHOOL PHOBIA

School phobia is a condition in which a child has a traumatic aversion to school, characterized by the development of physical symptoms before or at school in an attempt to be allowed to stay home or be sent home. (The word **phobia**, from the Greek word for fear, refers to an excessive or unfounded fear of someone or something.) It is thought that about 3% of children have school phobia, and the condition is three to nine times more common in boys than in girls (Pillitteri 1992).

School phobia may be a form of separation anxiety in which the child has fear of separation from or has not successfully dealt with separation from the parent (usually the mother). Factors associated with school phobia include difficulty in making the adjustment to school and doing school tasks; difficulty with the teacher; feelings of ridicule, humiliation, or embarrassment; fear of having to speak in front of others; fear of tests; feelings of losing the parent's attention to younger siblings; and parental fears of "losing" the child or overprotectiveness, which may be imparted to the child.

Symptoms may include irritability, nausea, abdominal pain, headache, leg pain, or dizziness. In class, the child may be tense, tremulous, and perspire. Symptoms are absent on weekends and holidays and often decrease if the parent is present in the class. A behavioral description by teacher and parent is important because children with school phobias may be anxious and timid away from home and controlling and obstinate in the home. Tests are performed to rule out physical causes for the child's symptoms.

Treatment includes listening to the child's story and being consistent with responses. It may be that this behavior is the child's way of breaking away from conformity or a rigid mold or of dealing with family problems by displacing them to the school setting. Treatment approaches might include a modified systematic desensitization plan in which a therapist works with the child in the classroom or counseling with the child and parents or family.

EATING DISORDERS

Eating disorders are conditions in which a person uses food in a dysfunctional way, most often as a source of emotional nurturance. These disorders are most likely to occur during crisis periods when the person feels overwhelmed or during periods of significant change. Eating disorders may be linked to an underlying depression. They may also represent a person's attempt to gain some control over changing and extraordinary events by engaging in behaviors that he or she, and no one else, can control (McCoy 1985).

Early diagnosis and treatment of these disorders is important to minimize or prevent harmful effects on the body and address self-esteem and body-image issues.

Obesity. Obesity is a condition in which a person's weight is 20% to 30% or more above his or her "ideal" weight for sex, height, and age (Haber et al. 1992, Townsend 1993). Overweight, in contrast, is described as a condition in which the person is 10% over the ideal weight. Because the height and weight of children vary, obesity and overweight are often difficult to define. In addition, a person can be overweight and at the same time malnourished because the foods consumed lack nutritional value.

Various factors have been proposed as causes of obesity, including genetic predisposition, excessive numbers of fat cells, and body build. Obesity often begins in infancy when a parent overfeeds the infant. Cultural influences, misconceptions such as "a fat baby is a healthy baby," attempts to quiet an infant, and lack of knowledge are some of the reasons given for overfeeding at this age. Because needs and habits developed in infancy continue for a lifetime, prevention during this period is important.

Boys tend to be overweight during the school-age years; girls after puberty. (Girls also tend to try to control their weight through fad diets and dysfunctional eating patterns; see later discussion of anorexia nervosa and bulimia nervosa.) Physiological complications of obesity in school-age children and adolescents include hypertension and elevated total cholesterol, along with poor self-esteem and body-image disturbances. Obese children are often excluded from activities or even taunted about their appearance and may become withdrawn and socially isolated as a consequence.

Treatment focuses on dietary planning to meet the nutritional needs of the growing child while ensuring necessary caloric restrictions. School-age children should be encouraged to achieve short-term dietary goals and to engage in preferred physical exercises and activities. The child's dietary program should be supervised by a physician and dietician who understand the metabolic and psychological impact of weight loss (Rudolph et al. 1991). Parents play an important role in the treatment success of the child. Having obese parents makes it more difficult for the child to succeed. Consistency of approach, support, and acknowledgment of the child's successes in meeting goals are important aspects of the treatment plan.

ADOLESCENT

EATING DISORDERS

Anorexia Nervosa. Anorexia nervosa is a condition of self-starvation based on an unrealistic fear of being fat. The disorder occurs predominantly in adolescent and young adult females. Total body weight is 20% to 40% below normal, Figure 30–5 (Pillitteri 1992, Varcarolis 1990). Death may occur in prolonged, severe cases from self-starvation itself or as a result of complications such as electrolyte imbalances, cardiovascular problems and arrhythmias, and renal impairment.

The typical adolescent with anorexia is described as a compliant, "model" child and a high achiever who receives attention for these behaviors. The parents are demanding (usually the father, regarding expectations for achievement) and controlling (usually the mother). The adolescent attempts to control the environment, body, and other people, but does not truly succeed at having control over his or her own self.

The adolescent is obsessed with food, although often giving the appearance of not being interested in eating. Symptoms usually include amenorrhea, lanugo, dry skin, and bruising. Body image is distorted, so that the excessively thin adolescent looking in the mirror sees a reflection that is fat. Characteristically, the adolescent refuses to admit that anything is wrong and does not think treatment is necessary.

Treatment requires a multidimensional, coordinated, and consistent approach. An approach that facilitates trust is an essential part of treatment. Establishing trust may not be easy because of the often manipulative behavior of the anorexic patient. Staff may have difficulty coping with mixed feelings that are often generated by working with these patients.

Depending on the severity of the illness, the adolescent may be hospitalized to manage physiological aspects of the disorder. The treatment plan may include short-term separation from the family, a prescribed dietary regimen, psychotherapy that includes individual and family counseling, weighing several times weekly (observing for extra clothing or hiding of objects that might increase the weight), observance of mealtimes, limitation of exercise and activity, and providing opportunities for the adolescent to verbalize loss, fears, and anxiety. Long-term management is required to monitor the success of behavioral modification and weight gain.

Bulimia Nervosa. Bulimia nervosa is characterized by a cycle of abnormal consumption of food (**binging**) — as much as 3,000 to 5,000 calories at one time — followed by self-induced vomiting or use of diuretics or laxatives (**purging**). Like anorexia, bulimia affects primarily adolescent and young adult females. The

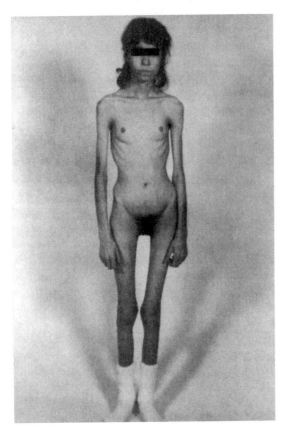 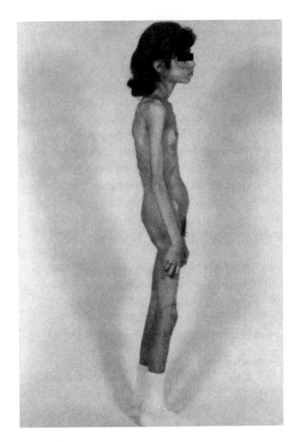

Figure 30–5 *Physical manifestations of extreme wasting in an adolescent with anorexia nervosa (From R. P. Rawlings, S. R. Williams, and C. K. Beck.* Mental Health-Psychiatric Nursing, *3rd ed. St. Louis, MO: Mosby-Year Book, 1992)*

adolescent has an overconcern about weight and attempts to maintain weight through the binge-purge behaviors. Psychological factors associated with bulimia include a belief of not "measuring up," feeling inadequate, and not feeling accepted by the peer group.

Because the adolescent with bulimia usually maintains a weight within normal limits, the disorder is often difficult to diagnose. The adolescent may hide food, be dishonest or lie about the behavior, and eat normally in front of others. Symptoms include muscle wasting, dark circles under the eyes, and dental caries or loss of dental enamel caused by vomiting of stomach acids.

The adolescent may be unable to stop eating once binging starts, with the cycle ending in depression and sleep. As behavior interferes with normal daily activities, the adolescent becomes more isolated. Cardiovascular complications as well as gastrointestinal problems (such as parotitis, gastritis, ulcers, hernias, and bowel and liver problems) may result. The stomach may become very large, distended, and even rupture (Mitchell 1989). In severe cases, the disorder may be fatal.

Treatment focuses on increasing the adolescent's self-esteem and, through a long-term process, changing the bulimic lifestyle and thinking patterns. The treatment program requires a consistent approach; supportive environment; and multidisciplinary team to address the physiological, emotional, and behavioral components of the disorder.

DEPRESSION

Description. Depression can occur in children of any age but is most common in adolescents. Teenagers who suffer from feelings of low self-esteem, pronounced **dysphoria** (anguish), and distorted and disturbed thinking are at greatest risk for depression. Contributing factors in adolescent depression are a sense of loss (of childhood, of love), feelings of failure or lack of control, and threats to self-esteem. Other factors may include a family move, separation, divorce, death, or loss of a boyfriend or girlfriend.

Symptoms. Symptoms of depression in children and adolescents include listlessness and **anhedonia** (absence of pleasurable feelings; lack of interest in activities); impaired school work; preoccupation with morbid thoughts; irritability and even hostility; and somatic symptoms such as headaches, stomach aches, muscle aches, and changes in eating and sleeping patterns. The adolescent may act out these feelings, sometimes in the form of delinquency. At other times, there may be withdrawal and isolation. The use and abuse of substances (alcohol and drugs, both prescription and illegal) may occur. The adolescent may also engage in high-risk activities that result in frequent injuries. Thoughts of suicide are always a possibility.

Treatment. The treatment program includes providing a safe, predictable, controlled, and controllable (by the individual) environment for the adolescent. Promotion of self-esteem and the development of coping skills, including learning to make choices, are essential parts of the treatment plan. Continued assess-

ment of behavior changes and suicide risk is necessary.

Open communication allows for expression of feelings and assists the adolescent to express feelings, learn to cope, and to understand himself or herself. Many parents have difficulty understanding that adolescents go through stages, such as being tired or sleeping much of the time (related to physiological changes) and need to be with peer groups in order to become healthy, functioning adults.

Nursing Care. The nurse needs to be supportive of the adolescent as well as understanding and supportive of parents. Listening and providing information about the normal development and expected tasks of adolescence may be helpful for both parents and the adolescent. Knowledge of what to expect often eases the pressures that parents feel about their child and their insistence that the adolescent should act in certain ways.

SUICIDE

Suicide has become the second leading cause of death in adolescents and young adults aged 15 to 24 years, after accidents (Townsend 1993). Since the early 1960s, suicides in this age group increased 300% (Townsend 1993). Among suggested underlying causes are: increased life stresses (related to the assumption of adult responsibilities), factors such as those discussed above for depression, feelings of rejection, confusion about life and personal circumstances, failure to meet self and parental expectations, lack of purpose, and lack of coping skills to deal with these situations.

Adolescents at risk for suicide may demonstrate warning signs such as sleep and eating disorders (often with severe weight loss in a short amount of time); behavioral changes (often abrupt); changes in mood (including abrupt elevation of mood after a depressed mood and affect); changed or lack of interest in friends, family, school, and life; expressed feelings of helplessness, hopelessness, and worthlessness; expressed intent to commit suicide; giving away valued possessions; increased use of illegal drugs or substances; and high-risk activities.

A thorough assessment of the adolescent's symptoms, feelings, thoughts, and behaviors is necessary. Assessment must include environmental aspects, such as recent changes in the adolescent's or family's life; relationships; impulsivity and decision-making capability; and risk factors such as previous attempts, attempts by other family members, and suicide of a peer. Children and adolescents are often impulsive and may act on their feelings and thoughts without regard to the consequence (that death is permanent). *These symptoms must be taken seriously!* The adolescent should be asked directly whether he or she is considering suicide and then asked if he or she has a plan. This approach does not create thoughts of suicide; in fact, the adolescent may be relieved that someone is inquiring.

Depending on the seriousness of the threat, treatment of an adolescent at risk for suicide may include hospitalization. Adolescents with suicidal symptoms and risk factors require immediate intervention and referral to a mental health care professional with expertise in this area. Probably the single most important factor in reducing the possibility of suicide is the formation and continuation of a relationship with a supportive, concerned person.

SUBSTANCE ABUSE

Description. Substance abuse is the use of any **psychoactive** (mind-altering) substance in a manner other than that prescribed by cultural standards or in ways that impair a person's ability to function. Psychoactive substances include alcohol, prescription drugs (amphetamines, barbiturates), and illicit drugs (marijuana, cocaine/crack, heroin, phencyclidine [PCP], and LSD).

Many adolescents experiment with drugs or alcohol; experimentation is not considered abuse. It may occur or be precipitated by the need to be a part of a group, for "kicks," because of peer pressure ("Just try it"), to test one's own capabilities, or as an escape from problems and overwhelming stress. Continued experimentation, however, may lead to regular use, resulting in physical and psychological dependency, tolerance, habituation, and addiction. Regular substance use has many long-term implications, including unexpected overdose and possible death.

Symptoms. Symptoms depend on the particular substance abused. Characteristic physical findings include reddened eyes, euphoria, loss of appetite and weight loss, wearing long sleeves (to hide needle marks), blackouts, sweating, nervousness, and lethargy. Long-term effects of commonly used drugs and substances are listed in Figure 30–6.

Treatment. An important part of the treatment of the adolescent is to provide an environment that is safe and supportive of the individual. Chemical dependency programs for adolescents that provide a structured, predictable environment and assist the adolescent to learn new coping skills, behaviors, and attitudes while encouraging the development of self-esteem have the best long-term results. Trusting relationships with staff are most important. The recovery process is slow, requiring long-term management. Health care team members need to be nonjudgmental and caring.

Support groups (Tough Love for parents, Alcoholics Anonymous for teens [Al-anon, Alateen], Cocaine Anonymous, Narcotics Anonymous) and family counseling can provide a support system for the adolescent and family. Prevention education programs such as D.A.R.E. (Drug Abuse Resistance Education), M.A.D.D. (Mothers Against Drunk Driving), and S.A.D.D. (Students Against

EFFECTS OF SUBSTANCE ABUSE	
Drug/Substance	**Effects of Long-Term Use**
Alcohol	Gastritis; peptic ulcer disease; increased risk for depression, suicide, and automobile accidents; blackouts; cirrhosis
Cocaine Crack	Chronic sinus and upper respiratory congestion; nose bleeds; chronic cough; anorexia or weight loss
Inhalants	Liver or kidney damage (depends on substance abused)
LSD	Flashbacks; psychoses, depression, and personality changes
Marijuana	Apathy, passivity, and decreased motivation; impaired ability to concentrate and memorize new information; increased risk for respiratory cancers
PCP	Psychotic states; increased capacity for aggressive and violent behavior

Figure 30–6 (Based on information in E. G. Bennett and D. Woolf. Substance Abuse: Pharmacologic, Developmental and Clinical Perspectives, 2nd ed. Albany, NY: Delmar Publishers, 1991, and A. D. Hoffman and D. E. Greydanus. Adolescent Medicine, 2nd ed. Norwalk, CT: Appleton and Lange, 1989)

Driving Drunk) that focus on drug and alcohol awareness have been implemented in schools and communities. The goals of these programs are to provide general education about drugs, teach antidrug attitudes, stress the importance of personal values, teach decision-making skills, and teach social skills (Bennett and Woolf 1991).

Nursing Care. The role the nurse plays in providing care to children and adolescents who are substance abusers will depend on the hospital or facility in which he or she is employed. Nurses who care for adolescent substance abusers must become familiar with (1) their own feelings about the use of psychoactive substances and (2) their feelings about the use and abuse of substances by children and adolescents.

It is most important for the nurse to be nonjudgmental and understanding while being able to: (1) identify the problem, (2) communicate about the problem, (3) educate the adolescent and family, (4) counsel the adolescent and family, and (5) refer the adolescent and family for treatment.

Areas for assessment include parental substance abuse, family dynamics, availability of prescription drugs and alcohol in the home, support systems, and ways of handling problems and conflicts. Always be alert to behaviors that could indicate potential substance abuse and report them to nursing managers and physicians.

Review Questions

A. Multiple choice. Select the best answer.

1. Which characteristics suggest that an infant is experiencing failure to thrive syndrome?
   a. stomach aches, high-pitched crying, uneven growth spurts
   b. apathy, avoidance of eye contact, delayed development
   c. stranger anxiety, rocking motions, sucking reflexes
   d. muscle tension, cooing, eye contact with parent

2. Nursing interventions to increase parent bonding might include:
   a. encouraging parents to talk to the infant
   b. showing parents what is wrong with their parenting skills
   c. feeding the infant when the parents visit
   d. showing parents how to weigh the infant

3. When parents ask the nurse what to do about their hyperactive child, the most helpful response would be:
   a. indulge the child when the behavior begins to be unmanageable
   b. discuss the child's behavior with the child to help the child decide how to stop the activity
   c. limit environmental stimuli, distractions, and choices given the child
   d. tell the child he or she is overstimulated and out of control

4. A mother whose child has school phobia might be advised to
   a. ignore complaints and expressions of fear by the child
   b. keep the child at home when there are physical symptoms
   c. have the child walk to school with another child
   d. work with school staff to desensitize the child's anxiety

5. Parents of a 14-year-old girl who has been diagnosed with anorexia nervosa would most likely tell the nurse:
   a. "We found her to be such an active, impish child."
   b. "She's always made us so proud of her until now."
   c. "We had trouble getting her to eat the right foods as a child."
   d. "She had difficulty getting along in grade school."

6. The highest priority for treatment of an adolescent hospitalized with anorexia nervosa related to extremely low weight is to
   a. establish rapport with the patient and family to gain their trust
   b. teach the patient the basics of good nutrition
   c. follow the prescribed plan to restore nutritional balance
   d. discuss the importance of adhering to the treatment plan

7. Which question would elicit the most information about the status of an adolescent who has been treated for bulimia nervosa?
   a. "What's happening in your life with people and activities?"
   b. "How are you managing your diet since you began the treatment program?"
   c. "What have been the fluctuations in your weight over the past three to six months?"
   d. "Are you continuing to follow the treatment plan developed when you were hospitalized?"

8. An 11-year-old middle-school child doesn't want to go to school, isn't interested in school or after-school activities, and admits that when she watches television she doesn't remember the programs. This is an example of
   a. morbid preoccupation
   b. listlessness
   c. isolation
   d. anhedonia

9. Tim, a 15-year-old high school sophomore, has been engaging in reckless behaviors since he broke up with his girlfriend last month. Which of the following questions is essential for assessment at this time?
   a. "Why are you doing all of these activities?"
   b. "What have you been doing since the breakup with your girlfriend?"
   c. "How are you doing?"
   d. "Are you thinking about suicide?"

10. Joan, a 13-year-old freshman whose parents have recently divorced, has been seen smoking marijuana cigarettes and says she "had a few beers" over the weekend. An intervention plan for Joan would include
    a. monitoring symptoms daily to determine if there is substance abuse
    b. finding out what her perceptions are about her family situation
    c. reporting her behavior and comments to the school psychologist for testing
    d. calling the parent with whom Joan lives to find out whether the parent is aware of the situation

SUGGESTED ACTIVITIES

• Observe a child with attention deficit hyperactive disorder. Review normal growth and development responses. Then observe a child of the same age who does not have ADHD. Describe differences in behavior relevant to the disorder.

• Given the importance of being direct and, at the same time, sensitive to an adolescent, formulate questions to ask regarding substance use. An example might be, "When you are with friends, do you drink alcohol or use drugs?" Or, being more direct (and assuming that an adolescent experiments with drugs), "What drugs have you tried?"

• Investigate resources in your community that an adolescent might turn to for help with (1) feelings of distress or despair, (2) suicidal thoughts, and (3) use or abuse of alcohol and other substances (drugs). (One place to begin is in the telephone book.) Which would you give as a resource or referral?

Bibliography

American Psychiatric Association. *Diagnostic and Statistical Manual of Mental Disorders*, 3rd ed, revised (DSM-III-R). Washington, D.C.: American Psychiatric Association, 1987.

Bennett, E. G., and D. Woolf. *Substance Abuse: Pharmacologic, Developmental and Clinical Perspectives*, 2nd ed. Albany, NY: Delmar Publishers, 1991.

Bouchard, C. Genetic influences on body composition and regional fat distribution. *Contemporary Nutrition* 15, no. 10 (1990).

Carpenito, L. *Nursing Diagnosis: Application to Clinical Practice*, 4th ed. Philadelphia: J. B. Lippincott, 1992.

Davies, J., and E. Janosik. *Health and Psychiatric Nursing*. Boston: Jones and Bartlett, 1991.

Haber, J., A. McMahan, P. Price-Hoskins, and B. Sideleau. *Comprehensive Psychiatric Nursing*. St. Louis, MO: Mosby-Year Book, 1992.

Hoffman, A. D., and D. E. Greydanus. *Adolescent Medicine*, 2nd ed. Norwalk, CT: Appleton and Lange, 1989.

Jacques, J., and N. Snyder. Newborn victims of addiction. *RN* (April, 1991): 47–53.

Levy, G., and J. Hickey. Fighting the battle against drugs. *RN* (April, 1991): 30–47.

Lucas, A. Update and review of anorexia nervosa. *Contemporary Nutrition* 14, no. 9 (1989).

McCoy, K. *Coping with Teenage Depression*. New York: Dutton, 1985.

McEnany, G. Managing mood disorders. *RN* (September, 1990): 28–33.

Mitchell, J. Bulimia nervosa. *Contemporary Nutrition* 14, no. 10 (1989).

Olds, S., M. London, and P. Ladewig. *Maternal-Newborn Nursing*, 4th ed. Redwood City, CA: Addison-Wesley, 1992.

Pillitteri, A. *Maternal and Child Health Nursing*. Philadelphia: J. B. Lippincott, 1992.

Roth, G. *When Food Is Love*. New York: Plume Books, 1991.

Rudolph, A. M., J. I. E. Hoffman, and C. D. Rudolph. *Rudolph's Pediatrics*, 19th ed. Norwalk, CT: Appleton and Lange, 1991.

Smith, M., and F. Lifshitz. Failure to thrive. *Contemporary Nutrition* 15, no. 5 (1990).

Townsend, M. *Psychiatric Mental Health Nursing: Concepts of Care*. Philadelphia: F. A. Davis, 1993.

Varcarolis, E. *Foundations of Psychiatric and Mental Health Nursing*. Philadelphia: W. B. Saunders, 1990.

Wong, D. *Whaley & Wong's Essentials of Pediatric Nursing*, 4th ed. St. Louis, MO: Mosby-Year Book, 1993.

BOYS: BIRTH TO 36 MONTHS
PHYSICAL GROWTH
NCHS PERCENTILES*

NAME _____ RECORD # _____

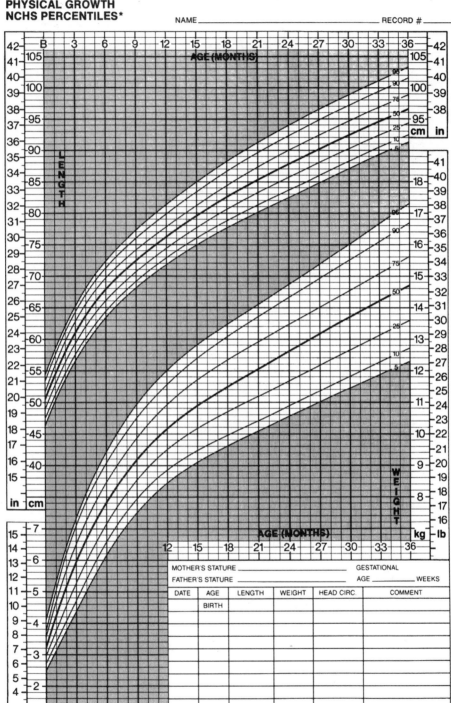

*Adapted from: Hamill PVV, Drizd TA, Johnson CL, Reed RB, Roche AF, Moore WM: Physical growth: National Center for Health Statistics percentiles. AM J CLIN NUTR 32:607-629, 1979. Data from the Fels Longitudinal Study, Wright State University School of Medicine, Yellow Springs, Ohio.

© 1982 Ross Laboratories

MOTHER'S STATURE _____ GESTATIONAL
FATHER'S STATURE _____ AGE _____ WEEKS

DATE	AGE	LENGTH	WEIGHT	HEAD CIRC.	COMMENT
	BIRTH				

BOYS: BIRTH TO 36 MONTHS
PHYSICAL GROWTH
NCHS PERCENTILES*

NAME _____ RECORD # _____

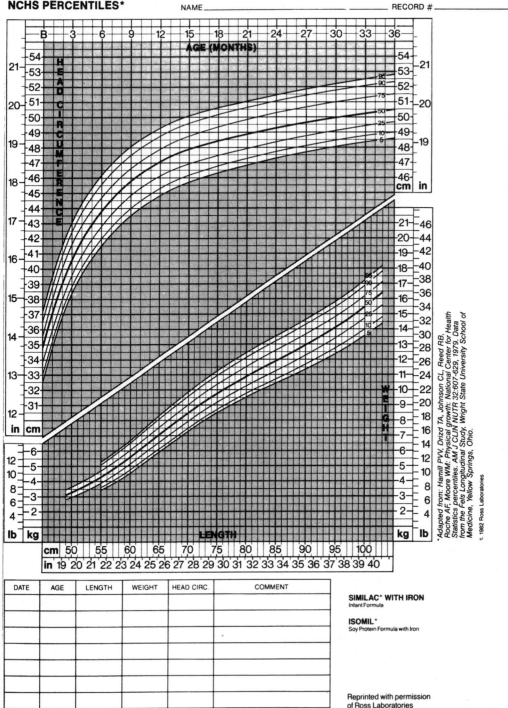

*Adapted from: Hamill PVV, Drizd TA, Johnson CL, Reed RB, Roche AF, Moore WM: Physical growth: National Center for Health Statistics percentiles. AM J CLIN NUTR 32:607-629, 1979. Data from the Fels Longitudinal Study, Wright State University School of Medicine, Yellow Springs, Ohio.

© 1982 Ross Laboratories

DATE	AGE	LENGTH	WEIGHT	HEAD CIRC.	COMMENT

SIMILAC® WITH IRON
Infant Formula

ISOMIL®
Soy Protein Formula with Iron

Reprinted with permission
of Ross Laboratories

GIRLS: BIRTH TO 36 MONTHS
PHYSICAL GROWTH
NCHS PERCENTILES*

NAME _____ RECORD # _____

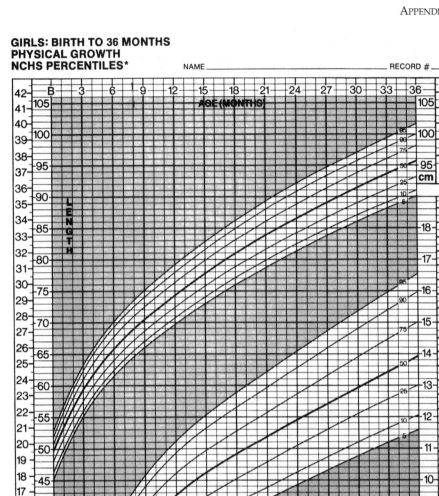

MOTHER'S STATURE _____ GESTATIONAL

FATHER'S STATURE _____ AGE _____ WEEKS

DATE	AGE	LENGTH	WEIGHT	HEAD CIRC.	COMMENT
	BIRTH				

* Adapted from: Hamill PVV, Drizd TA, Johnson CL, Reed RB, Roche AF, Moore WM: Physical growth: National Center for Health Statistics percentiles. AM J CLIN NUTR 32:607-629, 1979. Data from the Fels Longitudinal Study, Wright State University School of Medicine, Yellow Springs, Ohio.

© 1982 Ross Laboratories

GIRLS: BIRTH TO 36 MONTHS
PHYSICAL GROWTH
NCHS PERCENTILES*

NAME _____ RECORD # _____

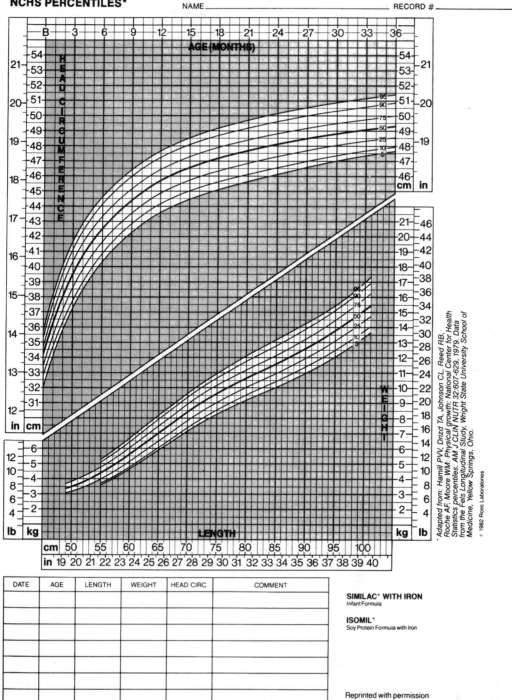

DATE	AGE	LENGTH	WEIGHT	HEAD CIRC.	COMMENT

SIMILAC* WITH IRON
Infant Formula

ISOMIL*
Soy Protein Formula with Iron

Reprinted with permission
of Ross Laboratories

*Adapted from: Hamill PVV, Drizd TA, Johnson CL, Reed RB, Roche AF, Moore WM: Physical growth: National Center for Health Statistics percentiles. AM J CLIN NUTR 32:607-629, 1979. Data from the Fels Longitudinal Study, Wright State University School of Medicine, Yellow Springs, Ohio.

© 1982 Ross Laboratories

BOYS: 2 TO 18 YEARS
PHYSICAL GROWTH
NCHS PERCENTILES*

NAME _____ RECORD # _____

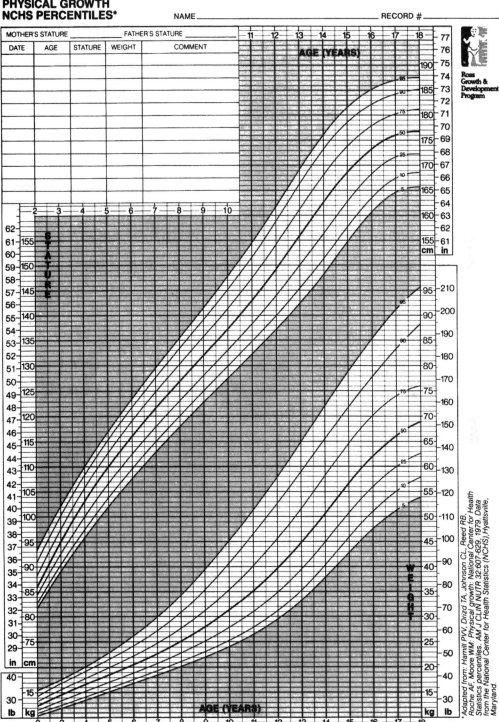

*Adapted from: Hamill PVV, Drizd TA, Johnson CL, Reed RB, Roche AF, Moore WM: Physical growth: National Center for Health Statistics percentiles. AM J CLIN NUTR 32:607-629, 1979. Data from the National Center for Health Statistics (NCHS), Hyattsville, Maryland.

© 1982 Ross Laboratories

Ross
Growth &
Development
Program

GIRLS: 2 TO 18 YEARS
PHYSICAL GROWTH
NCHS PERCENTILES*

NAME _____ RECORD # _____

*Adapted from: Hamill PVV, Drizd TA, Johnson CL, Reed RB, Roche AF, Moore WM: Physical growth: National Center for Health Statistics percentiles. AM J CLIN NUTR 32:607-629, 1979. Data from the National Center for Health Statistics (NCHS), Hyattsville, Maryland.

© 1982 Ross Laboratories

NANDA Approved Nursing Diagnoses

This list represents the NANDA-approved nursing diagnoses for clinical use and testing (1994).

PATTERN 1: EXCHANGING

	1.1.2.1	Altered Nutrition: More than Body Requirements
	1.1.2.2	Altered Nutrition: Less than Body Requirements
	1.1.2.3	Altered Nutrition: Potential for More than Body Requirements
*	1.2.1.1	Risk for Infection
*	1.2.2.1	Risk for Altered Body Temperature
	1.2.2.2	Hypothermia
	1.2.2.3	Hyperthermia
	1.2.2.4	Ineffective Thermoregulation
	1.2.3.1	Dysreflexia
	1.3.1.1	Constipation
	1.3.1.1.1	Perceived Constipation
	1.3.1.1.2	Colonic Constipation
	1.3.1.2	Diarrhea
	1.3.1.3	Bowel Incontinence
	1.3.2	Altered Urinary Elimination
	1.3.2.1.1	Stress Incontinence
	1.3.2.1.2	Reflex Incontinence
	1.3.2.1.3	Urge Incontinence
	1.3.2.1.4	Functional Incontinence
	1.3.2.1.5	Total Incontinence
	1.3.2.2	Urinary Retention
	1.4.1.1	Altered (Specify Type) Tissue Perfusion (Renal, Cerebral, Cardiopulmonary, Gastrointestinal, Peripheral)
	1.4.1.2.1	Fluid Volume Excess
	1.4.1.2.2.1	Fluid Volume Deficit
*	1.4.1.2.2.2	Risk for Fluid Volume Deficit
	1.4.2.1	Decreased Cardiac Output
	1.5.1.1	Impaired Gas Exchange
	1.5.1.2	Ineffective Airway Clearance
	1.5.1.3	Ineffective Breathing Pattern
	1.5.1.3.1	Inability to Sustain Spontaneous Ventilation
	1.5.1.3.2	Dysfunctional Ventilatory Wean-ing Response (DVWR)
*	1.6.1	Risk for Injury
	1.6.1.1	Risk for Suffocation
*	1.6.1.2	Risk for Poisoning
*	1.6.1.3	Risk for Trauma
*	1.6.1.4	Risk for Aspiration
*	1.6.1.5	Risk for Disuse Syndrome
	1.6.2	Altered Protection
	1.6.2.1	Impaired Tissue Integrity
	1.6.2.1.1	Altered Oral Mucous Membrane
	1.6.2.1.2.1	Impaired Skin Integrity
*	1.6.2.1.2.2	Risk for Impaired Skin Integrity
#	1.7.1	Decreased Adaptive Capactiy: Intracranial
#	1.8	Energy Field Disturbance

PATTERN 2: COMMUNICATING

	2.1.1.1	Impaired Verbal Communication

PATTERN 3: RELATING

	3.1.1	Impaired Socal Interaction
	3.1.2	Social Isolation
#	3.1.3	Risk for Loneliness
	3.2.1	Altered Role Performance
	3.2.1.1.1	Altered Parenting
*	3.2.1.1.2	Risk for Altered Parenting
#	3.2.1.1.2.1	Risk for Altered Parent/Infant/Child Attachment
	3.2.1.2.1	Sexual Dysfunction
	3.2.2	Altered Family Processes
	3.2.2.1	Caregiver Role Strain
*	3.2.2.2	Risk for Caregiver Role Strain
#	3.2.2.3.1	Altered Family Process: Alcoholism
	3.2.3.1	Parental Role Conflict
	3.3	Altered Sexuality Patterns

PATTERN 4: VALUING

	4.1.1	Spiritual Distress (Distress of the Human Spirit)
#	4.2	Potential for Enhanced Spiritual Well-Being

PATTERN 5: CHOOSING

	5.1.1.1	Ineffective Individual Coping
	5.1.1.1.1	Impaired Adjustment
	5.1.1.1.2	Defensive Coping
	5.1.1.1.3	Ineffective Denial
	5.1.2.1.1	Ineffective Family Coping: Disabling
	5.1.2.1.2	Ineffective Family Coping: Compromised

New diagnoses added in 1994.
* Diagnoses with modified label terminology in 1994.

LENGTH AND WEIGHT CONVERSIONS							
Length				**Weight**			
in.	cm	cm	in.	lb	kg	kg	lb
1	2.5	1	0.4	1	0.5	1	2.2
2	5.1	2	0.8	2	0.9	2	4.4
4	10.2	3	1.2	4	1.8	3	6.6
6	15.2	4	1.6	6	2.7	4	8.8
8	20.3	5	2.0	8	3.6	5	11.0
12	30.5	6	2.4	10	4.5	6	13.2
18	45.7	8	3.1	20	9.1	8	17.6
24	61.0	10	3.9	30	13.6	10	22.1
30	76.2	20	7.9	40	18.1	20	44.1
36	91.4	30	11.8	50	22.7	30	66.2
42	106.7	40	15.7	60	27.2	40	88.2
48	121.9	50	19.7	70	31.8	50	110.3
54	137.2	60	23.6	80	36.3	60	132.3
60	152.4	70	27.6	90	40.9	70	154.4
66	167.6	80	31.5	100	45.4	80	176.4
72	182.9	90	35.4	150	68.1	90	198.5
78	198.1	100	39.4	200	90.8	100	220.5
1 in. = 2.54 cm		1 cm = 0.3937 in.		1 lb = 0.454 kg		1 kg = 2.205 lb	

Temperature Conversion
(Celcius and Fahrenheit)

°C	°F	°C	°F
34.0	93.2	38.2	100.8
34.2	93.6	38.4	101.1
34.4	93.9	38.6	101.5
34.6	94.3	38.8	101.8
34.8	94.6	39.0	102.2
35.0	95.0	39.2	102.6
35.2	95.4	39.4	102.9
35.4	95.7	39.6	103.3
35.6	96.1	39.8	103.6
35.8	96.4	40.0	104.0
36.0	96.8	40.2	104.4
36.2	97.2	40.4	104.7
36.4	97.5	40.6	105.1
36.6	97.9	40.8	105.4
36.8	98.2	41.0	105.8
37.0	98.6	41.2	106.2
37.2	99.0	41.4	106.5
37.4	99.3	41.6	106.9
37.6	99.7	41.8	107.2
37.8	100.0	42.0	107.6
38.0	100.4	42.2	108.0

$°C = (°F - 32) \div 1.8$ $°F = (°C \times 1.8) + 32$

Glossary

ABO incompatibility: a hemolytic disease caused by the presence of naturally occurring antigens of blood group A, B, or AB

acquired heart disease: a heart condition that occurs after birth as a result of complications of another disease

active immunity: an immune response that occurs when an individual forms antibodies or antitoxins against specific antigens, either by exposure to the infectious agent or by introduction of the antigen; also called humoral immunity

acyanotic heart disease: condition usually associated with defects that increase the flow of blood to the lungs

adolescence: the period of increased physical growth and development, characterized by the development of primary and secondary sex characteristics, occurring between the ages of 12 and 19 years

adolescent growth spurt: a period of accelerated growth affecting practically all skeletal and muscular growth in an adolescent; typically lasts about 2 years

agranulocytes: a type of white blood cell; specifically, lymphocytes and monocytes

allergen: a substance capable of inducing hypersensitivity

allergic shiner: dark circles under the eyes or discolorations greater than usual; a symptom of allergic rhinitis

amenorrhea: permanent or temporary suppression of menstruation

anaphylaxis: the generalized systemic response of a sensitized individual to a specific antigen; can result in life-threatening symptoms, including respiratory distress and shock

anhedonia: absence of pleasurable feelings in acts that normally give pleasure; lack of interest in activities

anovulatory menstruation: menstruation that occurs despite a failure of the ovary to release an ovum

anoxia: reduction of oxygen in body tissue

anticipatory grieving: the process by which parents begin to work through their grief in accepting the loss of their child; increases in intensity until the child's death

anticipatory guidance: a form of teaching that provides information to help parents understand their children's behavior and improve their parenting skills

Apgar scoring system: guide to evaluation of the infant's condition at birth

apical pulse: the pulse heard at the apex of the heart

apnea: temporary cessation of respirations

asphyxia neonatorum: failure of the newborn to breathe spontaneously

assessment: nursing process step in which the nurse collects subjective and objective data about a patient

attachment: an enduring affectional tie one person forms for another; the emotional ties from infant to parent

485

automatisms: involuntary movements that look purposeful

bacterial endocarditis: a bacterial infection of the valves or the inner lining of the heart

Ballard scale: assessment tool used to estimate a newborn's gestational age based on maturity level

barrier: a method to prevent exposure to infectious agents in blood or other body fluids of patients; involves use of gloves, gown, mask, and protective eyewear

beneficence: striving to do good and to avoid or prevent harm

bilirubin: a red bile pigment from the hemoglobin of erythrocytes

binging: abnormal consumption of food

blended family: family in which two custodial parents bring children from previous marriages into one new household

bonding: a gradually unfolding emotional attachment to another person; the emotional ties from parent to infant

cardiopulmonary resuscitation (CPR): a technique that provides basic life support to a victim who is unable to breathe or pump sufficient blood through the body

causative agent: an organism that causes a disease; also called a pathogen

cephalocaudal: the process in which maturation begins at the head and moves toward the toes

cerebral injury: damage to brain tissue

chain of infection: the process by which infectious diseases are transmitted in human beings

chest retractions: see-saw type of respiration typical of infant with respiratory distress syndrome

child abuse: the intentional physical or emotional maltreatment or neglect of children

circumcision: surgical excision of the foreskin of the penis

cleft lip: failure of the soft or bony tissue in the lip to unite during fetal development

cleft palate: failure of the soft or bony tissue in the palate to unite during fetal development

cognitive development: intellectual development encompassing a wide variety of mental abilities, including learning, language, memory, reasoning, and thinking

colostrum: the thin yellowish fluid released by the breasts during the latter part of pregnancy and for the first few days after delivery, before milk is released

coma: a state of unconsciousness in which a person cannot open the eyes, speak, obey commands, or be aroused by any measure

comedones: accumulation of keratin and sebum within the opening of a hair follicle; commonly called blackheads or whiteheads

communicable diseases: diseases spread from one person to another either directly or indirectly

congenital: existing at birth as a result of heredity or some other factor occurring during intrauterine development

congenital heart disease: a heart condition that arises during fetal development and is present at birth

congenital hip dysplasia: birth defect caused by improper embryonic development of the acetabulum (socket of the pelvis)

congestive heart failure: a condition in which the blood supply to the body is insufficient to meet metabolic demands

consolability: the ability of the newborn to calm down after fussiness

continuous positive airway pressure (CPAP): a treatment in which air is administered at a constant pressure to assist in ventilation of an infant with respiratory distress syndrome

cot death: *see* sudden infant death syndrome

cradle hold: a method of holding infant in which the infant's head rests in the bend of the nurse's elbow, with the back supported; the infant's thigh is held by the carrying arm

crib death: *see* sudden infant death syndrome

cryptorchidism: failure of one or both testes to descend into the scrotum

cyanosis: bluish discoloration of the skin due to insufficient oxygen in the blood

cyanotic heart disease: condition associated with defects that result in the mixing of unoxygenated blood with oxygenated blood, or a right to left shunt; skin has bluish tint because of the unoxygenated blood circulating through the body

dehydration: excessive loss of body fluid; fluid output exceeds fluid intake

demand feeding: feeding a baby when the infant signals hunger rather than on a time schedule

denial: defense mechanism in which one refuses to acknowledge a reality

dental caries: tooth decay

Denver II Developmental Screening Test: a screening test given to children between 1 month and 6 years of age to assess gross motor skills, fine motor skills, personal and social development, and language development

despair: the second phase in an infant's response to hospitalization, characterized by sadness, withdrawal, anger, and increasing protest

detachment: the third phase in an infant's response to hospitalization, usually occurring after prolonged separation, characterized by an apparent loss of interest in the parent

development: the qualitative, continuous process in which the child's level of functioning and progression of skills become more complex

diaphragmatic hernia: protrusion of some abdominal organs through an opening in the diaphragm into the left chest

differentiation: development into a more specialized or complex form; the progression from general and simple responses to more specific and complex responses as children mature

diplopia: double vision

direct contact: transmission of infection to a susceptible host through physical contact (body to body)

disbelief: inability of parents to believe (or admit) that their child has a serious disease or disability; often coupled with anger or guilt

Down syndrome: congenital disorder characterized by brain and body damage

dysmenorrhea: painful menstruation

dysphoria: a disorder of affect characterized by extreme anguish

dyspnea: difficult breathing

ecchymosis: a bruise

ego: according to Freud, the aspect of the personality that represents reason or common sense; its goal is to find a way to gratify the id

electrolytes: substances that when dissolved dissociate into ions carrying either a positive or negative charge

emotional abuse: any interaction over time that causes a child unnecessary psychological pain; can include excessive demands, verbal harassment, excessive yelling, belittling, teasing, or rejection

epilepsy: recurrent seizures, which may be idiopathic or a result of trauma, injury, or metabolic alterations

epispadias: the urethra opens on the upper surface of the penis

Erb's palsy: partial paralysis of the arm due to injury to the brachial plexus *erythroblastosis fetalis*: a hemolytic disease of the newborn

erythrocytes: red blood cells

eschar: the tough, leathery scab that forms over severely burned areas

essential amino acids: amino acids that cannot be manufactured by the body and must be provided in food

evaluation: nursing process step in which the nurse measures the care plan's success in achieving patient goals

exstrophy of the bladder: the interior of the bladder lies completely exposed through the abdominal opening

extended family: nuclear family and other relatives, such as aunts, uncles, and grandparents

extracellular fluid: fluid found outside the cells of the body

extrauterine life: life outside the uterus

failure to thrive: a disorder of infants and children under 2 years of age, characterized by a weight for age that is below the third percentile

family-centered care: care in which the health care team considers the child as part of a family, community, and culture

fatty acids: acids found in animal products, vegetable fats, and most oils; classified as saturated or unsaturated

fecalith: a hard, impacted fecal mass

fetal alcohol syndrome (FAS): a possible consequence if an expectant mother consumes alcohol during her pregnancy; symptoms include prenatal and postnatal growth retardation, neurological abnormalities, developmental delay, and facial dysmorphology

fidelity: faithfulness to promises and duties

fine motor skills: ability to coordinate the small muscle groups

fontanel: space or soft spot between the bones of the newborn's skull

food pyramid: guide for daily food planning, published by the U.S. Department of Agriculture

football hold: a method of holding infant in which the infant's body is supported on the nurse's forearm, with the infant's head and neck resting in the nurse's palm; the rest of infant's body is securely held between the nurse's body and elbow

fracture: a break in a bone, usually as a result of injury

galactosemia: inborn error of metabolism in which the body is missing the enzyme needed to convert galactose into glucose

gastric lavage: instillation of large amounts of warm normal saline through an orogastric tube into the patient's stomach until the return is clear

gavage feeding: feeding by means of a stomach tube

Gower's sign: self-climbing movement in which a child uses arm muscles to compensate for weak hip extensor muscles in rising to an upright position; characteristic symptom of Duchenne's muscular dystrophy

granulocytes: a type of white blood cell; specifically, neutrophils and eosinophils

gross motor skills: ability to control the large muscle groups

growth: the continuous and complex process in which the body and its parts increase in size

head circumference: size of head, measured at its greatest circumference, slightly above the eyebrows and pinna of the ears and around the occipital prominence at the back of the skull; usually measured in all children up to 3 years of age

Heimlich maneuver: method of dislodging food or other material from the throat of a choking victim; uses subdiaphragmatic abdominal thrusts to forcefully expel the material

hermaphroditism: condition in which a newborn possesses the gonads and genitals typical of both sexes

hiatal hernia: protrusion of the stomach through the esophageal hiatus

high-risk newborn: any neonate who is at risk for a serious condition or illness, or death

homeostasis: equilibrium of the internal environment

hospice care: provides holistic care and support for the patient with a terminal illness; goal is to enable the person to live life as fully as possible, free of pain, and with respect, choices, and dignity

host: person who harbors or nourishes an infectious organism

hydrocele: accumulation of fluid in a saclike cavity, especially in the tunica vaginalis; result of the failure of the processus vaginalis to close during fetal development

hydrocephalus: a condition characterized by abnormal accumulation of fluid in the cranial vault; accompanied by enlargement of the head

hyperbilirubinemia: excessive bilirubin in the blood

hyperlipidemia: an excess of lipids in the plasma

hypertension: high blood pressure

hypoalbuminemia: an abnormally low level of albumin in the blood

hypoglycemia: a deficiency of sugar in the blood

hypoproteinemia: a decreased amount of protein in the blood

hypospadias: the urethra terminates on the underside of the penis

hypovolemia: diminished blood flow

id: according to Freud, the aspect of the personality that represents one's desires; is present at birth and seeks immediate gratification under the pleasure principle

immune response: occurs when the body's lymphocytes are stimulated to produce antibodies that react with antigens

imperforate anus: the anal opening is abnormally closed

implementation: nursing process step in which the nurse puts the care plan into action through various interventions

incubator: an apparatus for maintaining a premature infant in an environment of proper temperature and humidity

indirect contact: transmission of infection to a susceptible host by means of an animate or inanimate object, which becomes a common source and can infect many people

infancy: the period of rapid growth and development occurring between birth and 1 year of age

infectious diseases: diseases caused by microorganisms that invade the body and then reproduce and multiply

inguinal hernia: protrusion of the intestine into the inguinal canal

insensible perspiration: loss of body fluid that is unnoticed; evaporation

integration: the process of combining simple movements or skills to achieve complex tasks

interstitial fluid: fluid found in the spaces between the cells and blood vessels; a type of extracellular fluid

intracellular fluid: fluid found within cells of the body

intravascular fluid: fluid found within the blood vessels; a type of extracellular fluid

intussusception: telescoping of the bowel

irritability: newborn characteristic evaluated according to the neonatal behavioral assessment scale; reflects how the newborn controls his or her own behavior

isolation: separation of infected individuals from those uninfected for the period of communicability of a particular disease; purpose is to interrupt the chain of infection by preventing the transmission of microbes

justice: treating all patients fairly in providing care and allocating resources

kerion: a boggy, pustular inflammation that usually develops in association with tinea infections

ketoacidosis: accumulation of ketones in the body, causing acidosis

ketonuria: loss of ketones in the urine

killed inactivated virus: form of vaccine in which the virus has been killed and therefore inactivated

lactose: a complex carbohydrate (disaccharide) obtained from milk

lanugo: fine, downy hair distributed over the newborn's body

large-for-gestational-age infant (LGA): an infant in the highest 10th percentile of weight for gestational age

laryngospasm: involuntary vibrating contractions of the muscles of the larynx

leukocytes: white blood cells

leukopenia: decrease in the number of white blood cells in the body

limb salvage: removal of a tumor without amputation

lipid: any one group of substances that include the fats, oils, and fat-like substances called sterols

live attenuated virus: form of vaccine in which the virus has been weakened

lordosis: abnormal increased curvature of the lumbar spine

low-birth-weight infant: an infant who weighs 1,500 to 2,000 g

magical thinking: belief that thoughts and deeds can cause an event to occur; characteristic of preschool children

malnutrition: condition resulting from inadequate intake of essential nutrients

meconium: greenish black, tarlike substance in the intestines of a full-term fetus; the newborn's first stools

menarche: the beginning of the menstrual function

meningocele: hernial protrusion of the meninges through a defect in the vertebral column

meningomyelocele: hernial protrusion of a part of the meninges and substance of the spinal cord through a defect in the vertebral column; also called myelomeningocele

menorrhagia: menstrual bleeding that is excessive, prolonged or both

menstruation: cyclic, physiological discharge of blood from a nonpregnant uterus, occurring at about four-week intervals

metrorrhagia: uterine bleeding that is unrelated to the menstrual period

milia: tiny, white pimples, especially on the newborn's nose and chin

Moro reflex: a reflex with stimulation in which the infant's arms are suddenly thrown out in an embrace attitude

myringotomy: surgical incision of the eardrum

narcosis: state of stupor or unconsciousness caused by drugs

nasal salute: wiping the nose with the heel of the hand; a symptom of allergic rhinitis

neglect: deliberate or unintentional lack of care for a child's basic needs that places the child's life or health in danger

neonatal behavioral assessment scale (NBAS): scale developed by Dr. T. Berry Brazelton to evaluate 27 newborn characteristics that fall into 4 categories

neonatal intensive care unit: hospital unit that specializes in the intensive care of high-risk newborns *nonessential amino acids*: amino acids that can be manufactured by the body and, therefore, do not need to be obtained from the diet

nuclear family: family in which a father, mother, and children share a common household

nursing care plan: written guide that includes nursing diagnoses, goals, and interventions and that directs individualized nursing care

nursing diagnosis: nursing process step in which the nurse identifies actual or potential health problems susceptible to nursing interventions

nursing process: problem-solving method for nurses that uses five steps: assessment, nursing diagnosis, planning, implementation, and evaluation

nutrients: foods or their components that are necessary for proper body function, including carbohydrates, protein, fats, minerals, and vitamins

occlusion therapy: closure or obstruction to prevent or improve a condition (e.g., wearing a patch over the stronger eye in strabismus and amblyopia)

oliguria: decreased urine output

omphalocele: protrusion of some abdominal contents into the umbilical cord's root, forming a sac covered with peritoneal membrane that lays on the abdomen

osmosis: the diffusion of solvent molecules through a semipermeable membrane, going from the side of lower concentration to that of higher concentration

pain management: control of pain through administration of medications at regular intervals and/or nonpharmacological methods such as distraction, hypnosis, imagery, and application of heat and cold

paresis: paralysis

passive immunity: an immune response that occurs when an individual receives ready-made antibodies from a human or animal that has been actively immunized against the disease

pathogen: *see* causative agent

pediatric nursing: health care profession that combines the science of health promotion and illness prevention with the art of caring for children and their families

personality: the pattern of characteristic thoughts, feelings, and behaviors that distinguishes one person from another

petechiae: pinpoint hemorrhages

phenylketonuria (PKU): disorder resulting from a congenital defect in phenylalanine metabolism; may cause brain damage unless a special diet is consumed

phobia: an excessive or unfounded fear of someone or something

photophobia: extreme sensitivity to light

phototherapy: treatment of disease by light rays; used to treat jaundice

physical abuse: deliberate physical maltreatment that causes injury to the body

physiological jaundice: mild yellowing of the newborn's skin and eyes occurring 3 to 5 days after birth and self-resolving

planning: nursing process step in which the nurse develops and prioritizes patient goals and then chooses interventions to help meet them

plasma: the liquid portion of blood, containing protein, clotting factors, and electrolytes

polydipsia: excessive thirst

polyphagia: markedly increased food intake

polyuria: excessive urine output

portal of entry: the method by which an infectious organism enters a host; may occur through breaks in the skin or mucous membranes, ingestion, inhalation, or across the placenta in utero

portal of exit: the method by which an infectious organism leaves the reservoir; occurs through bodily secretions

postoperative care: physical and emotional care that occurs in the postanesthesia room and the nursing unit during recovery from a surgical procedure

postoperative exercises: actions performed after surgery, such as coughing, deep breathing, and ambulating, to stimulate circulation and respiration, thereby preventing atelectasis and blood stasis

postterm infant: an infant born after 42 weeks' gestation

preoperative care: emotional and physical care given in preparation for upcoming surgery

preoperative checklist: steps of the preoperative process, used in preparing a patient for surgery

preoperative teaching: teaching before surgery, designed to reduce preoperative anxiety and promote a positive outcome

prepubertal growth spurt: a growth spurt that begins at about age 7, preceding the true growth spurt of adolescence

preschool: a period in which physical growth slows and stabilizes, occurring between 3 and 6 years of age

preterm infant: an infant born before 37 weeks' gestation

primary irritant: an agent that produces irritation (contact dermatitis) on the first exposure to it

primary (deciduous) teeth: first teeth; children have 20 primary teeth, usually by age 33 months

prodromal phase: the earliest phase of a developing disease or condition

protest: the initial phase in an infant's response to hospitalization in which the infant cannot be consoled and refuses any attention except from the parent

proximodistal: the process in which development proceeds from the center of the body outward toward the extremities

pseudohermaphroditism: condition in which a newborn has the external sex organs of one sex and the gonads of the other sex

pseudohypertrophy: seeming enlargement

psychoactive: affecting the mind or behavior; mind-altering, as in psychoactive drugs

puberty: period of time between the ages of 9 and 14½ years in girls and 10½ and 16 years in boys; an increased amount of sex hormones is usually released into the bloodstream at this time as secondary sex characteristics develop

purging: self-induced vomiting or use of diuretics or laxatives to rid the body of ingested food

pyloric stenosis: a constriction at the junction of the stomach and the small intestine

Recommended Dietary Allowances: guidelines for the intake of essential nutrients from infancy through adulthood

rescue breathing: breathing for a victim who is unable to breathe on his/her own because of unconsciousness or airway obstruction; part of CPR procedure

reservoir: the place where an organism grows and reproduces; serves as a source from which others can be infected; can be someone with the disease, someone carrying the disease, an animal, or the environment

respect for persons: support for a patient's right to autonomy, confidentiality, refusal of treatment, and truthfulness

respiratory distress syndrome (RDS): condition in which alveoli of lungs fail to expand due to lack of surfactant; also called hyaline membrane disease

respite care: temporary care of patient to relieve family or care provider

retraction: a visible drawing in of the soft tissues of the chest, often a sign of severe distress

RhoGAM: solution of gamma globulin containing Rh antibodies

ritualistic behavior: repetitive actions, often connected with mealtime, especially in toddlers

rituals: a series of repetitive acts performed as part of daily living for the child (e.g., story before bedtime, afternoon nap, snack time); provide comfort and stability for the child

school age: a period of slow, steady growth occurring between 6 and 12 years of age

scoliosis: a lateral S-shaped curvature of the spine, occurring most often in adolescent girls

sealants: thin, plastic coatings to protect the teeth, particularly the molars, from bacteria

secondary (permanent) teeth: permanent teeth that emerge starting at about age 6 years and continuing through childhood and early adulthood

sensible perspiration: loss of body fluid that can be noticed; sweating

separation anxiety: responses of distress and apprehension in a child on being removed from parents, home, or familiar surroundings; common in toddlers

sexual abuse: sexual contact between a child, aged 16 years or younger, and another person in a position of authority, no matter what the age, in which the child's participation has been obtained through force, threats, bribes, or gifts; can include intercourse, masturbation, fondling, exhibitionism, sodomy, or prostitution

sexual maturity: stage reached after the adolescent growth spurt ends; principal sign in girls is menstruation; principal sign in boys is presence of sperm in urine

Silverman-Anderson Index: a means of continuous evaluation of an infant's respiratory status

single-parent family: family in which one parent assumes essentially all responsibility for maintaining a home and raising children

sinus arrhythmia: normal cycle of irregular heart rhythm associated with respiration; heart rate is faster on inspiration and slower on expiration

sleep apnea: cessation of breathing for brief periods during sleep

small-for-gestational-age infant: an infant in the lowest 10th percentile of weight for gestational age

social responsiveness: newborn's ability to respond to parents and other external stimuli; evaluated according to the neonatal behavioral assessment scale

socialization: process by which the family teaches its children about society's rules, language, values, and acceptable behaviors

spina bifida occulta: malformation of the spine in which the posterior portion of the laminae of the vertebrae fails to close; defect only in the vertebrae

sprains: injuries caused by overstretching of a muscle

status epilepticus: series of generalized tonic-clonic seizures in which child does not regain consciousness between seizures

steatorrhea: presence of fat in the stool

stepfamily: family in which the custodial parent and children reside in a household with the parent's new spouse

strains: injuries caused by pulling of a ligament

stressors: adverse physical, mental, or emotional stimuli that cause anxiety for the child or parents, often creating situations beyond their ability to cope

stridor: high-pitched, noisy sound or wheezing created by narrowing of the airway, often caused by foreign-body aspiration

substance abuse: use of any mind-altering substance in socially inappropriate ways or in ways that impair the ability to function

sudden infant death syndrome (SIDS): the sudden death of an infant under 1 year of age that remains unexplained after a complete autopsy investigation and review of the history; leading cause of death in children aged 1 to 12 months in the United States

superego: according to Freud, the aspect of the personality that incorporates "shoulds" and "should nots" into one's personal value system; the conscience

surfactant deficiency: an insufficiency of the agent that stabilizes alveolar sacs by lowering surface tension; this agent is necessary for normal respiratory function

susceptible host: a person at risk for contracting an infectious disease

suture: junction between bones of the skull; also refers to sewing together an incision

sweat test: diagnostic test that analyzes the sodium and chloride content of a child's sweat; used to diagnose cystic fibrosis

talipes: clubfoot; a foot or feet may turn in any abnormal direction

teething: tooth eruption

temperament: a person's style of approaching other people and situations

thrombocytes: platelets

thrush: fungal infection in the mouth

toddlerhood: a period of slower growth occurring between 1 and 3 years of age

torticollis: condition in which the head tilts to one side; caused by shortening of the sternocleidomastoid muscle

total parenteral nutrition (TPN): the provision of all the nutrients directly into the veins through a surgically inserted catheter; also called hyperalimentation

toxoid: form of vaccine in which the agent has been treated to destroy its toxic qualities

traction: use of weights and pulleys to realign bone fragments, reduce dislocations, immobilize fractures, provide rest for an extremity, help prevent contracture deformities, and allow preoperative and postoperative positioning and alignment

transmission: spread of pathogens, either by direct or indirect contact, by airborne spread, by inanimate objects, or by vectors

trigger: stimulus (substance or condition) that precedes an asthmatic episode or allergic reaction

triglycerides: compounds consisting of three fatty acids combined with glycerol

two-career family: family in which both parents work outside the home

tympanometry: measurement of internal ear pressure

umbilical hernia: protrusion of part of an organ (usually intestine) through the wall of the umbilical ring

upright hold: a method of holding infant in which the infant is held upright against the nurse's chest and shoulder; infant's buttocks are supported by one of the nurse's hands, with the other hand and arm supporting the infant's head and shoulders

urinary stasis: condition in which flow of urine is interrupted

vaccine: an active immunizing agent that incorporates an infectious antigen

vernix caseosa: a cheeselike substance that may appear on the newborn's skin

very-low-birth-weight infant: an infant who weighs less than 1,500 g

vesicoureteral reflux: abnormal backflow of urine from the bladder to the ureters

visual acuity: clarity or clearness of sight; refractive ability

visual field: an area within which stimuli will produce the sensation of sight

weaning: discontinuing the breast feeding of an infant with substitution of other feeding methods

Index

Note: Page numbers in **bold** type reference non-text information.